Study Guide

Pharmacology
A Nursing Process Approach

7th Edition
Revised Reprint

Joyce LeFever Kee, MS, RN
Associate Professor Emerita
School of Nursing
College of Health Sciences
University of Delaware
Newark, Delaware

Evelyn R. Hayes, PhD, MPH, FNP-BC
Professor
School of Nursing
College of Health Sciences
University of Delaware
Newark, Delaware

Linda E. McCuistion, PhD, RN
Professor
South University, Richmond Campus
Glen Allen, Virginia

Study Guide prepared by

Nancy Haugen, PhD, RN
Associate Professor and ABSN Program Chair
School of Nursing
Samuel Merritt University
Oakland, California

ELSEVIER
SAUNDERS

ELSEVIER
SAUNDERS

3251 Riverport Lane
Maryland Heights, Missouri 63043

STUDY GUIDE FOR PHARMACOLOGY: ISBN: 978-1-4557-4218-9
A NURSING PROCESS APPROACH

ISBN: 978-1-4557-4218-9

Senior Editor: Lee Henderson
Senior Developmental Editor: Jennifer Ehlers
Developmental Editor: Kelly McGowan
Publishing Services Manager: Jeff Patterson
Senior Project Manager: Clay S. Broeker

Printed in the United States of America

Last digit is the print number: 9 8 7 6 5 4 3 2 1

Preface

This comprehensive *Study Guide* is designed to provide the learner with clinically based situation practice problems and questions. This book accompanies the text *Pharmacology: A Nursing Process Approach,* seventh edition, and may also be used independently of the text.

Opportunities abound for the enhancement of critical thinking and decision-making abilities. Hundreds of study questions and answers are presented on nursing responsibilities in therapeutic pharmacology. For example, Chapter 4 details the principles of medication administration. Chapter 5 is composed of six sections, each devoted to a specific area of medications and calculations. Multiple practice opportunities are provided in the areas of measurement, methods of drug calculations, calculation of oral and injectable dosages (including pediatrics), and calculation of intravenous fluids. Each chapter follows a new format that includes study questions (including multiple choice, matching, word searches, crossword puzzles, and completion exercises), NCLEX review questions (including alternate item format questions), critical thinking exercises, and case studies.

There are more than 160 drug calculation problems and questions, many relating to actual client care situations and enhanced with real drug labels. The learner is also expected to recognize safe dosage parameters for the situation. The combination of the instructional material in the text and the multiplicity of a variety of practice problems in this *Study Guide* preclude the need for an additional drug dosage calculation book.

The nursing process is used throughout the client situation-based questions and critical thinking exercises. Chapters have questions that relate to assessment data, including laboratory data and side effects, planning and implementing care, client/family teaching, cultural and nutritional considerations, and effectiveness of the drug therapy regimen.

Because of the ever-expanding number of drugs available, pharmacology can be an overwhelming subject. To help students grasp essential content without becoming overwhelmed, chapters have been divided into multiple smaller sections. The result is a layout that is user-friendly. In addition, one new chapter has been added, covering questions related to medication safety.

Answers to all questions are presented in the Answer Key. Additional resources may be found in the appendices, including a basic math review and a prototype drug chart format for your use.

The *Study Guide* is part of a comprehensive pharmacology package, including the textbook and Instructor and Student Resources available on the companion Evolve website. This package and each of its components were designed to promote critical thinking and learning. We are excited about this edition of the *Study Guide* because it offers the learner a variety of modalities for mastering the content.

Acknowledgments

We extend most sincere appreciation to the many professionals who facilitated the development of this *Study Guide for Pharmacology: A Nursing Process Approach*, seventh edition. We extend a special thank you to Nancy Haugen, PhD, RN, who revised this new edition. We also thank the following for their past assistance with questions for individual chapters: Margaret Barton-Burke, PhD, RN; Joseph Boullata, PharmD, BCNSP; Michelle M. Byrne, MS, PhD, CNOR; Robin Webb Corbett, PhD, RN, C; Sandy Elliott, CNM, MSN; Linda Goodwin, RNC, MEd; Judith W. Herrman, PhD, RN; Kathleen J. Jones, RN-C, MS, ANP; Robert J. Kizior, BS, RPh; Paula R. Klemm, PhD, RN, OCN; Anne E. Lara, RN, MS, AOCN, APRN,BC; Linda Laskowski-Jones, RN, MS, APRN, BC, CEN; Ronald J. Lefever, RPh; Patricia S. Lincoln, BSN, RN; Patricia O'Brien, MA, MSN; Laura K. Williford Owens, PharmD; Lisa Ann Plowfield, PhD, RN; Larry D. Purnell, PhD, RN, FAAN; Nancy C. Sharts-Hopko, RN, PhD, FAAN; Jane Purnell Taylor, RN, MS; Lynette M. Wachholz, MN, APRN, IBCLC; and Gail Wilkes, MS, RNC, AOCN.

We are indebted to the students and clients we have had the privilege of knowing during our many years of professional nursing practice. From you we have learned many important aspects about the role of therapeutic pharmacology in nursing practice.

To the staff at Elsevier, especially Lee Henderson, Senior Editor; Jennifer Ehlers, Senior Developmental Editor; Clay Broeker, Senior Project Manager; and Jeff Patterson, Publishing Services Manager, we thank you for your reviews and suggestions.

Joyce LeFever Kee
Evelyn R. Hayes
Linda E. McCuistion

Contents

1 Drug Action: Pharmaceutic, Pharmacokinetic, and Pharmacodynamic Phases

Study Questions

Crossword puzzle: Use the definition to determine the pharmacologic term.

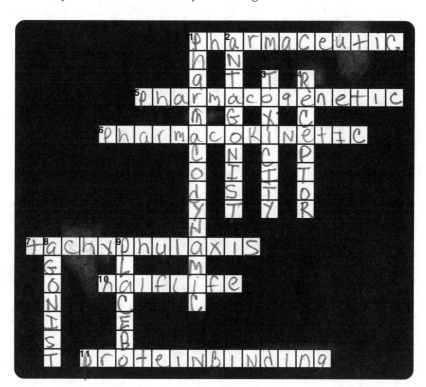

Across

1. Dissolution of the drug
5. Effect of drug action because of hereditary influence *pharmacogenetic*
6. Four processes of drug movement to achieve drug action .
7. Drug tolerance to repeated administration of a drug *Tachyphulaxis*
10. One-half of the drug concentration to be eliminated *half life*
11. Drug bound to protein *Protein Bindg*

Down

1. Effect of drug action on cells *pharmacodynamic*
2. Drug that blocks a response *antagonist*
3. Toxic effect as a result of drug dose or therapy *toxicity*
4. Located on a cell membrane to enhance drug action *receptor*
8. Drug that produces a response *agonist*
9. Psychologic benefit from a compound *placebo*

Match the following terms with their descriptions.

E 12. Protein-bound drug
D 13. Unbound drug
B 14. Hepatic first pass
A 15. Dissolution
F 16. Passive absorption
C 17. Nonselective receptors

a. Breakdown of a drug into smaller particles
b. Proceeds directly from intestine to the liver
c. Drugs that affect various receptors
d. Free active drug causing a pharmacologic response
e. Causes inactive drug action/response
f. Drug absorbed by diffusion
g. Drug requiring a carrier for absorption

NCLEX Review Questions

Select the best response.

18. Which drug form is most rapidly absorbed from the gastrointestinal (GI) tract?
    a. tablet
    b. enteric-coated tablet
    c. suspension
    d. poultice

19. Mark on the diagram below where enteric-coated tablets are absorbed.

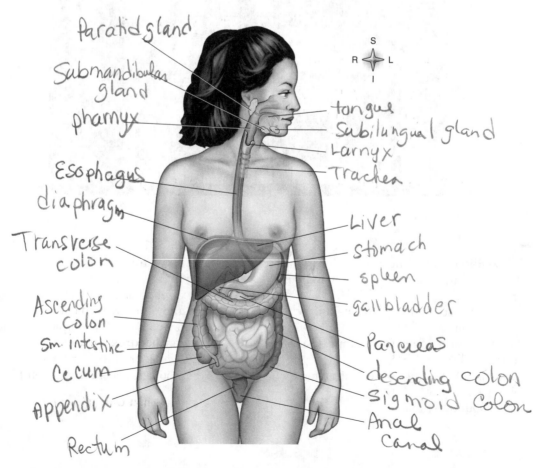

Paratid gland
Submandibular gland
pharnyx
Esophagus
diaphragm
Transverse colon
Ascending Colon
Sm. intestine
Cecum
Appendix
Rectum

tongue
Subilungual gland
Larnyx
Trachea
Liver
stomach
spleen
gallbladder
Pancreas
desending colon
Sigmoid Colon
Anal Canal

20. Usually food has what effect on drug dissolution and absorption?
    a. enhances
    b. interferes with
    c. does not affect
    d. catalytic

21. Which statement places the four processes of pharmacokinetics in the correct sequence?
    a. absorption, metabolism , distribution, excretion
    b. distribution, absorption, metabolism, excretion
    c. distribution, metabolism, absorption, excretion
    d. absorption, distribution, metabolism, excretion

22. Which type of drug passes rapidly through the GI membrane?
    a. lipid-soluble and ionized
    b. lipid-soluble and nonionized
    c. water-soluble and ionized
    d. water-soluble and nonionized

23. Which factors most commonly affect a drug's action?
    a. poor circulation, pain, stress, hunger, fasting
    b. stress, hunger, weather, pH of the drug
    c. poor circulation, hunger, stress, BMI
    d. BMI, pH of drug, stress, poor circulation

24. A client is taking a drug that is highly protein-bound. Several days later, the client takes a second drug that is 90% protein-bound. What happens to the first drug?
    a. The first drug remains highly protein-bound.
    b. The first drug becomes increasingly inactive.
    c. More of the first drug is released from the protein and becomes more pharmacologically active.
    d. The first drug is excreted in the urine.

25. Which body organ is the major site of drug metabolism?
    a. kidney
    b. liver
    c. lung
    d. skin

26. What route of drug absorption has the greatest bioavailability?
    a. oral
    b. intramuscular
    c. subcutaneous
    d. intravenous

27. Which statement is the best description of a drug's serum half-life?
    a. the time required for half of a drug dose to be absorbed
    b. the time required after absorption for half of the drug to be eliminated
    c. the time required for a drug to be totally effective
    d. the time required for half of the drug dose to be completely distributed

28. The client is taking a drug with a half-life of 24 to 30 hours. How often should this drug be administered to maintain the appropriate serum drug levels?
    a. three times a day
    b. twice a day
    c. once a day
    d. every other day

29. Which type of drug can be eliminated through the kidneys?
    a. lipid-soluble
    b. water-soluble
    c. protein-bound
    d. long half-life

30. A client has a renal disorder. Her creatinine clearance is 40 mL/min. What should happen to her drug dosage?
    a. It should be increased.
    b. It should be decreased.
    c. It should remain unchanged.
    d. The drug should be discontinued.

31. Which is the best determinant of the biologic activity of a drug?
    a. the fit of the drug at the receptor site
    b. the misfit of the drug at the receptor site
    c. inability of the drug to bind to a specific receptor
    d. ability of the drug to be rapidly excreted

32. Which type of drug prevents or inhibits a cellular response?
    a. antagonists
    b. agonists
    c. depressants
    d. antiseptics

33. A receptor located in different parts of the body may initiate a variety of responses depending on its anatomic site. Which type of receptor responds in this manner?
    a. nonselective
    b. instigating a drug-enzyme interaction
    c. initiating a primary response
    d. nonspecific

34. Which indicator measures the margin of safety of a drug?
    a. therapeutic range
    b. therapeutic index
    c. duration of action
    d. biologic half-life

35. A client is taking a medication that requires plasma/serum drug level monitoring. To avoid drug toxicity, how often should blood levels be drawn?
    a. yearly
    b. daily
    c. at periodic intervals
    d. weekly

36. The nurse has just given a client his prescribed drugs. Which measurement checks for the highest plasma/serum concentration of the drug?
    a. peak level
    b. trough level
    c. half-life
    d. minimum effective concentration

37. Before administering a medication, the nurse should check a drug reference book or the drug pamphlet to obtain pertinent data. Which data should be noted? (Select all that apply.)
    a. protein-binding effect
    b. half-life
    c. therapeutic range
    d. maximum effective concentration

38. Which type of physiologic effect is not related to the desired effect(s) that are predictable or are associated with the use of a specific drug?
    a. severe adverse reactions
    b. side effects
    c. synergistic effects
    d. toxic effects

39. The nurse is giving a large initial dose of a drug to rapidly achieve minimum effective concentration in the plasma. What is this type of dosage called?
    a. therapeutic dose
    b. toxic dose
    c. loading dose
    d. peak dose

40. A time-response curve evaluates parameters of a drug's action. Which parameters are part of a time-response curve? (Select all that apply.)
    a. therapeutic range
    b. onset of action
    c. peak action
    d. duration of action

41. Which nursing intervention concerning drug therapy should the nurse implement? (Select all that apply.)
    a. assessing for side effects of drugs, especially those that are nonselective
    b. checking drug reference books for dosage ranges, side effects, protein-binding percentage, and half-life
    c. teaching the client to wait a week after the occurrence of signs and symptoms to see if they disappear
    d. checking the client's serum therapeutic range of drugs that are more toxic or have a narrow therapeutic range

Critical Thinking Exercises

Complete the following.

42. Medications given intramuscularly are best absorbed when given in the ___Deltoid___.

43. To avoid medication toxicity, the nurse should check the ___protein binding %___ of all drugs given to a client.

44. The main route of drug elimination is though the kidneys. Other areas that eliminate drugs from the body include: ___breast milk___, ___bile___, ___feces___, ___sweat___, ___vaginal___, ___saliva___, and ___lungs___.

45. The four categories of drug action are ___Irratation___, ___Killing of organisms___, ___depression___, and ___replacement___.

Match the term with its appropriate descriptor.

___D___ 46. Onset
___C___ 47. Peak action
___A___ 48. Duration of action
___B___ 49. Therapeutic index

a. Length of time a drug has a pharmacologic effect
b. The margin of safety of a drug
c. Occurs when a drug has reached its highest plasma concentration
d. Time it takes a drug to reach minimum effective concentration

Case Study

Select the best answer.

J.R., an older client, has been taking digoxin 0.25 mg daily and warfarin (Coumadin) 5 mg daily for several months. She reports that large purple spots (purpura) have developed on her hands, arms, and ankles. She tells the nurse that she has never had these types of spots before.

1. What is the most probable cause of this client's purpura?
    a. Her digoxin dosage is too high for her age and she has become toxic.
    b. She is taking two protein-binding medications that cause more free warfarin to be available.
    c. She has a bleeding disorder that she has not reported in her health history.
    d. She has complications from Raynaud's syndrome.

2. What are nursing actions that should be implemented in the care of this client? (Select all that apply.)

    a. Inform the health care provider of her condition.

    b. Be sure the appropriate lab tests have been completed.

    c. Protect the client from injury or increased bleeding.

    d. Reassure her that no long-term complications will occur.

3. J.R. wants to know what is going to happen concerning medications. What is the nurse's best response?

    a. "We are going to monitor your medications and wait for the bruises to disappear."

    b. "We will discontinue the warfarin, as that is the cause of the 'spots' on your hands and arms."

    c. "We need to elevate your legs as poor circulation is responsible for the 'spots' on your ankles."

    d. "We will monitor your drug levels and adjust the dosages based on the lab results."

4. J.R.'s urine output has decreased. What changes, if any, should be made to her medications?

    a. The medication dosage should be increased.

    b. The medication dosage should be decreased.

    c. The medication dosage should not be changed.

    d. The medications she is taking should be discontinued.

2 Nursing Process and Client Teaching

Study Questions

Match the step of the nursing process in Column II with the phrases in Column I.

Column I

A 1. Nursing diagnosis
A 2. Current health history
B 3. Goal-setting
A 4. Client's environment
C 5. Action to accomplish goals
A 6. Drug allergies and reactions
D 7. Referral
C 8. Client/significant other education
C 9. Use of teaching drug cards
A 10. Laboratory test results
D 11. Effectiveness of health teaching and drug therapy

Column II

a. Assessment
b. Planning
c. Implementation/intervention
d. Evaluation

Match the clinical manifestations in Column I with the data type in Column II.

Column I

B 12. Productive cough
A 13. Pain in left ear
B 14. Lab values
A 15. Nausea
B 16. Heart rate
A 17. Client perception of drug's effectiveness
A 18. Reported allergies

Column II

a. Subjective — client tells you
b. Objective — you observe

NCLEX Review Questions

Select the best response.

19. *Risk for injury* is included in which phase of the nursing process?
    a. assessment
    b. potential nursing diagnoses
    c. planning
    d. implementation

20. *Obtain client's weight to be used for future comparison* is included in which phase of the nursing process?
    a. assessment
    b. potential nursing diagnoses
    c. planning
    d. evaluation

21. *The client will receive adequate nutritional support through enteral feedings* is included in which phase of the nursing process?
    a. assessment
    b. potential nursing diagnoses
    c. planning
    d. implementation

22. *The client will be free from hyperactivity* is included in which phase of the nursing process?
    a. assessment
    b. potential nursing diagnoses
    c. planning
    d. evaluation

23. *Instruct client to avoid caffeine-containing foods* is included in which phase of the nursing process?
    a. potential nursing diagnoses
    b. planning
    c. implementation
    d. evaluation

24. *Evaluate effectiveness of drug therapy* is included in which phase of the nursing process?
    a. assessment
    b. potential nursing diagnoses
    c. implementation
    d. evaluation

25. *Sleep pattern disturbance* is included in which phase of the nursing process?
    a. assessment
    b. potential nursing diagnoses
    c. planning
    d. implementation

26. *Advise client to report adverse reactions such as nausea and severe vomiting to health care provider; drug choice or dosage may need modification* is included in which phase of the nursing process?
    a. assessment
    b. potential nursing diagnoses
    c. planning
    d. implementation

27. *Anxiety* is included in which phase of the nursing process?
    a. potential nursing diagnoses
    b. planning
    c. implementation
    d. evaluation

28. *Instruct client not to discontinue medication abruptly* is included in which phase of the nursing process?
    a. assessment
    b. potential nursing diagnoses
    c. planning
    d. implementation

29. The nurse is developing a teaching plan for the client. Which of the following are suggested to be included? (Select all that apply.)
    a. Actively involve client.
    b. Provide written instructions at appropriate level for client.
    c. Consider using a variety of media.
    d. Discourage questions from client and family.
    e. Provide for return demonstration.

30. The nurse is administering medications to a client. As part of the plan of care, the nurse must develop a nursing diagnosis specific to medication administration. Which nursing diagnoses would be most appropriate for a client taking multiple medications? (Select all that apply.)
    a. Alteration in comfort
    b. Potential for injury
    c. Knowledge deficit
    d. Ineffective self-health maintenance

31. The nurse is teaching a client how to self-administer insulin and heparin. Which statements are parts of an effective goal statement? (Select all that apply.)
    a. The goal should state expected outcomes.
    b. The goal should be developed by the nurse.
    c. The goal should be measurable and realistic.
    d. The goal should be client-centered.

32. Which is the best goal for a client learning self-administration of insulin?
    a. The client will have a basic understanding of medication administration at discharge.
    b. The client will understand how to test blood glucose levels.
    c. The client will know what to do if an insulin reaction is experienced.
    d. The client will demonstrate appropriate self-administration of insulin prior to discharge.

33. The nurse is developing a teaching plan for a client who will be discharged using an inhaler. What teaching strategies should the nurse include in the teaching/learning plan? (Select all that apply.)
    a. Discuss side effects and diet required while taking the prescribed medication.
    b. Have the client provide a return demonstration of how to use the inhaler.
    c. Provide the client with written administration instructions at discharge.
    d. Provide time for questions and involvement of significant other in the teaching sessions.

34. Which factors are commonly associated with nonadherence with a drug therapy plan? (Select all that apply.)
    a. forgetfulness
    b. knowledge deficit
    c. motivation
    d. side effects
    e. language barrier

3 Medication Safety

Study Questions

Match the statement in Column I with the nursing implication of drug administration in Column II.

Column I

C __ 1. Right route
F __ 2. Right client
J __ 3. Right time
G __ 4. Right documentation
A __ 5. Right assessment
H __ 6. Right drug
B __ 7. Right dose
D __ 8. Right to education
E __ 9. Right to refuse
I __ 10. Right evaluation

Column II

a. Measurement of a client's apical pulse
b. Amount of medication given as prescribed
c. Medication given IM as prescribed
d. Teaching a client about possible side effects of the medication
e. The client refuses to take medication
f. Verification of client ID
g. Nurse charts that client pain was decreased after drug administration
h. Client receives the prescribed medication
i. Nurse checks the blood pressure following blood pressure medication administration
j. Drug given at the time prescribed

Match the term in Column I with the definition in Column II.

Column I

D __ 11. Absorption
F __ 12. Distribution
E __ 13. Metabolism
B __ 14. Toxicity
A __ 15. Additive effect
C __ 16. Tolerance

Column II

a. Combination of two drugs may be greater than effects of a single drug
b. More prevalent in old and young, and those with liver or renal impairment
c. Client's ability to respond to a drug decreases over time with repeated administration
d. Affected by the route of administration
e. Age, weight, and liver function affect drug biotransformation
f. Protein binding modifies distribution of a drug

Match the letter in Column II with the correct response in Column I.

Column I

Column II

A 17. Drugs poured by others

a. Do not administer

A 18. Client states that drug is different than usual

b. Do administer

B 19. Offer ice to numb taste buds for distasteful drugs

A 20. Drugs transferred from one container to another

B 21. Record fluids taken with medications on the intake and output sheet

A 22. Medications left with visitors

Match the pregnancy category with the correct definition. p.31

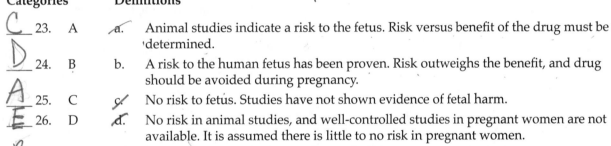

Categories   **Definitions**

C 23. A   a. Animal studies indicate a risk to the fetus. Risk versus benefit of the drug must be determined.

D 24. B   b. A risk to the human fetus has been proven. Risk outweighs the benefit, and drug should be avoided during pregnancy.

A 25. C   c. No risk to fetus. Studies have not shown evidence of fetal harm.

E 26. D   d. No risk in animal studies, and well-controlled studies in pregnant women are not available. It is assumed there is little to no risk in pregnant women.

B 27. X   e. A risk to the human fetus has been proven. Risk versus benefit of the drug must be determined. It could be used in life-threatening situations.

NCLEX Review Questions

Select the best response.

28. The order to *give multivitamins ii caps PO daily* is an example of what category of drug order?

    a. STAT
    b. standing
    c. single
    d. PRN

29. A client has an order to receive Demerol 100 mg, IM, STAT. This is an example of what category of drug order?

    a. PRN
    b. standing
    c. STAT
    d. single

30. When the nurse calculates the dosage for a client's cardiac medication, the drug dose is "large." Which is the best initial action for the nurse to take?

    a. Check the client's name band and give the medication.
    b. Check the calculations.
    c. Call the health care provider.
    d. Withhold the medication and document as not given.

31. The client's medication was taken from an open vial in the refrigerator. Which is the best action for the nurse to take before putting the medication back into the refrigerator?

 a. date and time vial opened; initials

 b. date and time vial opened and client's name

 c. date and number of remaining doses

 d. date and initials

32. The client has refused to take a medication. Which action should the nurse take first?

 a. Call the health care provider.

 b. Document the reason not taken.

 c. Contact the supervisor.

 d. Reinforce the importance of taking medication.

33. Which abbreviations are not allowed by the Joint Commission? (Select all that apply.)

 a. IM

 b. U

 c. IU

 d. trailing zero

 e. q.d.

34. The "right to education" includes which actions? (Select all that apply.)

 a. the client receives correct information about the drug and how it relates to the situation

 b. possible side effects

 c. laboratory monitoring

 d. data collected before administration of drug

 e. evaluation of the client's response

4 Medication Administration

Study Questions

Complete the following.

1. ___enteric coated___ and ___time released___ capsules must be swallowed whole to be effective.

2. Handheld nebulizers deliver a very ___fine___ spray of medication.

3. When giving a client a medication via hand nebulizer, the client should be placed in ___semi-high Fowlers___ position.

4. A nasogastric tube should be flushed with ___50___ mL of water following medication administration.

5. Following insertion of a rectal suppository, the client should remain in a side-lying position for ___20___ minutes.

Match the route in Column I with the correct length of needle in Column II.

Column I

_C_ 6. Subcutaneous

_A_ 7. Intradermal

_B_ 8. IM

Column II

a. ⅜ to ⅝ inches in length

b. 1- to 1½-inch needle

c. ½ to ⅝ inches in length

Complete the following.

9. The injection site that is well-defined by bony anatomic landmarks is ___gluteal___.

10. The preferred site for intramuscular injections for infants and children is ___Vastus laterilis___

11. The site that is easily accessible but not suitable for repeated injections or injections of more than 2 mL is ___deltoid___.

12. The preferred site for the Z-track technique is ___gluteal___.

13. The site (not visible to the client) that has the danger of injury if incorrect technique is used is ___dorso gluteal or sciatica___

NCLEX Review Questions

Select the best response.

14. For clients who are vomiting or comatose, medication administration is contraindicated via which route?
    a. intravenous
    b. intradermal
    c. oral
    d. suppository

15. When administering ear drops, the client should be sitting with the head tilted toward which side?
    a. affected
    b. unaffected

16. In an adult, gently pull the auricle in which direction before instilling ear drops?
    a. up and back
    b. down and back
    c. forward and back
    d. forward and up

17. When is the best time to administer ear drops?
    a. When the medication is at room temperature.
    b. Immediately after removal from the refrigerator.
    c. When the medication is slightly heated.
    d. Right before the client eats.

18. Which is the best site for an IM injection to be given to a 6-month-old infant?
    a. ventrogluteal
    b. deltoid
    c. dorsogluteal
    d. vastus lateralis

19. The client is 10 months old and is receiving an IM injection. Which is the best site to give this injection?
    a. ventrogluteal
    b. deltoid
    c. dorsogluteal
    d. vastus lateralis

20. The client is being discharged on new medications. Which statement made by the client would indicate that more teaching is required?
    a. "I can take any OTC medication or herbal preparation that I think would be helpful."
    b. "I need to make sure I keep my appointments with my health care provider."
    c. "I need to report any side effects to my health care provider."
    d. "I will contact my pharmacy if I am going out of town to ensure that I have enough medication."

21. The nurse is teaching the client about newly prescribed medications. What should be included in the teaching? (Select all that apply.)
    a. information about potential food-drug interactions
    b. information about alcohol use while taking medications
    c. written discharge instructions about medications
    d. information about storing medications in original containers

22. The client is taking a steroid via a metered dose inhaler. What is the most important thing she must do following medication administration?
    a. wash hands
    b. suck on hard candy
    c. rinse out the mouth
    d. blow the nose

23. The nurse is administering a medication via the Z-track method. Which site is best for administration of medication by this method? (Select all that apply.)
    a. ventrogluteal
    b. dorsogluteal
    c. deltoid
    d. vastus lateralis

5 Medications and Calculations

Introduction

The medications and calculations chapter in this Study Guide is subdivided into six sections: (5A) Systems of Measurement; (5B) Methods for Calculation; (5C) Calculations of Oral Dosages; (5D) Calculations of Injectable Dosages; (5E) Calculations of Intravenous Fluids; and (5F) Pediatric Drug Calculations. Before reading and working the drug calculation problems, the student or nurse may find it helpful to review Appendix A: Basic Math Review, located near the end of this book.

Numerous drug labels appear in the drug calculation problems. The purpose is to familiarize the user with reading drug labels and calculating drug dosages from the information provided on the drug labels.

Drug calculation practice problems in each of the six sections provide an opportunity for the user to gain skill and competence in collecting and organizing the required data. Practice problems have examples of the administration of medications via a variety of routes, including both oral and parenteral (subcutaneous, intramuscular, and intravenous).

It is recommended that the user first read the practice problem and estimate an answer. The user should select one of the four methods (basic formula, ratio and proportion, fractional equation, or dimensional analysis) for drug calculations that are presented in the textbook. After completing the required calculations, the user can compare the estimate with the calculated answer. In the event of a discrepancy, the user should review both the thought process used in answering the problem and the actual mathematical calculation. It may be necessary to review the related section in Chapter 5 of the textbook. Practice problems provide reinforcement for the user to gain expertise in the process of actually calculating drug dosages.

Section 5A—Systems of Measurement with Conversion

Metric and Household Systems

Match the term in Column I with the appropriate abbreviation in Column II.

Column I		Column II	
B 1.	Gram	a.	T
F 2.	Milligram	b.	g
G 3.	Liter	c.	mL
C 4.	Milliliter	d.	gr
K 5.	Kilogram	e.	fl oz
L 6.	Microgram	f.	mg
M 7.	Nanogram	g.	L or l
R 8.	Meter	h.	fl dr
D 9.	Grain	i.	minim
E 10.	Fluid ounce	j.	gtt
H 11.	Fluid dram	k.	kg
Q 12.	Quart	l.	mcg
P 13.	Pint	m.	ng
I 14.	Minim	n.	t
O 15.	Cup	o.	c
A 16.	Tablespoon	p.	pt
N 17.	Teaspoon	q.	qt
J 18.	Drops	r.	m

Complete the following.

19. The most frequently used conversions within the metric system are:
    a.   1 g = __1000__ mg
    b.   1 L = __1000__ mL
    c.   1 mg = __1000__ mcg

Complete the unit equivalent for the following measurements. kg – g – mg – mcg

20. 3 grams = __3000__ milligrams *mcg*   3,000

21. 1.5 liters = __15000__ milliliters *mL*   1,5000

22. 0.1 gram = __100__ milligrams *mg*   0.1000   0.100

23. 2500 milliliters = __2.5__ liters *L*   2.500

24. 250 milliliters = __0.25__ liter *L*   0.250

25. 500 milligrams = __0.5__ gram *g*   0.500

26. 2 quarts = __4__ pints *pt*   1 qt = 2 pints

27. 2 pints = __32__ fluid ounces   16 × 2

28. 1½ quarts = __48__ fluid ounces ←

29. 32 fluid ounces = __2__ pints

30. 2 fluid ounces = _____ fluid drams

(handwritten notes at top right:)
16.oz in pt

2pts in 1qt
32oz
16
48

Metric, Apothecary, and Household Systems

31. When converting a unit of measurement from one system to another, convert to the unit on the drug container.

Example:

Order: V-Cillin K 0.5 g, PO, q8h.

Available:

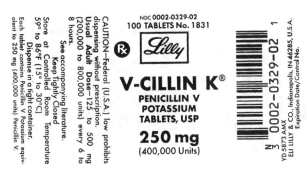

Convert __grams__ to __milligrams__

Convert the following units of measurement to metric, apothecary, and household equivalents. Refer to Table 5A-3 in the textbook as needed.

32. 1 g = __1000__ mg, or _____ gr

33. _____ g = 500 mg, or _____ gr

34. 0.1 g = _____ mg, or _____ gr

35. 1 gr = _____ mg

36. 0.4 mg = _____ gr

37. _____ L = 1000 mL, or _____ qt

38. 240 mL = _____ fl oz, or _____ glass

39. 30 mL = _____ oz, or _____ T, or _____ t

40. 5 mL = _____ t

41. 1 mL = _____ m, or _____ gtt

42. 3 T = _____ oz, or _____ t

43. 5 oz = _____ mL, or _____ T

Section 5B—Methods for Calculation

Select the best response.

1.   Before calculating drug dosages, all units of measurement must be converted to one system. Which system should the nurse use?

    a.   Any one he or she prefers.

    b.   One that fits with how he or she will administer the drug.

    c.   One that is easy to convert to.

    (d.)   The one on the drug label.

Interpretation of Drug Label

Give information concerning the following drug label.

Trade or Brand name

Brand name

2.   What is the brand name of this drug?

    a.   Ampicillin

    (b.)   Principen

3.   What is the generic name of this drug?

    (a.)   Ampicillin

    b.   Principen

4.   What is the dosage of this drug? _250mg pr 5mL_

5.   What is the form of this drug?

    a.   tablet

    b.   liquid

    c.   capsule

    (d.)   suspension

$K_g - g - mg - mcg$

Methods for Drug Calculation

Use the basic formula, ratio and proportion, or dimensional analysis methods to calculate the following drug problems.

6.   Order: Norvir (ritonavir) 0.2 g, PO, b.i.d.

      Available:

      0.200

      NDC 0074-9492-54
      84 Capsules

      Do not accept if seal over
      bottle opening is broken or
      missing.

      NORVIR™
      RITONAVIR CAPSULES
      100 mg

      Dispense in a USP tight,
      light-resistant container.

      Each capsule contains:
      100 mg ritonavir.

      $\dfrac{0.2g}{100mg}\quad \dfrac{200\,mg}{100\,mg}$
      $= 2\ Cap$

      Caution: Federal (U.S.A.) law prohibits
      dispensing without prescription.

      See enclosure for
      prescribing information.

      ©Abbott
      Abbott Laboratories
      North Chicago,
      IL 60064, U.S.A.

      Store in refrigerator between
      36° - 46°F (2° - 8°C). Protect from light.
      02-7878-2/R2
      Exp.
      Lot
      TM-Trademark

      A.   Is conversion needed to give this medication?
            a.   No; it may be administered in grams.
            b.   No; the pill may be broken if needed.
            c.   Yes; it should be converted to grains.
            d.   Yes; it should be converted to milligrams.
      B.   How much of this medication should the nurse administer?
            a.   1 capsule
            b.   2 capsules
            c.   3 capsules
            d.   4 capsules

7.   Order: Benadryl (diphenhydramine) 25 mg, PO, q6h, PRN.
      Available: Benadryl 12.5 mg/5 mL

      $\dfrac{25mg}{12.5mg} \times 5mL$
      $2 \times 5 = 10mL$

      A.   Is conversion needed to give this drug?
            a.   No; it can be administered in milligrams as ordered.
            b.   No; the capsule may be broken if needed.
            c.   Yes; it should be converted to grains.
            d.   Yes; it should be converted to grams.
      B.   How many mL should the nurse give? Calculate the drug problem using the method selected.
            a.   5 mL
            b.   10 mL
            c.   15 mL
            d.   20 mL

Kg - g - mg - mcg

8. Order: Biaxin (clarithromycin) 0.25 g, PO, b.i.d.

Available:

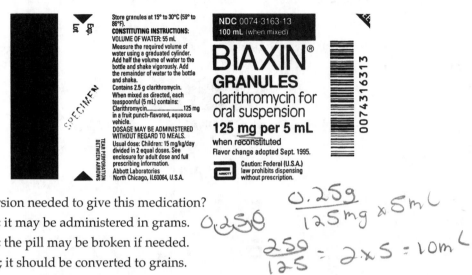

A. Is conversion needed to give this medication?

a. No; it may be administered in grams.

b. No; the pill may be broken if needed.

c. Yes; it should be converted to grains.

(d.) Yes; it should be converted to milligrams.

0.25g

$\dfrac{0.25g}{125mg} \times 5mL$

$\dfrac{25g}{125} = 2 \times 5 = 10mL$

B. How many mL should be administered?

a. 5 mL

(b) 10 mL

c. 15 mL

d. 20 mL

9. Order: hydroxyzine (Vistaril) 100 mg, IM, q6h.

Available:

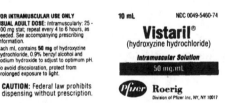

100 mg

$\dfrac{100mg}{50mg/mL}$

2

How many mL should be administered?

a. ½ mL

b. 1 mL

c. 1½ mL

(d.) 2 mL

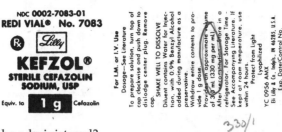

$Kg - g - mg - mcg$

10.   Order: cefazolin (Kefzol) 500 mg, IM, q8h.

Available: (NOTE: Redi-vial container has diluent in a separate compartment of the vial. Push plug to release diluent for reconstitution.)

$$\frac{500mg}{1g}\qquad\frac{500mg}{1000m}$$

$$1.000$$

$$\frac{500m}{330mg}\times 1 \qquad \frac{0.5}{1.5\,mL}$$

$$330/1$$

How many mL should be administered?

a.   1 mL

b.   1.5 mL

c.   2 mL

d.   2.5 mL

Additional Dimensional Analysis

11.   Order: Precose (acarbose) 50 mg, PO, t.i.d.

Available:

$$\frac{50mg}{25mg}=2$$

A.   How many tablets should be administered?

a.   1 tablet

b.   2 tablets

c.   3 tablets

d.   4 tablets

B.   Which drug label(s) should be selected?

a.   25 mg per tablet

b.   100 mg per tablet

Kg – g – mg – mcg

12. Order: Losartan potassium (Cozaar) 0.1 g, daily.

Available:

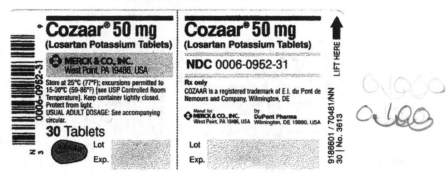

0.1000
0.100

How many tablets should the client receive per day?

a.   1 tablet

b.   2 tablets

c.   3 tablets

d.   4 tablets

$$\frac{0.1\,g}{50\,mg} \quad \frac{100}{50} = 2$$

Section 5C—Calculations of Oral Dosages

Drug calculation problems include oral dosages for adults.

1. Order: benztropine (Cogentin) 1 mg, PO, daily.

Available:

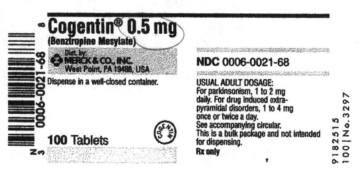

How many tablets should be administered?

a.   1 tablet

b.   1½ tablets

c.   2 tablets

d.   2½ tablets

$$\frac{1\,mg}{0.5\,mg} = 2$$

2.   Order: codeine sulfate 60 mg, PO, q6h, PRN.

Available: Tablets are available in two forms (see drug labels).

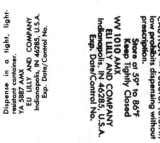 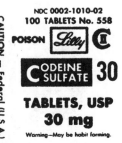

A.   Which form should be used? Why?

a.   15 mg tablets; the client will take more pills

b.   30 mg tablets; the client will take fewer pills

c.   15 mg tablets; the client will take fewer pills

d.   30 mg tablets; the client will take more pills

B.   How many tablets should be administered?

a.   1 tablet

b.   1½ tablets

c.   2 tablets

d.   2½ tablets

3.   Order: propranolol (Inderal) 15 mg, PO, q6h.

Available: propranolol 10 mg and 20 mg tablets.

A.   Which tablet strength should be administered?

a.   10 mg tablets

b.   20 mg tablets

B.   How many tablets should be administered?

a.   1 tablet

b.   1½ tablets

c.   2 tablets

d.   2½ tablets

4. Order: penicillin V potassium 250 mg, PO, q6h.

    Available: (NOTE: The generic name of the drug may be given instead of the brand name. Check the label for both names.)

    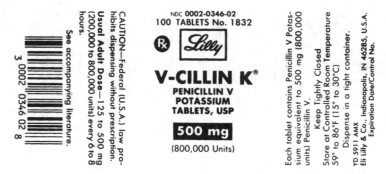

    How many tablets should be administered?

    a. ½ tablet
    b. 1 tablet
    c. 1½ tablets
    d. 2 tablets

5. Order: cimetidine (Tagamet) 600 mg, PO, hour of sleep.

    Available:

    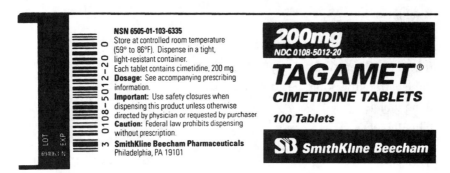

    How many tablets should be administered?

    a. 1 tablet
    b. 2 tablets
    c. 3 tablets
    d. 4 tablets

6.   Order: verapamil 60 mg, PO, q.i.d.

Available:

NDC 0005-3447-23

Verapamil HCl Tablets

120 mg

CAUTION: Federal law prohibits dispensing without prescription.

100 TABLETS STANDARD *Lederle* PRODUCTS

Each tablet contains 120 mg of verapamil hydrochloride
USUAL ADULT DOSAGE: See accompanying circular for complete directions for use. This package not for household dispensing.
Store at Controlled Room Temperature 15-30°C (59-86°F).
Dispense in a tight, light resistant container using a child-resistant closure.
Control No.   Exp. Date

LEDERLE LABORATORIES DIVISION
American Cyanamid Company
Pearl River, NY 10965   24256   D1

NDC 0005-3446-43

Verapamil HCl
Tablets **80 mg**

CAUTION: Federal law prohibits dispensing without prescription.

100 TABLETS *Lederle*

Each tablet contains 80 mg of verapamil hydrochloride.
USUAL ADULT DOSAGE: See accompanying circular.
Store at controlled room temperature 15-30°C (59-86°F). Dispense in a tight, light resistant container using a child-resistant closure.
LEDERLE LABORATORIES DIVISION   25985 D3
American Cyanamid Company, Pearl River, NY 10965

Control No.   Exp. Date

N 3 0005-3446-43 6

A.   Which strength of verapamil should be selected?

a.   120 mg tablet

b.   80 mg tablet

B.   Tablets are scored. How many tablets should be administered?

a.   ½ tablet

b.   1 tablet

c.   1½ tablets

d.   2 tablets

7.   Order: Artane SR 10 mg, PO, daily.

Available:

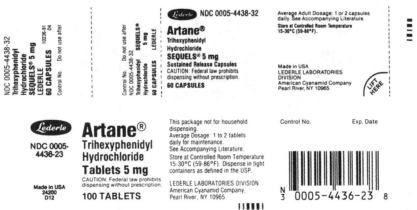

A.   Which container of Artane 5 mg should be selected?

a.   5 mg sustained release tablets

b.   5 mg tablets

B. How many tablet(s)/sequel(s) should be administered?

    a. ½ tablet

    b. 1 tablet

    c. 1½ tablets

    d. 2 tablets

8. Order: trazodone (Desyrel) 150 mg, PO, daily.

Available: Desyrel in 50 mg tablets and 100 mg tablets.

A. How many tablets should be administered if the 50 mg (strength) tablet is used?

    a. 1 tablet

    b. 2 tablets

    c. 3 tablets

    d. 4 tablets

B. How many tablets should be administered if the 100 mg tablet is used?

    a. ½ tablet

    b. 1 tablet

    c. 1½ tablets

    d. 2 tablets

9. Order: Coumadin (warfarin) 7.5 mg, PO, daily.

Available: (NOTE: Tablet is scored.)

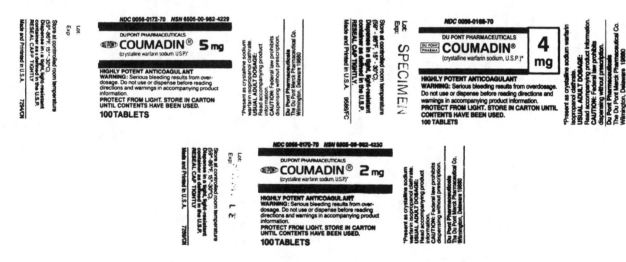

A. Which container of Coumadin should be selected?

    a. Coumadin 2 mg

    b. Coumadin 4 mg

    c. Coumadin 5 mg

B. How many tablets should be administered?

    a. ½ tablet

    b. 1 tablet

    c. 1½ tablets

    d. 2 tablets

10.   Order: lithium carbonate, 300 mg, PO, t.i.d.

Available: lithium carbonate in 150 and 300 mg capsules, and 300 mg tablets. The client's lithium level is 1.8 mEq/L (normal value is 0.5-1.5 mEq/L). What is the best action by the nurse?

a.   Give 150 mg (half the dose).

b.   Give 300 mg tablet and not the capsule.

c.   Advise the client not to take the dose for a week.

d.   Withhold the drug and contact the health care provider.

11.   Order: Coreg (carvedilol) 25 mg, PO, b.i.d.

Available:

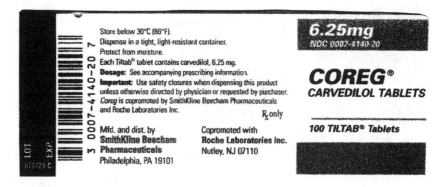

A.   How many tablets should be administered per dose?

a.   3 tablets

b.   4 tablets

c.   5 tablets

d.   6 tablets

B.   How many tablets should the client receive in 24 hours?

a.   4 tablets

b.   6 tablets

c.   8 tablets

d.   10 tablets

12. Order: azithromycin (Zithromax) 400 mg, daily first day, then 200 mg, daily next 4 days.
    Available:

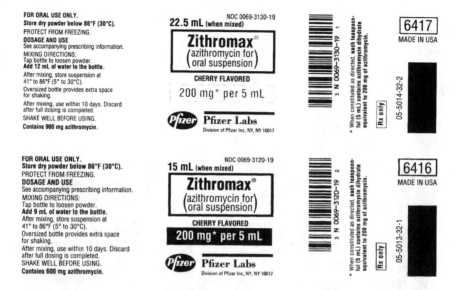

A. How many mL should be administered the first day?

    a. 10 mL/day

    b. 15 mL/day

    c. 20 mL/day

    d. 25 mL/day

B. How many mL should be administered per day for the next 4 days?

    a. 5 mL/day

    b. 8 mL/day

    c. 10 mL/day

    d. 15 mL/day

13.   Order: Artane (trihexyphenidyl) Elixir 1 mg, PO, b.i.d.

Available: Artane 2 mg/5 mL.

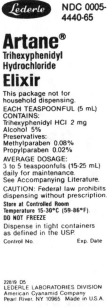

What amount should be administered?

a.   1/2 teaspoon

b.   2 teaspoons

c.   3 teaspoons

d.   4 teaspoons

14.   Order: doxycycline (Vibra-Tabs), 0.2 g, PO first day, then 0.1 g, PO daily for 6 days.

Available:

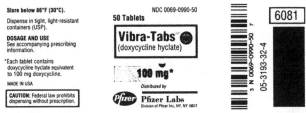

How many tablets should the client receive the first day, then how many tablets per day for 6 days?

a.   2 for the first day and then 2 tablets for each of the following days

b.   2 for the first day and then 1 tablet for each of the following days

c.   3 for the first day and then 2 tablets for each of the following days

d.   3 for the first day and then 1 tablet for each of the following days

15. Order: digoxin 0.25 mg, PO, daily.

    Available: Lanoxin (digoxin) 0.125 mg tablets. The drug comes in 0.25 mg tablets, but that strength of tablet is not available.

    How many tablets should be administered?
    a. 1 tablet
    b. 1½ tablets
    c. 2 tablets
    d. 2½ tablets

16. The client is concerned as she receives the pills because they are a different color and a different amount from what she takes daily. When the client questions the tablets, what is the nurse's best response?
    a. "Please don't worry; it is because we use generic drugs."
    b. "Please don't worry; I calculated this carefully and it is your regular dose."
    c. "We don't have the 0.25 mg tablets available, so you must take two pills of a different strength."
    d. "You are right, this is the wrong dosage. I will be right back with the correct one."

17. Order: Augmentin, 400 mg, PO, q6h.

    Available:

    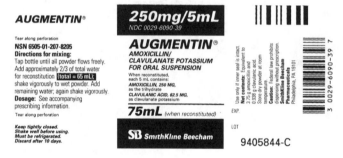

    How many mL should be administered?
    a. 4 mL
    b. 8 mL
    c. 12 mL
    d. 16 mL

18. Order: cefadroxil (Duricef) 1 g, PO, daily.

    Available:

    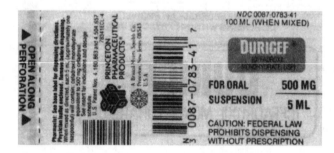

    How many mL should be administered?
    a. 5 mL
    b. 10 mL
    c. 15 mL
    d. 20 mL

19. Order: prazosin (Minipress) 10 mg, PO, daily.

    Available: prazosin 1 mg, 2 mg, and 5 mg tablets.

    Which tablet should be selected, and how many should be administered?

    a.   The 1 mg tablet; 5 pills should be given.

    b.   The 5 mg tablets; 2 pills should be given.

    c.   The 5 mg tablets; 5 pills should be given.

    d.   The 2 mg tablets; 3 pills should be given.

20. Order: carbidopa-levodopa (Sinemet), 12.5-125 mg, PO, b.i.d.

    Available: Sinemet 25-100 mg, 25-250 mg, and 10-100 mg tablets.

    Which tablet should be selected, and how many should be administered?

    a.   The 25-100 mg tablet; ½ tablet should be given.

    b.   The 25-100 mg tablet; 1 tablet should be given.

    c.   The 10-100 mg tablet; 2 tablets should be given.

    d.   The 10-100 mg tablet; 1 tablet should be given.

    e.   The 25-250 mg tablet; ½ tablet should be given.

    f.   The 25-250 mg tablet; 1 tablet should be given.

21. Order: Ceclor 150 mg, PO, q8h.

    Available:

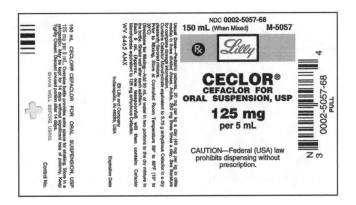

    How many mL should the client receive per dose?

    a.   4 mL

    b.   6 mL

    c.   8 mL

    d.   10 mL

22. Order: ampicillin (Principen) 0.5 g, PO, q6h.

    Available:

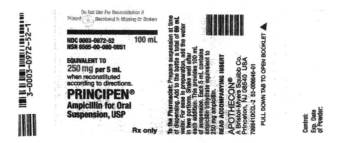

    How many mL should the client receive per dose?
    a.   10 mL
    b.   15 mL
    c.   20 mL
    d.   25 mL

Section 5D—Calculations of Injectable Dosages

Select the best response.

1. What are the methods for administering medications by parenteral routes? (Select all that apply.)
   a. via a nasogastric tube
   b. subcutaneous
   c. intramuscular
   d. intradermal
   e. intravenous
   f. any liquid medication via all routes

2. What are the routes of administration for insulin and heparin? (Select all that apply.)
   a. oral
   b. intramuscular
   c. subcutaneous
   d. intravenous
   e. intradermal

3. Vials are glass containers with (self-sealing rubber tops/tapered glass necks). Vials are usually (discarded/reusable if properly stored). (Circle correct answers.)

4. Before drug reconstitution, the nurse should check the drug circular and/or drug label for instructions. After a drug has been reconstituted and additional dose(s) are available, what should the nurse write on the drug label? (Select all that apply.)
   a. the health care provider's order
   b. date to discard
   c. initials
   d. what it is reconstituted with

5.   A tuberculin syringe (is/is not) used for insulin administration. (Circle correct answer.)

6.   Insulin syringes are calibrated in (units/mL). (Circle correct answer.)

7.   After use of a prefilled cartridge and Tubex injector, which piece(s) of equipment should be discarded?
      a.   cartridge
      b.   Tubex injector
      c.   cartridge and Tubex injector
      d.   neither cartridge nor Tubex injector

8.   The nurse is preparing an IM injection for an adult. What should be used for the needle gauge and length?
      a.   20, 21 gauge; ½, ⅝ inch in length
      b.   23, 25 gauge; ½, ⅝ inch in length
      c.   19, 20, 21 gauge; 1, 1½, 2 inches in length
      d.   25, 26 gauge; 1, 1½ inches in length

9.   Which two parts of a syringe must remain sterile?
      a.   outside of syringe and plunger
      b.   tip of the syringe and plunger
      c.   both the tip and outside of the syringe
      d.   tip and outside of syringe and plunger

10.   Subcutaneous injections can be administered at which degree angle(s)?
      a.   10-degree and 15-degree angles
      b.   45-degree, 60-degree, and 90-degree angles
      c.   45-degree angle only
      d.   90-degree angle only

11.   The nurse calculates the drug dosage to be 0.25 mL. What type of syringe should be selected?
      a.   3 mL syringe
      b.   insulin syringe
      c.   tuberculin syringe
      d.   10 mL syringe

12.   To mix 4 mL of sterile saline solution in a vial containing a powdered drug, which size syringe should be selected?
      a.   tuberculin syringe
      b.   insulin syringe
      c.   3 mL syringe
      d.   5 mL syringe

Determine how many mL to give.

13. Order: heparin 3000 units, subQ, q6h.
    Available:

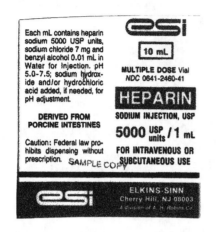 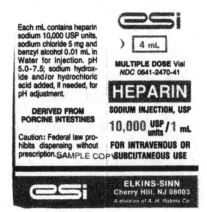

A. Which heparin should be selected?
    a. The 10,000 unit vial
    b. The 5000 unit vial

B. How many mL should be administered?
    a. 0.2 mL
    b. 0.4 mL
    c. 0.6 mL
    d. 0.8 mL

14. Order: codeine ½ gr q4-6h, subQ, PRN.
    Available: Prefilled drug cartridge contains 60 mg/1 mL.
    How many mL should be administered?
    a. ½ mL
    b. 1 mL
    c. 1½ mL
    d. 2 mL

15.   Order: morphine sulfate 1/6 gr subQ, STAT.

Available:

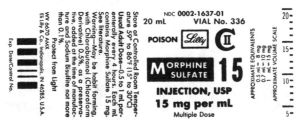

How many mL would you give?

a.   0.5 mL

b.   0.6 mL

c.   0.7 mL

d.   0.8 mL

16.   Order: Humulin L insulin 36 units, subQ, qAM.

Available:

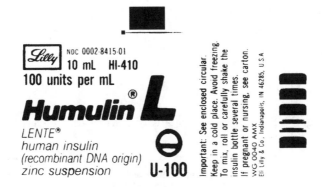

Indicate on the insulin syringe the amount of insulin to be withdrawn.

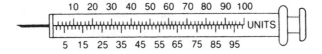

17. Order: regular insulin 8 units and NPH 44 units, subQ, qAM.

    Available: (NOTE: These insulins can be mixed together in the same insulin syringe.)

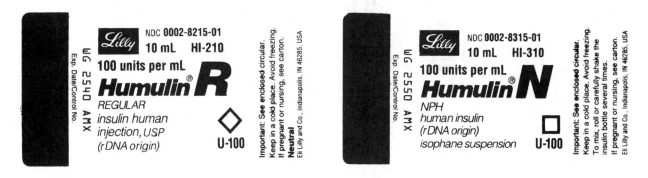

Indicate on the insulin syringe the amount of each insulin to be withdrawn.

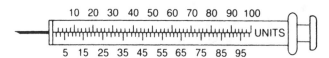

Which insulin should be drawn up first?

a.   Either one can be drawn first

b.   The NPH insulin

c.   The regular insulin

d.   Neither; they should not be given together

18. Order: digoxin 0.25 mg, IM, STAT. (NOTE: Usually digoxin is administered intravenously; however, in this problem, IM is indicated.)

    Available:

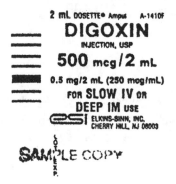

How many mL should be administered?

a.   ½ mL

b.   1 mL

c.   1½ mL

d.   2 mL

19. Order: vitamin B$_{12}$ (cyanocobalamin) 400 mcg, IM, daily for 5 days.

Available:

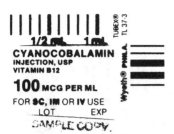   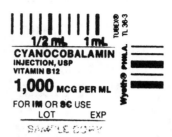

A. Which prefilled cartridge should be selected?

    a. Select the 1000 mcg cartridge.

    b. Select the 100 mcg cartridge.

B. How many mL should be administered?

    a. 0.4 mL

    b. 0.6 mL

    c. 0.8 mL

    d. 1 mL

20. Order: clindamycin 300 mg, IM, q6h.

Available:

How many mL should be administered?

a. 1 mL

b. 2 mL

c. 3 mL

d. 4 mL

21. Order: meperidine (Demerol) 60 mg, IM, and atropine 0.5 mg, IM, preoperatively.

    Available: (NOTE: These drugs are compatible and can be mixed in the same syringe.)

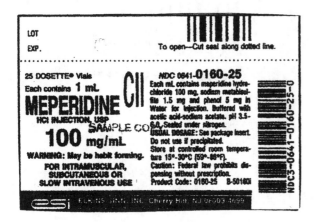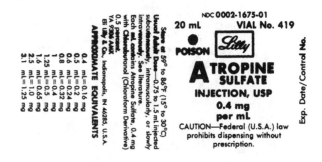

    A. How many mL of meperidine should be discarded?

       a. 0.2 mL

       b. 0.3 mL

       c. 0.4 mL

       d. 0.5 mL

    B. How many mL of meperidine and how many mL of atropine should be administered?

       a. meperidine 0.4 mL and atropine 1.25 mL

       b. meperidine 0.6 mL and atropine 0.7 mL

       c. meperidine 0.6 mL and atropine 1.25 mL

       d. meperidine 0.4 mL and atropine 0.7 mL

22. Order: naloxone (Narcan) 0.8 mg, IM, for narcotic-induced respiratory depression. Repeat in 3 minutes if needed.

    Available:

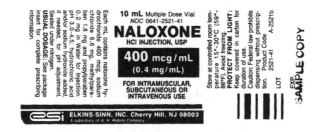

How many mL should be administered?

    a. 1 mL

    b. 2 mL

    c. 3 mL

    d. 4 mL

23. Order: hydroxyzine (Vistaril) 35 mg, IM, preoperatively.

    Available:

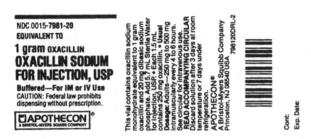

    How many mL should be administered?

    a.   0.25 mL

    b.   0.5 mL

    c.   0.7

    d.   0.9 mL

24. Order: oxacillin sodium 500 mg, IM, q6h.

    Available: Drug in powdered form. (NOTE: Convert to the unit system on the bottle.)

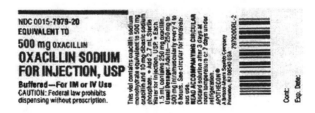

    How many mL should be administered?

    a.   2 mL

    b.   3 mL

    c.   4 mL

    d.   5 mL

25. Order: oxacillin sodium 300 mg, IM, q6h.

    Available:

    A.   The nurse must add _____ mL of sterile water to yield _____ mL of drug solution.

    B.   How many mL should be administered?

        a.   0.5 mL

        b.   1 mL

        c.   1.8 mL

        d.   2 mL

26.   Order: nafcillin (Nafcil) 250 mg, IM, q4h.

Available:

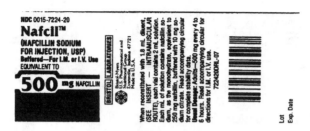

A.   The nurse must add _____ mL of diluent to yield _____ mL of drug solution.

B.   How many mL should be administered?

   a.   1 mL

   b.   2 mL

   c.   3 mL

   d.   4 mL

27.   Order: trimethobenzamide (Tigan) 100 mg, IM, STAT.

Available: trimethobenzamide (Tigan) ampule, 200 mg/2 mL.

How many mL should be administered?

a.   0.3 mL

b.   0.5 mL

c.   0.8 mL

d.   1 mL

28.   Order: chlorpromazine (Thorazine) 20 mg, deep IM, t.i.d.

Available:

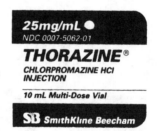

How many mL should be administered?

a.   0.3 mL

b.   0.5 mL

c.   0.8 mL

d.   1 mL

29. Order: ticarcillin (Ticar) 400 mg, IM, q6h.

    Available:

    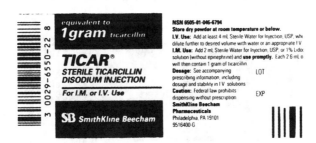

    A.   The nurse must add _____ mL of diluent to yield _____ mL of drug solution.

    B.   How many mL should be administered?

         a.   0.4 mL

         b.   1 mL

         c.   1.4 mL

         d.   2 mL

30. Order: cefonicid (Monocid) 750 mg, IM, daily.

    Available:

    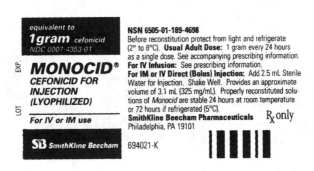

    A.   How many grams is 750 mg?

         a.   0.25 g

         b.   7.5 g

         c.   0.75 g

         d.   75 g

    B.   How many mL of diluent should be injected into the vial? (See drug label.)

         a.   1 mL

         b.   1.5 mL

         c.   2 mL

         d.   2.5 mL

    C.   How many mL of cefonicid should the client receive per day?

         a.   1.3 mL

         b.   2.3 mL

         c.   3.3 mL

         d.   4.3 mL

31.   Order: cefotetan disodium (Cefotan) 750 mg, IM, q12h.

Available: (NOTE: Mix 2 mL of diluent; drug solution will equal 2.4 mL.)

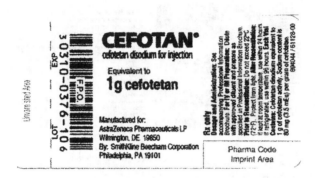

How many mL should be administered per dose?

a.   1 mL

b.   1.8 mL

c.   2.0 mL

d.   2.8 mL

32.   Order: Unasyn (ampicillin sodium/sulbactam sodium) 1 g, IM, q6h.

Available: (NOTE: Mix 2.2 mL of diluent; drug solution will equal 2.6 mL.)

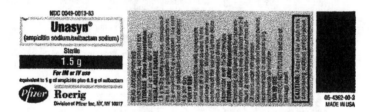

How many mL should be administered per dose?

a.   1.3 mL

b.   1.4 mL

c.   1.7 mL

d.   1.0 mL

Section 5E—Calculations of Intravenous Fluids

Select the best response.

1.   The health care provider orders the type and amount of intravenous (IV) solutions per 24 hours. What should the nurse use to calculate the IV flow rate? (Select all that apply.)

a.   drop factor

b.   amount of fluid to be infused

c.   time of administration

d.   weight of the client

2. When should drugs such as potassium chloride (KCl) and multiple vitamin solutions be injected into the IV bag or bottle?
   a. As soon as the order is written.
   b. When one-half of the bag has been administered.
   c. Before the infusion is started.
   d. Just after the infusion has been started.

Complete the following.

3. Macrodrip infusion sets deliver _____ gtt/mL; microdrip infusion sets deliver _____ gtt/mL.

4. If the infusion rate is less than 100 mL/hr, the preferred IV set is (macrodrip/microdrip). (Circle correct answer.)

5. KVO means _____. The preferred size of IV bag for KVO is (1000 mL/500 mL/250 mL). (Circle correct answer.)

Give the abbreviations for the following solutions.

6. 5% dextrose in water: _____

7. Normal saline solution or 0.9% sodium chloride (NaCl): _____

8. 5% dextrose in ½ normal saline solution (0.45% NaCl): _____

9. 5% dextrose in lactated Ringer's: _____

Complete the following.

10. Intermittent IV administration is prescribed when a drug is administered in a (small/large) volume of IV fluid over a (long/short) period of time. (Circle correct answers.)

11. The Buretrol is a (calibrated cylinder with tubing/small IV bag of solution with short tubing). It is used in (continuous IV drug administration/intermittent IV drug administration). (Circle correct answers.)

12. The pump infusion regulator that delivers mL/hr is a (volumetric/nonvolumetric) IV regulator. (Circle correct answer.)

13. Patient-controlled analgesia (PCA) is a method used to administer drugs intravenously. The purpose/objective is to provide _____.

Continuous Intravenous Administration

Select step method I, II, or III from the text to calculate the continuous IV flow rate. Memorize the step method.

14. Order: 1 liter or 1000 mL of D_5W to infuse over 6 hours.

Available: Macrodrip set: 10 gtt/mL.

The IV flow rate should be regulated as _____ gtt/min.

15. Order: 1000 mL of D_5 ½ NS with multiple vitamins and KCl 10 mEq to infuse over 8 hours.

Available: Macrodrip set: 15 gtt/mL

KCl (potassium chloride) 20 mEq/10 mL ampule

Multiple vitamin (MVI) vial

A.   When should KCl and MVI be injected into the IV bag?

   a.   As soon as the order is written.

   b.   When half of the bag has been administered.

   c.   Before the infusion is started.

   d.   Just after the infusion has been started.

B.   Calculate the IV flow rate in gtt/min. _____

16. Order: 1 L of 0.9% NaCl (normal saline solution) to infuse over 12 hours.

Available: Macrodrip set: 10 gtt/mL

Microdrip set: 60 gtt/mL

A.   Which IV set should be used?

   a.   Macrodrip set

   b.   Microdrip set

B.   Calculate the IV flow rate in gtt/min according to the IV set selected. _____

17. Order: 2.5 L of IV fluids to infuse over 24 hours. This includes 1 L of D_5W, 1 L of D_5 ½ NS, and 500 mL of 5% D/LR.

Available: The three above solutions.

   a.   One liter is equal to _____ mL.

   b.   Total number of mL of IV solutions to infuse in 24 hours is _____ mL.

   c.   Approximate amount of IV solution to administer per hour is _____ mL.

   d.   Which type of IV set would you select? _____

   e.   Calculate the IV flow rate according to the IV set you selected. _____ gtt/min

18. A liter of IV fluid was started at 7:00 AM and was to run for 8 hours. The IV set delivers 10 gtt/mL. At 12:00 PM, only 500 mL were infused.

A.   How much IV fluid is left?

   a.   100 mL

   b.   200 mL

   c.   300 mL

   d.   400 mL

   e.   500 mL

B.   Recalculate the flow rate for the remaining IV fluids. Keep in mind that if the client has a cardiovascular problem, rapid IV flow rate may not be desired. _____

Intermittent Intravenous Administration

(NOTE: Only add the volume of drug solution ≥ 5 mL to IV fluid to determine final drip rate.)

19. Order: cimetidine (Tagamet) 200 mg, IV, q6h.

    Available:

    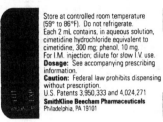 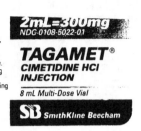

    Set and solution: Buretrol (calibrated cylinder set) with drop factor 60 gtt/mL; 500 mL of NSS.

    Instruction: Dilute cimetidine 200 mg in 50 mL of NSS and infuse in 20 minutes.

    How much cimetidine will be infused per mL?

    a.   2 mg
    b.   3 mg
    c.   4 mg
    d.   5 mg

    IV flow calculation (determine gtt/min):

    a.   50 gtt/min
    b.   100 gtt/min
    c.   150 gtt/min
    d.   200 gtt/min

20. Order: cefamandole (Mandol) 500 mg, IV, q6h.

    Available:

    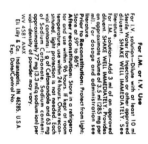 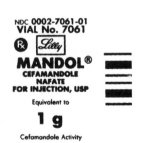

    How many mL of diluent should be added? _____

    Drug solution equals: _____

    Set and solution: Calibrated cylinder with drop factor, 60 gtt/mL; 500 mL of D₅W.

    Instruction: Dilute cefamandole 500 mg reconstituted solution in 50 mL of D₅W and infuse in 30 minutes.

    IV flow calculation (determine gtt/min):

    a.   100 gtt/min
    b.   110 gtt/min
    c.   120 gtt/min
    d.   130 gtt/min

21. Order: nafcillin (Nafcil) 1000 mg, IV, q6h.

    Available:

    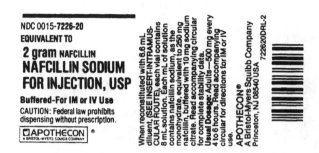

    How many mL of diluent should be added? _____

    Drug solution equals: _____

    Set and solution: Secondary set with drop factor 15 gtt/mL; 100 mL of D$_5$W.

    Instruction: Dilute nafcillin 1000 mg in 100 mL of D$_5$W and infuse in 40 minutes.

    IV flow calculation (determine gtt/min):

    a. 20-22 gtt/min

    b. 37-38 gtt/min

    c. 50-53 gtt/min

    d. 68-69 gtt/min

22. Order: kanamycin (Kantrex) 250 mg, IV, q6h.

    Available:

    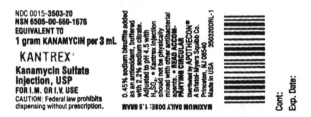

    Set and solution: Secondary set with drop factor 15 gtt/mL; 100 mL of D$_5$W.

    Instruction: Dilute kanamycin 250 mg in 100 mL of D$_5$W and infuse in 45 minutes.

    Drug calculation (convert to the unit on the drug label):

    a. 250 mg = 1 g

    b. 250 mg = 0.5 g

    c. 250 mg = 0.25 g

    d. 250 mg = 0.15 g

    IV flow calculation (determine gtt/min):

    a. 25-27 gtt/min

    b. 33-34 gtt/min

    c. 51-54 gtt/min

    d. 75-76 gtt/min

23. Order: ticarcillin (Ticar) 750 mg, IV, q4h.

Available:

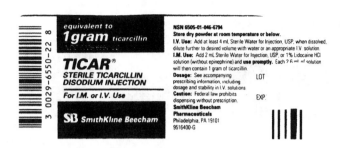

How many mL of diluent would you add? _____

Drug solution equals: _____

Set and solution: Buretrol set with drop factor 60 gtt/mL; 500 mL of D_5W.

Instruction: Dilute ticarcillin 750 mg solution in 75 mL of D_5W and infuse in 30 minutes.

Drug calculation (convert to the unit on the drug label):

a. 1 mL of ticarcillin

b. 2 mL of ticarcillin

c. 3 mL of ticarcillin

d. 4 mL of ticarcillin

IV flow calculation (determine gtt/min):

a. 100 gtt/min

b. 135 gtt/min

c. 150 gtt/min

d. 175 gtt/min

Volumetric IV Regulator

24. Order: Septra (trimethoprim 80 mg and sulfamethoxazole 400 mg), IV, q12h.

Available: Septra (trimethoprim 160 mg and sulfamethoxazole 800 mg/10 mL).

Set and solution: Volumetric pump regulator and 125 mL of D_5W.

Instruction: Dilute Septra 80/400 mg in 125 mL of D_5W and infuse in 90 minutes.

Drug calculation:

a. 5 mL

b. 10 mL

c. 12 mL

d. 15 mL

Volumetric pump regulator (How many mL/hr?):

a. 50 mL/hr

b. 72 mL/hr

c. 87 mL/hr

d. 94 mL/hr

25. Order: doxycycline (Vibramycin) 75 mg, IV, q12h.

    Available: Add 8 mL of diluent = 10 mL.

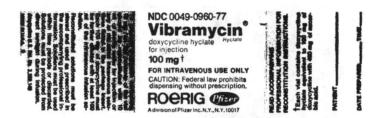

How many mL would equal the Vibramycin 75 mg? _____

Set and solution: Volumetric pump regulator; 100 mL of D_5W.

Instruction: Dilute Vibramycin 75 mg solution in 100 mL of D_5W and infuse in 1 hour.

Volumetric pump regulator (How many mL/hr?):

a. 75 mL/hr

b. 95 mL/hr

c. 108 mL/hr

d. 118 mL/hr

26. Order: amikacin sulfate 400 mg, IV, q12h.

    Adult weight: 64 kg

    Adult drug dosage: 7.5 mg/kg/q12h

    Available:

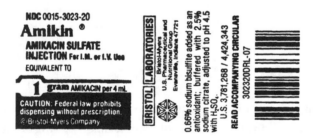

How many mL would equal amikacin 400 mg? _____

Set and solution: Volumetric pump regulator; 125 mL of D_5W.

Instruction: Dilute amikacin 400 mg in 125 mL of D_5W and infuse in 1 hour.

Volumetric pump regulator (How many mL/hr?):

a. 100 mL/hr

b. 125 mL/hr

c. 150 mL/hr

d. 200 mL/hr

27.   Order: minocycline 75 mg, IV, q12h.

Available: Add 5 mL of diluent.

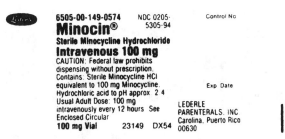

Set and solution: Volumetric pump regulator; 500 mL of D_5W.

Instruction: Dilute minocycline 75 mg in 500 mL of D_5W and infuse in 2 hours.

How many mL would equal minocycline 75 mg?

a.   1.25 mL

b.   2.50 mL

c.   3.75 mL

d.   4.00 mL

Volumetric pump regulator (How many mL/hr?):

a.   150 mL/hr

b.   200 mL/hr

c.   250 mL/hr

d.   300 mL/hr

28.   Order: cefepime hydrochloride (Maxipime) 500 mg, IV, q12h.

Available:

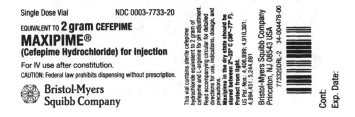

Set and solution: Calibrated cylinder set with drop factor.

Instruction: 60 gtt/mL; 100 mL of D_5W.

The drug label does not indicate the amount of diluent to use. This may be found in the pamphlet insert. Usually, if 2.6 mL of diluent is injected, the amount of drug solution should be 3.0 mL. If 3.4 or 3.5 mL of diluent is injected, the amount of drug solution should be 4.0 mL.

How many mL of drug solution should the client receive?

a.   1 mL

b.   2 mL

c.   3 mL

d.   4 mL

29. Order: Unasyn (ampicillin sodium/sulbactam sodium) 1.5 g, IV, q6h.

Available: (NOTE: Mix 3 g in 10 mL of diluent.)

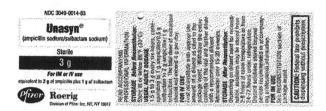

Set and solution: Buretrol or like set with drop factor of 60 gtt/mL; 500 mL of D_5W.

Instruction: Dilute Unasyn 1.5 g solution in 100 mL of D_5W and infuse in 30 minutes.

Drug calculation:

a.   2.5 mL

b.   5.0 mL

c.   7.5 mL

d.   10 mL

IV flow calculation (determine gtt/min):

a.   175 gtt/min

b.   210 gtt/min

c.   225 gtt/min

d.   250 gtt/min

30. Order: Mefoxin (cefoxitin) 500 mg, IV, q6h.

Available: (NOTE: Mix 1 g in 10 mL of diluent.)

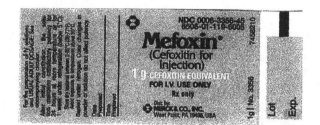

Set and solution: Volumetric pump regulator; 60 gtt/mL; 100 mL of D_5W.

Instruction: Dilute Mefoxin 500 mg in 100 mL of D_5W and infuse in 45 minutes.

Drug calculation:

a.   2.5 mL

b.   5.0 mL

c.   7.5 mL

d.   10 mL

IV flow calculation (determine gtt/min):

a.   120 gtt/min

b.   140 gtt/min

c.   180 gtt/min

d.   200 gtt/min

Section 5F—Pediatric Drug Calculations

Orals

1. Order: penicillin V potassium (V-Cillin K) 200,000 units, PO, q6h.

    Child weighs 46 pounds or 21 kg.

    Child's drug dosage: 25,000-90,000 units/kg/day in 3-6 divided doses.

    Available: (NOTE: The dosage per 5 mL is in mg and units.)

    Is the prescribed dose safe?

    a. No

    b. Yes

    How many mL should the child receive for each dose?

    a. 1.5 mL

    b. 2.0 mL

    c. 2.5 mL

    d. 3.0 mL

2. Order: cefuroxime axetil (Ceftin), 200 mg, PO, q12h.

    Child's age: 8 years; weight: 75 pounds.

    Child's drug dosage (3 months-12 years): 10-15 mg/kg/day.

    Available:

    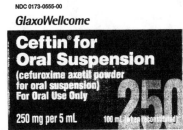

    Is the prescribed dose safe?

    a. No

    b. Yes

    How many mL should the child receive per dose?

    a. 1.0 mL

    b. 2.0 mL

    c. 3.0 mL

    d. 4.0 mL

3.   Order: amoxicillin 75 mg, PO, q6h.

Child weighs 5 kg.

Child's drug dosage: 50 mg/kg/day in divided doses.

Available:

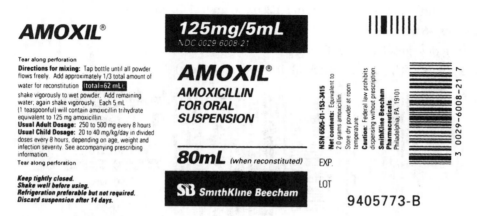

Is the prescribed dose safe?

a.   No

b.   Yes

According to the drug order, how many mg should the child receive per day (24 hours)?

a.   250 mg

b.   300 mg

c.   350 mg

d.   400 mg

4. Order: acetaminophen 250 mg, PO, PRN.

    Available: 160 mg/5 mL.

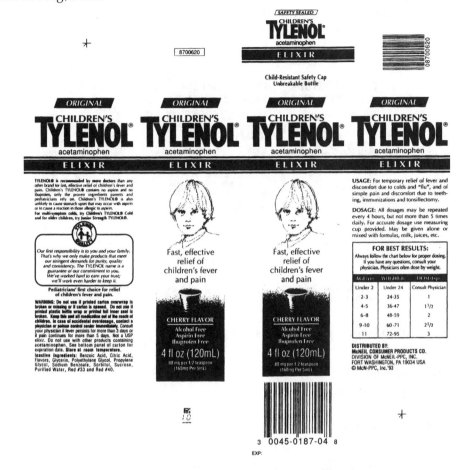

How many mL should be administered? (Round off numbers when necessary.)

a.   4 mL

b.   6 mL

c.   8 mL

d.   10 mL

e.   12 mL

5. Order: cloxacillin 100 mg, PO, q6h.

    Child weighs 8 kg.

    Child's drug dosage: 50-100 mg/kg/day in 4 divided doses.

    Available: cloxacillin (Tegopen), 125 mg/5 mL.

    Is the prescribed dose safe?

a.   Yes

b.   No

How many mL should the child receive per dose?

a.   2 mL

b.   4 mL

c.   6 mL

d.   8 mL

e.   10 mL

6.   Order: erythromycin suspension 160 mg, PO, q6h.

Child weighs 25 kg.

Child's drug dosage: 30-50 mg/kg/day in divided doses, q6h.

Available:

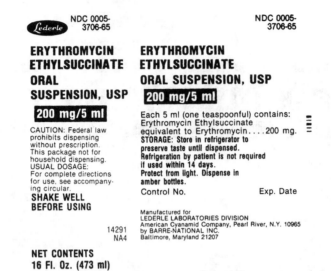

Is the prescribed dosage within dose parameters?

a.   Yes, the dosage is safe.

b.   No, the dosage is too low.

c.   No, the dosage is too high.

7.   Order: cefaclor (Ceclor) 75 mg, PO, q8h.

Child weighs 22 pounds.

Child's drug dosage: 20-40 mg/kg/day in 3 divided doses.

Available:

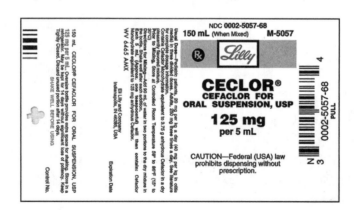

How many mL per dose should be given?

a.   2 mL

b.   3 mL

c.   4 mL

d.   5 mL

e.   6 mL

8. Order: Augmentin 150 mg, PO, q8h.

    Child weighs 26 pounds.

    Child's drug dosage: 40 mg/kg/day in 3 divided doses.

    Available:

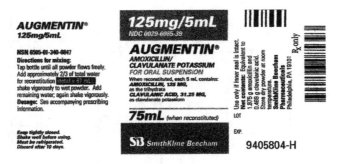

    How many kg does the child weigh?

    a.   10 kg

    b.   12 kg

    c.   14 kg

    d.   15 kg

    Is the prescribed dosage within dose parameters?

    a.   Yes, the dosage is safe.

    b.   No, the dosage is too low.

    c.   No, the dosage is too high.

    How many mL of Augmentin should the child receive per dose?

    a.   2 mL

    b.   3 mL

    c.   4 mL

    d.   5 mL

    e.   6 mL

9. Order: phenytoin (Dilantin).

    Child's weight is 50 pounds; height is unknown.

    Child's BSA is _____ m². Use the center graph of the nomogram (next page) because the height is unknown.

    Child's drug dosage: 250 mg/m² in 3 divided doses.

    Available: Dilantin 30 mg/5 mL.

    How many mL should be given per dose? Round off numbers.

    a.   8 mL

    b.   10 mL

    c.   12 mL

    d.   14 mL

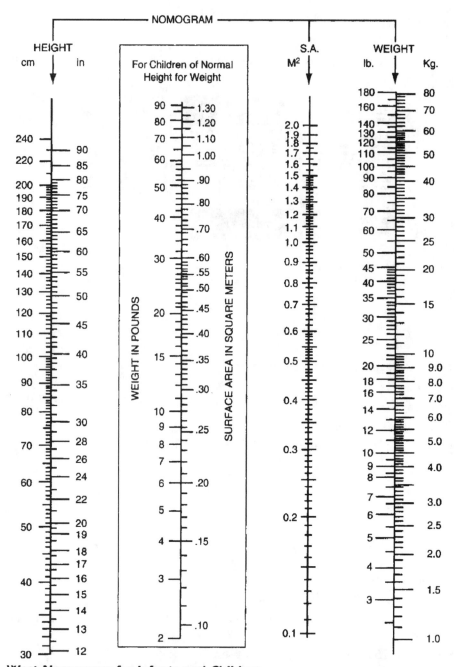

─── NOMOGRAM ───

HEIGHT

cm	in

For Children of Normal Height for Weight

S.A.
M²

WEIGHT

lb.	Kg.

WEIGHT IN POUNDS

SURFACE AREA IN SQUARE METERS

West Nomogram for Infants and Children

Directions: (1) Find height. (2) Find weight. (3) Draw a straight line connecting the height and weight. Where the line intersects on the SA column is the body surface area (m²). (Modified from data by Boyd E, West CD. In Behrman RE, Kliegman RM, Jensen HB: *Nelson Textbook of Pediatrics*, ed 18, Philadelphia, 2007, Saunders.)

Injectables

10. Order: ampicillin (Polycillin-N) 100 mg, IM, q6h.

Child's weight: 26 pounds. (Convert pounds to kilograms [kg].)

Child's drug dosage: 25-50 mg/kg/day.

Available:

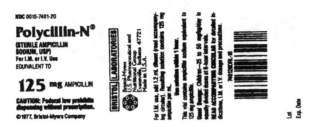

Is the drug dose safe?

a.   Yes

b.   No

How many mL per dose should the child receive?

a.   1 mL

b.   10 mL

c.   15 mL

d.   20 mL

11. Order: pentobarbital (Nembutal) 25 mg, IM, preoperatively.

Child's weight: 40 pounds. (Convert pounds to kilograms.)

Child's drug dosage: 3-5 mg/kg

Available: Nembutal 50 mg/mL

Is the drug dose safe and effective?

a.   Yes

b.   No

How many mL per dose should the child receive?

a.   0.25 mL

b.   0.5 mL

c.   0.75 mL

d.   1.0 mL

12. Order: kanamycin (Kantrex) 50 mg, IM, q12h.

Child's weight: 10 kg.

Child's drug dosage: 15 mg/kg/day in 2 divided doses.

Available:

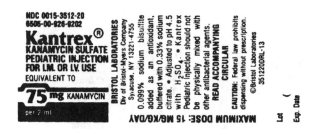

Is the drug dose safe?

a.   Yes

b.   No

How many mL per dose should the child receive?

a.   1.1 mL

b.   1.3 mL

c.   1.6 mL

d.   1.9 mL

13. Order: amikacin sulfate (Amikin) 50 mg, IM, q12h.

Child's weight: 9 kg.

Child's drug dosage: 5 mg/kg/q8h **OR** 7.5 mg/kg/q12h.

Available:

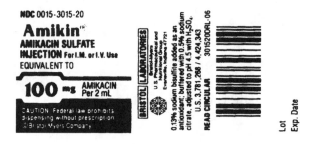

Is the drug dose safe?

a.   Yes

b.   No

How many mL per dose should the child receive?

a.   0.5 mL

b.   1. mL

c.   1.6 mL

d.   2.0 mL

14.   Order: cefazolin sodium (Kefzol) 125 mg, IM, q6h.

Child's weight: 48 pounds.

Child's drug dosage: 25-50 mg/kg/day in 3-4 divided doses.

Available:

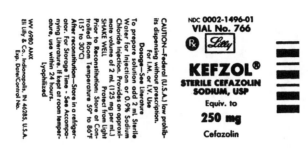

The nurse must add _____ mL of diluent to yield _____ mL of drug solution.

Is the drug dose safe?

a.   Yes

b.   No

How many mL per dose should the child receive?

a.   0.5 mL

b.   1 mL

c.   1.6 mL

d.   2.0 mL

15.   Order: tobramycin (Nebcin) 25 mg, IM, q8h.

Child's weight: 22 kg.

Child's drug dosage: 3-5 mg/kg/day in 3 divided doses.

Available:

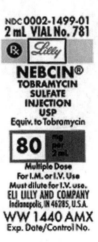

Is the drug dose safe?

a.   Yes

b.   No

How many mL per dose should the child receive?

a.   0.3 mL

b.   0.6 mL

c.   0.9 mL

d.   1.3 mL

6 The Drug Approval Process

Study Questions

Crossword puzzle: Use the definitions to determine the correct terms.

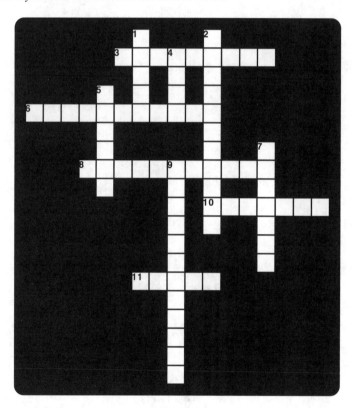

Across

3. Derived from the foxglove plant
6. A drug dose that results in the client's death
8. Omitting a drug dose that results in the client's death
10. Schedule II drug—American
11. Owned by the manufacturer

Down

1. Approval seal of reputable online pharmacies
2. Giving the right drug by the wrong route that results in the client's death
4. Toxic to children in large doses
5. Schedule I drug—Canadian
7. Nonproprietary name
9. Schedule III drug—Canadian

Match the act or amendment in Column I with the description in Column II.

Column I

____ 12. Kefauver-Harris Amendment
____ 13. Food, Drug, and Cosmetic Act
____ 14. Drug Regulation Reform Act
____ 15. Durham-Humphrey Amendment

Column II

a. Determine which drugs can be sold with or without a prescription
b. Resulted from thalidomide tragedy of the 1950s
c. Resulted in increased approval rate for drugs to treat AIDS and cancer
d. Empowered the FDA to monitor and regulate manufacture and marketing of drugs

NCLEX Review Questions

Select the best response.

16. What resource provides the basis for standards in drug strength and composition throughout the world?
    a. *U.S. Pharmacopeia/National Formulary*
    b. *Physicians' Desk Reference*
    c. *Drug Facts and Comparisons*
    d. *International Pharmacopeia*

17. What is the current authoritative source for drug standards?
    a. nurse practice acts
    b. *U.S. Pharmacopeia/National Formulary*
    c. *Physicians' Desk Reference*
    d. Controlled Substances Act

18. What is the primary purpose of federal legislation related to drug standards?
    a. Provide consistency.
    b. Establish cost controls.
    c. Ensure safety.
    d. Act as an information resource.

19. Which legislation gave the FDA a mandate to monitor and control the manufacture and marketing of drugs?
    a. Food, Drug, and Cosmetic Act of 1938
    b. Controlled Substances Act.
    c. Kefauver-Harris Amendment
    d. Durham-Humphrey Amendment

20. Which legislation identified those drugs that required a prescription and a new prescription for refill?
    a. Food, Drug, and Cosmetic Act of 1938
    b. Controlled Substances Act
    c. Kefauver-Harris Amendment
    d. Durham-Humphrey Amendment

21. The Kefauver-Harris Amendment was established to improve safety by requiring which information to be included in the drug's literature?
    a. recommended dose
    b. pregnancy category
    c. side effects and contraindications
    d. adverse effects and contraindications

22. What state law controls drug administration by nurses?
    a. nurse practice act
    b. FDA
    c. Food, Drug, and Cosmetic Act
    d. State Board of Nursing

23. Controlled substances are grouped in schedules/categories. What is the number of schedules?
    a. 3
    b. 5
    c. 7
    d. 9

24. Which Schedule drugs have accepted medical use?

    a.   I through IV

    b.   I through V

    c.   II through V

    d.   III through V

25. What is correct about Schedule drugs' potential for abuse?

    a.   V > IV

    b.   III > I

    c.   I > III

    d.   V > III

26. The client abuses LSD and heroin. To which schedule do these drugs belong?

    a.   I

    b.   II

    c.   III

    d.   IV

27. In which schedule category would the nurse find codeine that is included in cough syrup?

    a.   II

    b.   III

    c.   IV

    d.   V

28. In institutions/agencies, where must controlled substances be stored?

    a.   in a medicine cabinet

    b.   in a locked location

    c.   near the nurses' station

    d.   double wrapped and labeled

29. Drugs in Canada's Schedule F have moderate potential for abuse and require a prescription both for initial allocation and for refills. These drugs are similar to which Schedule in the United States?

    a.   II

    b.   III

    c.   IV

    d.   V

30. In Canada, OTC preparations are administered by what group of the respective provinces?

    a.   Pharmacy Acts

    b.   Canadian Food and Drug Act

    c.   1961 Narcotic Control Act

    d.   Health Protection Act

31. According to the FDA, drugs in which pregnancy category are considered not to present a risk to the fetus?

    a.   A

    b.   B

    c.   C

    d.   D

32. Which legislation decreased the time for approval of drugs used for treating AIDS and cancer?

    a.   Drug Regulation Act of 1992

    b.   Controlled Substances Act

    c.   Durham-Humphrey Amendment

    d.   Kefauver-Harris Amendment

33. Which drug resource is published annually and updated monthly?

    a.   *U.S. Pharmacopeia*

    b.   *Physicians' Desk Reference*

    c.   *American Hospital Formulary*

    d.   Internet Drug Index

34. What are advantages associated with use of generic drugs? (Select all that apply.)

    a.   lower cost

    b.   same active ingredients

    c.   different active ingredients

    d.   same price

35. What are disadvantages associated with generic drugs? (Select all that apply.)

    a.   less extensive testing

    b.   similar testing

    c.   variation in response

    d.   no disadvantages

36. The nurse must be alert for counterfeit prescription drugs. What are clues to identification of counterfeit products? (Select all that apply.)
    a. variation in labeling
    b. different taste
    c. different appearance
    d. different dose

37. Which are implications of HIPAA? (Select all that apply.)
    a. release of information only to client
    b. private area for pharmacy consultation
    c. client receives report of each visit
    d. client signs a copy of privacy statement

38. What amendment approved drugs safe for consumption that may be sold as OTC drugs?
    a. Durham-Humphrey
    b. Kefauver-Harris
    c. Drug Modernization
    d. Food, Drug, and Cosmetic Act

39. What amendment requires proof of efficacy and safety of the drug?
    a. Durham-Humphrey
    b. Kefauver-Harris
    c. Drug Modernization
    d. Food, Drug, and Cosmetic Act

7 Cultural and Pharmacogenetic Considerations

Study Questions

Match the term in Column I with its definition in Column II.

Column I

____ 1.   Assimilation
____ 2.   Complementary health practices
____ 3.   Pharmacogenetics
____ 4.   Ethnopharmacology
____ 5.   Traditional health practices
____ 6.   Pharmacodynamics

Column II

a.   Study of drug responses unique to an individual due to social, cultural, and biological phenomena

b.   The effect of a drug that varies from the predicted response due to genetic factors

c.   Drug concentrations and their effects on the body

d.   Include the use of teas, herbs, spices, and special foods

e.   Occurs when a less powerful group changes its ways to blend in with the dominant cultural group

f.   Combine traditional beliefs and mainstream health practices

NCLEX Review Questions

Select the best response.

7. Which statement reflects the physiologic response of African-American individuals to medications?

    a. They are less responsive to beta blockers than are European Americans and Hispanics.

    b. They are more responsive to beta blockers than are European Americans and Hispanics.

    c. They experience fewer toxic side effects with psychotropic medications than do European Americans.

    d. They experience fewer toxic side effects with antidepressant medications than do European Americans.

8. Many cultural groups have lactose intolerance. What would the nurse assess in a client experiencing this alteration?

    a. constipation

    b. palpitations

    c. elevated enzymes

    d. bloating

9. What communication action is part of the dominant culture in America?

    a. maintenance of eye contact

    b. use of traditional health care providers

    c. use of complementary/alternative medicine

    d. refusal to make eye contact

10. A client, age 22 years, is from the Caribbean. She is 6 months pregnant. At her parents' request, she eats red clay to provide minerals for the fetus, a practice she intends to continue. What would be the best action by the nurse?
    a. Insist that she stop the practice immediately.
    b. Determine the amount of clay she eats daily.
    c. Ask her to substitute corn starch for the clay.
    d. Double her daily iron supplement.

11. A client is newly diagnosed with diabetes and is taking an oral hypoglycemic. His healer has recommended that he drink sabila tea three times a day to improve his nutrition. What would be the nurse's best action?
    a. Encourage him to drink it four times a day.
    b. Discourage the practice; sabila tea potentiates oral hypoglycemics.
    c. Discourage the practice; sabila tea decreases the effects of oral hypoglycemics.
    d. Encourage him to drink the tea but also be sure he continues taking his oral hypoglycemic medication.

12. Which factors may affect clients' physiologic responses to medications? (Select all that apply.)
    a. genetics
    b. diet
    c. age
    d. values

13. Which factors may affect clients' adherence with medication prescriptions? (Select all that apply.)
    a. heredity
    b. poverty
    c. trust in health care provider
    d. access to health care

Case Study

Select the best answer.

A Chinese couple, Foua and Nao Liu, bring their 6-year-old daughter, Lia Liu, to the emergency department. The child had a pulmonary infection and was last seen in the emergency department 2 days ago. At that time, Lia was prescribed erythromycin 150 mg. She does not seem to be improving. The parents bring the bottle of liquid erythromycin with them in a plastic bag. Included in the bag is a porcelain soup spoon, which is about the size of a tablespoon. The instructions on the bottle read: Take 1 teaspoon every 6 hours for 10 days. The bottle is almost half empty.

1. If the parents do not make eye contact with the nurse, how should the nurse interpret this behavior?
    a. They are ignoring what is being said.
    b. They will not adhere to the treatment plan.
    c. They are demonstrating respect to someone considered knowledgeable.
    d. This is a way for them to listen more carefully to what is being said.

2. The parents have been giving Lia a tablespoon of erythromycin each time instead of a teaspoon. How much more erythromycin was the child receiving than prescribed?
    a. 1½ times the prescribed dosage
    b. 2 times the prescribed dosage
    c. 3 times the prescribed dosage
    d. 4 times the prescribed dosage

3. What should concern the nurse about this practice?
    a. Nothing should concern the nurse; it is a minor misunderstanding.
    b. The nurse should be very concerned because this client is being overdosed and it may cause liver impairment.
    c. The nurse should understand that this dose is on the high end of the regular range and may cause hearing problems.
    d. The nurse should realize that the parents did not comprehend the nurse's teaching, but the higher dose is not a big concern.

4. How might the use of a tablespoon versus a teaspoon have been prevented? (Select all that apply.)

  a. by giving the parents a teaspoon

  b. by having the parents demonstrate giving the correct dosage

  c. by providing clearly written instructions

  d. by having a translator present to provide information

5. If the parents speak only in the present tense, how will this affect the nursing care and discharge teaching?

  a. The nurse must present all the information by speaking in the present tense.

  b. The nurse must provide written instructions in the present tense.

  c. The nurse must realize that the parents may discontinue the medication once the child feels better.

  d. The nurse must be aware that the parents may give a larger dosage to enhance the healing process.

6. If the nurse needs an interpreter, who would be the "ideal" interpreter?

  a. a distant relative who speaks both languages

  b. a close family member who has some understanding of English

  c. a health care provider who speaks the clients' language

  d. anyone available on staff who speaks the client's language

8 Drug Interactions and Over-the-Counter Drugs

Study Questions

Crossword puzzle: Use the definition to determine the pharmacologic term.

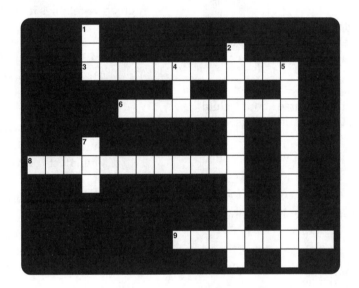

Across
3. No longer found in OTC weight loss drugs
6. Rate at which a drug gets into the body
8. How broadly a drug is found within the body
9. Elimination of a drug from the body

Down
1. Monitors safety of drugs
2. Break down a drug
4. Category of OTC drugs considered to be ineffective
5. When two drugs are given together, one can potentiate the other
7. Drugs obtainable without a prescription

Match the terms in Column I with the letter of the definition in Column II.

Column I

____ 10. Drug interaction
____ 11. Drug incompatibility
____ 12. Adverse drug reaction
____ 13. Pharmacokinetic interaction
____ 14. Pharmacodynamic interaction

Column II
a. Undesirable drug effect
b. Changes that occur in the absorption, distribution, metabolism, or excretion of one or more drugs
c. Altered effect of a drug as a result of interaction with other drugs
d. Reaction that occurs in vitro
e. Interaction that results in additive, synergistic, or antagonistic drug effects

Match the agents in Column I with the letter of the action in Column II.

Column I

____ 15.   Laxatives
____ 16.   Aspirin
____ 17.   Antacids
____ 18.   Food
____ 19.   Narcotics

Column II

a.   Decrease drug absorption
b.   Increase drug absorption
c.   Block drug absorption
d.   Change urine pH to alkaline
e.   Change urine pH to acidic
f.   Increase or decrease absorption
g.   Increase drug excretion

Select the best response.

E.J., 4 years old, is complaining of a sore throat, a cough productive of green sputum, and bilateral knee pain. His parent is about to administer several OTC preparations.

20.   What should concern the nurse about a child taking multiple OTC medications? (Select all that apply.)
   a.   The OTCs may interact with prescribed medications.
   b.   The OTCs should be taken with food.
   c.   The OTCs should never be taken with prescribed medications.
   d.   The OTC and prescription drugs should not be taken without consulting a health care provider.

Ms. Jones is a newly admitted client who is being treated with a ciprofloxacin for an infection. She regularly takes many medications, including digoxin, captropril, lorazepam, warfarin, aspirin, lovastatin, furosemide, antacids, and a laxative as needed. Questions 21-24 are specific to this case.

21.   Ms. Jones is taking ciprofloxacin for an infection. What should concern the nurse about the interaction of this medication with warfarin?
   a.   The ciprofloxacin has to be taken at a different time than the warfarin.
   b.   The ciprofloxacin increases the anticoagulant effects of warfarin.
   c.   The warfarin will increase the antibiotic effects of ciprofloxacin.
   d.   The medications will potentiate each other's effects.

22.   Ms. Jones says that she likes to eat lots of green vegetables including spinach and broccoli. What should concern the nurse about her diet and the types of anticoagulants she is taking?
   a.   The green vegetables are high in vitamin K, which increases the anticoagulant effects of warfarin.
   b.   The green vegetables are high in vitamin K, which decreases the anticoagulant effects of warfarin.
   c.   The green vegetables are low in vitamin K, which increases the anticoagulant effects of warfarin.
   d.   The green vegetables are low in vitamin K, which decreases the anticoagulant effects of warfarin.

23.   When questioned, Ms. Jones states that she takes a laxative at least four times a week. What should concern the nurse about the frequency of laxative use?
   a.   Laxatives slow down gastric emptying, which increases drug absorption.
   b.   Laxatives increase gastric emptying, which decreases drug absorption.
   c.   Laxatives impact the liver's metabolism of medications, thereby increasing their effects.
   d.   Laxatives impact the liver's metabolism of medications, thereby decreasing their effects.

24. Ms. Jones' lab values reveal that her serum potassium levels are low. Which of her medications, when taken regularly, can decrease serum potassium levels? (Select all that apply.)
    a. digoxin
    b. warfarin
    c. furosemide
    d. lovastatin

NCLEX Review Questions

Select the best response.

25. Which of the drug groups is primarily absorbed by the small intestine?
    a. barbiturates
    b. salicylates
    c. anticonvulsants
    d. xanthine derivatives

26. The client is receiving two analgesics for pain relief. Two drugs with similar action are administered to achieve which effects?
    a. additive
    b. synergistic
    c. agonistic
    d. antagonistic

27. The client had surgery yesterday. He is taking two drugs at the same time, a narcotic and an antihistamine. This is an example of which type of drug effects?
    a. additive
    b. synergistic
    c. agonistic
    d. antagonistic

28. When two drugs that have opposite effects are administered (e.g., stimulant and beta blocker), the drug effects are cancelled. This is an example of which type of drug effect?
    a. additive
    b. synergistic
    c. agonistic
    d. antagonistic

29. A major drug-food interaction occurs between monoamine oxidase (MAO) inhibitors and foods rich in which component?
    a. caffeine
    b. fiber
    c. tyramine
    d. acetylcholine

30. The client is taking digoxin and a diuretic. The nurse must be aware of digitalis toxicity and which of the following serum levels?
    a. potassium
    b. sodium
    c. calcium
    d. chloride

31. How are most drugs excreted from the body?
    a. through the lungs
    b. through the urine
    c. through the saliva
    d. through the feces

32. Based on review by the FDA, OTC drugs are assigned to one of how many categories?
    a. two
    b. three
    c. four
    d. five

33. Drugs not included in nonprescription products because they are unsafe or ineffective are assigned to which OTC category?
    a. I
    b. II
    c. III
    d. IV

34. Most drug-induced photosensitivity reactions can be avoided by which actions? (Select all that apply.)
    a. using sunscreen
    b. eating foods high in vitamin C
    c. wearing protective clothing
    d. avoiding excessive sunlight

35. Clients with impaired renal function should avoid which substance(s)? (Select all that apply.)

    a. aspirin

    b. acetaminophen

    c. Milk of Magnesia

    d. ibuprofen

36. The nurse is caring for a client receiving prescription drugs including an anticoagulant. The nurse is aware that anticoagulants have an increased effect with which drug(s)? (Select all that apply.)

    a. lovastatin

    b. aminoglycosides

    c. propranolol

    d. ibuprofen

    e. fibrates

37. The nurse is providing education to a client who is beginning to take an oral contraceptives. The client should be informed that many medications interfere with the actions of oral contraceptives. Which medications have been shown to decrease their effectiveness? (Select all that apply.)

    a. antacids

    b. laxatives

    c. antibiotics

    d. anticonvulsants

    e. calcium channel blockers

9 Drugs of Abuse

Study Questions

Crossword puzzle: Use the definitions to determine the correct terms.

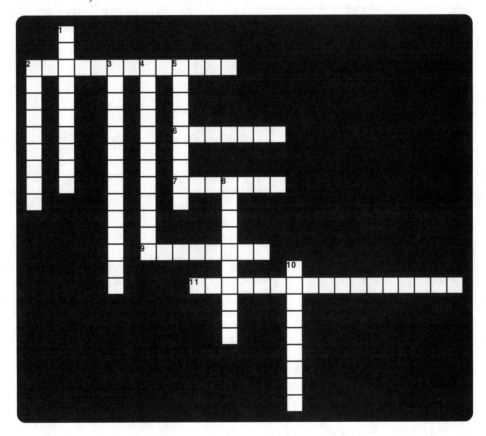

Across
2. Uncontrolled craving for a substance (2 words)
6. Return to drug use after a period of non-use
7. Most potent of the abused stimulants
9. Addictive agent in tobacco
11. A common cause of relapse (3 words)

Down
1. Recreational use of a chemical substance (2 words)
2. Overindulgence of a chemical substance resulting in negative functioning (2 words)
3. Treating an intoxicated client to remove drugs from the body
4. Under the influence or being affected by a drug
5. Need for larger doses of a drug to obtain original euphoria
8. Sustained avoidance of substance use
10. Antidepressant used to treat nicotine addiction

Match the term in Column I with the definition in Column II.

Column I

_____ 12.   Korsakoff's psychosis
_____ 13.   Wernicke's encephalopathy
_____ 14.   Cross-tolerance
_____ 15.   Withdrawal syndrome

Column II

a.   Inflammation of the brain from deficit of thiamine

b.   Short-term memory loss and inability to learn

c.   Can include gross tremors, seizures, and hallucinations

d.   Tolerance to one drug causes tolerance to another in the same category

NCLEX Review Questions

Select the best response.

16.   Several students are brought to the emergency department after their arrest for cocaine use. Which clinical manifestations most accurately describe the effects of cocaine?

   a.   insomnia and fine tremors
   b.   dilated pupils and diaphoresis
   c.   hypotension and tachycardia
   d.   depression and pinpoint pupils

17.   A cocaine-using client is also taking digoxin daily. What is the interaction of these two drugs?

   a.   no interaction
   b.   reciprocal increase in effects
   c.   bradycardia
   d.   dysrhythmias

18.   It is essential that nurses anticipate withdrawal syndrome in clients because alcohol withdrawal delirium can usually be prevented with the administration of which drugs?

   a.   naloxone (Narcan)
   b.   methadone (Dolophine)
   c.   disulfiram (Antabuse)
   d.   lorazepam (Ativan)

19.   Wernicke's encephalopathy is one of many effects of chronic alcohol use. What is the drug of choice to treat this condition?

   a.   IV thiamine
   b.   IV glucose
   c.   IV KCl
   d.   IV plasma expanders

20.   Which drug contains the only FDA-approved cannabis preparation?

   a.   dronabinol
   b.   lorazepam
   c.   methadone
   d.   naloxone

21.   The client has chosen to use nicotine lozenges to aid him with smoking cessation. What should be included in health teaching for this client?

   a.   Avoid food and drink for 15 minutes before taking the lozenge.
   b.   This product is not advised for those with asthma.
   c.   Chewing and swallowing the lozenge increases GI side effects.
   d.   Avoid food and drink for 15 minutes after taking the lozenge.

22.   What percentage of nurses abuse drugs and demonstrate related impaired practice?

   a.   3%-6%
   b.   7%-10%
   c.   11%-15%
   d.   >15%

23. The nurse is caring for a client experiencing withdrawal from alcohol. Which clinical manifestations are related to a major withdrawal syndrome? (Select all that apply.)

    a.   gross tremors

    b.   seizures

    c.   hyperreflexia

    d.   nausea

    e.   hallucinations

24. A health care provider just ordered Chantix for the client. Which are appropriate interventions to include in the care plan for this client? (Select all that apply.)

    a.   Set quit date with the client.

    b.   Instruct the client about nicotine replacement systems.

    c.   Provide the client with information on support groups.

    d.   Contact the client every 2 days.

    e.   Evaluate the effectiveness of the cessation plan.

10 Herbal Therapy with Nursing Implications

Study Questions

Match the description in Column I with the letter of the reference in Column II.

Column I

____ 1. "Reasonable certainty" reported on specific herbal remedy

____ 2. The authoritative source for therapeutic substances

____ 3. Supports study of alternative therapies

____ 4. Supportive of 1976 resolution for health care for world's population by 2000

____ 5. Plant-based remedies

____ 6. Two primary types of herbal monographs

____ 7. Clarified marketing regulations for herbal remedies

Column II

a. *United States Pharmacopeia*

b. World Health Organization

c. Phytomedicine

d. German Commission E

e. Office of Alternative Medicine

f. Dietary Supplement Health and Education Act of 1994

g. Therapeutic and qualitative

Complete the following word search. Clues are given in questions 8-13. Circle your responses.

```
P U R Y S T P J B W Q S A
I E H R Z X A J M I Y B N
T I N C T U R E Z P I I X
D A T W E X T R A C T S U
L D U E R E A O I L B X W
W V F D A O M T Y R N O L
N H R S Q U N U E Q P P I
W K L M P Z A H A R C U R
```

8. Adding a sweetener to an herb and cooking it results in a _____.

9. Soaking dried or fresh herbs in boiling water makes a _____.

10. A _____ is derived from soaking fresh or dried herbs in a solvent.

11. _____ have more reliable dosing by isolating certain components.

12. Soaking dried herbs in oil and heating for a long time results in an _____.

13. Enzyme activity may cause fresh _____ to decay in a few days.

Match the herb in Column I with the letter of its description in Column II.

Column I

____ 14. Ginkgo biloba
____ 15. Peppermint oil
____ 16. Yarrow
____ 17. Saw palmetto
____ 18. Kava kava
____ 19. Goldenseal
____ 20. Psyllium
____ 21. Echinacea
____ 22. Ginger
____ 23. St. John's wort

Column II

a. Provides muscle relaxation
b. Widely used as laxative and with Crohn's disease
c. Immune enhancer
d. May be helpful in Raynaud's and Alzheimer's diseases
e. Relief from stiffness and pain of osteoarthritis and rheumatoid arthritis
f. Tonic, astringent, and to relieve congestion of common cold
g. May be effective treatment for tension headache
h. Stops wound bleeding
i. "Herbal Prozac"
j. "Plant catheter"

Crossword puzzle: Use the definitions to determine the correct terms.

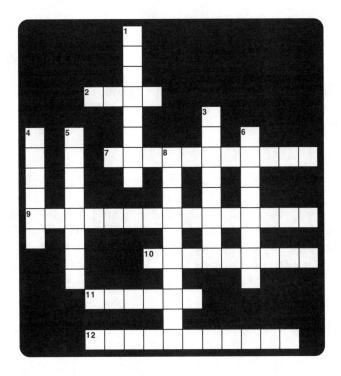

Across
2. Dries up mother's milk
7. Thought to decrease prostate size (2 words)
9. Natural estrogen promoter (2 words)
10. Helps prevent urinary tract infections
11. Increases immune function
12. Its extract may help to prevent liver damage (2 words)

Down
1. Used to treat menstrual cramps (2 words)
3. "Herbal valium"
4. Decreases nausea in pregnancy
5. May promote healthy vision
6. Used to relieve migraine headaches
8. Increases bile flow

NCLEX Review Questions

Select the best response.

24. Which herb is commonly used for external treatment of insect bites and minor burns?
    a.   feverfew
    b.   yarrow
    c.   aloe vera
    d.   licorice

25. Which popular herb is used for relief of digestive and gastrointestinal distress?
    a.   chamomile
    b.   licorice
    c.   St. John's wort
    d.   kava kava

26. What is the most the most commonly prescribed herbal remedy worldwide?
    a.   gingko biloba
    b.   echinacea
    c.   ginger
    d.   licorice

27. Which herb is a natural estrogen promoter and may lower the seizure threshold if taken with anticonvulsants?
    a.   ginger
    b.   psyllium
    c.   feverfew
    d.   evening primrose

28. Which herb is used for CNS sedation without loss of mental acuity or memory and has no risk of tolerance, and is used to treat anxiety and insomnia?
    a.   licorice
    b.   kava kava
    c.   peppermint
    d.   milk thistle

29. Health teaching for the client taking an anticoagulant would include information on which herbal product?
    a.   echinacea
    b.   garlic
    c.   evening primrose
    d.   sage

30. The nurse is concerned that the client is abusing ginseng. What should the nurse assess in a client with ginseng abuse syndrome? (Select all that apply.)
    a.   urinary retention
    b.   edema
    c.   insomnia
    d.   hypertonia

31. Which statements reflect prudent use of herbs? (Select all that apply.)
    a.   Herbs are fine to use when breastfeeding.
    b.   Do not take a large quantity of any one herbal product.
    c.   Give the herb time to work for a persistent symptom before seeking care from a health care provider.
    d.   Do not give herbs to infants or young children.
    e.   Brands of herbal products are interchangeable.

32. The nurse is caring for a client who takes a variety of herbal products and is starting a prescription antidiabetic medication. Which herbs will change the effect of the antidiabetic drug? (Select all that apply.)
    a.   cocoa
    b.   dandelion
    c.   evening primrose
    d.   feverfew
    e.   garlic

33. The client tells the nurse that he is taking ginkgo. Which medications have negative interactions with ginkgo? (Select all that apply.)
    a.   antiplatelet agents
    b.   nifedipine
    c.   omeprazole
    d.   theophylline
    e.   lithium

34. Which medication alterations are seen in combination with licorice? (Select all that apply.)
    a.   Antihypertensive's effects are decreased.
    b.   Corticosteroid's effects are increased.
    c.   Digoxin's effects are increased.
    d.   CNS depressant's effects are decreased.

Case Study

Select the best answer.

J.C., a 24-year-old teacher, visits his health care provider for a pre-employment physical examination. During the nursing history, J.C. tells the nurse that he has several questions about the use of herbs.

1. J.C. would like to know what to consider when deciding which types and brand of herbal supplements to purchase. What information should be received prior to purchasing any herbal supplements? (Select all that apply.)
   a. If J.C. is taking any prescription medications, he should check with his health care provider prior to taking any herbal supplements.
   b. Most herbs are prepared in such low doses there is essentially no risk when taking them.
   c. Herbal supplements are not regulated by the FDA and often contain additives and fillers.
   d. Purchase only preparations that have the plan and quantities listed on the package.

2. J.C. states that he has a friend who takes echinacea and St. John's wort and he is considering taking them as well. What is the specific information he should receive before taking these herbs? (Select all that apply.)
   a. Echinacea is recommended to boost the immune system on a short-term basis, only about 8 weeks.
   b. If J.C. is taking prescription medications, he should check with his health care provider first.
   c. These two herbs should never be taken together as they have an additive effect on each other.
   d. Taking these medications together can increase an individual's risk for depression and suicide.

3. J.C. informs the nurse that he wants to lose weight and is considering taking ma huang for weight loss and as an energy booster. What comment by J.C. indicates a need for further education?
   a. "I know the herb has to be taken with caution due to its side effects such as palpitations and possible stroke."
   b. "I should not have to worry because this herb will increase my energy without making me jittery."
   c. "I should notify my health care provider that I am taking this herb and if I experience any adverse reactions."
   d. "I might want to consider trying something else for weight loss because I already have heart problems."

4. J.C. has one last question. He states that he experiences nausea when flying and wants to know if there are any herbs he can take to decrease it. Which herb has been shown to be effective with nausea?
   a. garlic
   b. feverfew
   c. ginger
   d. milk thistle

11 Pediatric Pharmacology

Study Questions

Complete the following.

1. Infants have _____ protein sites than adults, so _____ dosages of medications are needed.

2. The degree and rate of absorption of medications within a pediatric client are based on _____, _____, and _____.

3. Gastric pH does not reach adult acidity until between _____ and _____ year(s) of age.

4. Distribution of a medication throughout the body is impacted by _____, _____, _____, and effectiveness of various barriers to medication transport.

5. Until about the age of _____, the pediatric client requires a _____ dose of water-soluble medications to achieve therapeutic levels.

Match the child's age group in Column I with a cognitive element to consider when administering medications in Column II.

Column I

____ 6.   Infant
____ 7.   Toddler
____ 8.   Preschool
____ 9.   School-age
____ 10. Adolescent

Column II

a. Allow some choice
b. Involvement in administration process
c. Contract regarding plan of care
d. Simple explanation
e. Minimum restraint

NCLEX Review Questions

Select the best response.

11. The nurse is administering an acidic medication to a 2-week-old infant. What is the impact of the client's age on the absorption of this medication?

    a.   increase
    b.   decrease
    c.   no effect
    d.   protective

12. A 2-year-old child is to receive a water-soluble medication. Based on the nurse's knowledge of medication distribution, how may the dosage need to be modified for this client in order to reach therapeutic levels?

    a.   increased
    b.   decreased
    c.   no change
    d.   alternate route

13. The blood-brain barrier in infants allows medication into the nervous system more easily than in adults. Which outcome is more likely in children?
    a. more side effects
    b. increased protection
    c. toxicity
    d. quicker recovery

14. What is the rate of absorption of topical drugs by children compared with adults?
    a. faster
    b. slower
    c. no difference
    d. depends on age

15. What are the components of pharmacokinetics? (Select all that apply.)
    a. absorption
    b. distribution
    c. onset
    d. metabolism
    e. excretion

16. What strategies should be implemented to involve parents and other significant family members in the administration of medications to pediatric clients? (Select all that apply.)
    a. restraining the child
    b. administering the medication
    c. evaluating the effectiveness of the medication
    d. providing comfort to the child after medication administration
    e. preparing the medication for the nurse to administer

17. The nurse is teaching a group of parents how to administer medications to their children. Which elements of medication administration should be included in the teaching? (Select all that apply.)
    a. Lightly restrain the child, do not use force.
    b. Praise the child after successful administration.
    c. Never threaten or shame the child into taking the medication.
    d. Never tell the child what to expect, just give the medication.

Case Study

Select the best answer.

A nurse on a busy pediatric unit needs to provide medications for five clients. These five clients include a 10-month-old receiving oral elixir antibiotics for an ear infection, a 10-year-old receiving subcutaneous insulin for diabetes mellitus, a 4-year-old receiving a topical anesthetic in preparation for insertion of an IV, a 2-year-old receiving eye drops for an infection, and a 16-year-old receiving intramuscular pain medication on a one-time basis.

1. What are the ways to most successfully administer the oral medications to the 10-month-old client?
    a. Forcefully restrain the child prior to giving the medication.
    b. Enlist the parents' support in giving the medication.
    c. Use a spoon to administer the medication.
    d. Mix the medication in water or saline.

2. What is the best method of administering a topical anesthetic in preparation for an IV insertion? (Select all that apply.)
    a. Enlist the parent to restrain the child prior to medication administration.
    b. Have the child participate in the medication administration.
    c. Allow the child to cover it with a opaque dressing.
    d. Provide a simple explanation of what you will be doing.

3. One of the clients will be discharged on medications. What information should be supplied to the parents in order to provide for safe, effective care? (Select all that apply.)
    a. Appropriate medication dosage, route and time of administration.
    b. Side effects that may be seen with this medication and which to report to the health care provider.
    c. Precautions that should be noted while the child is taking the medication.
    d. The child may take OTC medications without contacting the health care provider.

12 Geriatric Pharmacology

Study Questions

Crossword puzzle: Use the definitions to determine the correct terms.

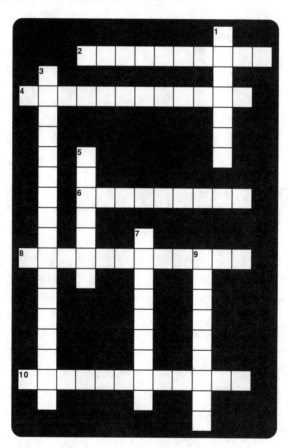

Across

2. Affected by alkaline GI pH found in older persons
4. Affected by loss of binding proteins
6. Type of drugs usually prescribed for heart failure or hypertension
8. Taking multiple medications together
10. Not taking medications as prescription indicates

Down

1. Long-term use of this drug must be monitored due to its narrow therapeutic range
3. Drug metabolism that occurs in the liver and contributes to clearance of drugs
5. Major organ involved in drug excretion
7. 75% of nursing home residents take this type of drug
9. Taking medications as prescribed

NCLEX Review Questions

Select the best response.

11. What is an indicator of the glomerular filtration rate and the normal value (mL/min) for an adult?
    a. creatinine clearance: 80-130
    b. SGOT: 4-12
    c. troponin: 80-120
    d. urea: 1.2-4.5

12. The best antihypertensive agents for older persons have a low incidence of which change occurring?
    a. electrolyte imbalance
    b. central nervous system side effects
    c. loss of appetite
    d. vision changes

13. Digoxin (Lanoxin), a cardiac glycoside, has a long half-life. In older adults, especially those more than 80 years old, digoxin accumulation might cause which alteration?
    a. weakness
    b. increased appetite
    c. urinary retention
    d. digitalis toxicity

14. An older client is taking an antidepressant. The dose is decreased by what percentage when compared to the dose for middle-aged adults?
    a. 10-30
    b. 30-50
    c. 50-70
    d. 70-90

15. Which drug would have fewer adverse and toxic effects?
    a. fat-soluble, half-life of 50 hours
    b. fat-soluble, 90% protein-bound
    c. half-life of 4 hours, 50% protein-bound
    d. half-life of 30 hours, 90% protein-bound

16. Which organs are especially significant in drug therapy of the older client and should be monitored?
    a. kidney and pancreas
    b. kidney and liver
    c. liver and pancreas
    d. kidney and lungs

17. A client reports dizziness every morning when he gets out of bed. What alteration is the client probably experiencing?
    a. bradycardia
    b. orthostatic hypotension
    c. intermittent claudication
    d. hyperventilation

18. What changes should the nurse recommend for the client to decrease the dizziness he experiences when he gets out of bed?
    a. Take his pulse rate before getting out of bed.
    b. Take deep breaths.
    c. Move a chair close to the bed.
    d. Change position slowly.

19. Following hospitalization, the client receives a home visit from the nurse. The client asks if she should continue to take the medications she took before hospitalization. What is the most appropriate response?
    a. "Yes, you should continue to take the drugs that you took before going to the hospital."
    b. "You should take one-half the dosage of each drug that you took prior to hospitalization."
    c. "You should take only the drugs that have been prescribed on discharge and not drugs that you took prior to hospitalization unless otherwise indicated."
    d. "You should continue to take those drugs that have been helpful to you."

20. The client says that before her hospitalization, she was taking digoxin 0.125 mg per day. The new prescription is digoxin 0.25 mg per day. The client wants to know what she should do. What is the nurse's best response?
    a. "You should take digoxin 0.125 mg per day."
    b. "You should take digoxin 0.25 mg per day."
    c. "You should take digoxin 0.125 mg in the morning and 0.25 mg in the evening."
    d. "You should take both doses of digoxin at least 1 hour apart."

21. A client says that he has problems opening the bottle tops of the drugs. What is the nurse's best response?
    a. "Please ask your pharmacist to place the drugs in bottles with non-child–proof caps."
    b. "Please put your medications in glass cups and place them in the cabinet."
    c. "Please put your drugs in individual envelopes."
    d. "Please ask a family member to help with your daily medication regimen."

22. A client is to take newly prescribed drugs at different times. The client has vision problems. What should the nurse suggest so that the client can comply with the medication regimen?
    a. "Line up the bottles of medications on a table and take them in that order."
    b. "Obtain a daily (preferably) or weekly pill container from the drugstore and fill the container the day or week before with the drugs."
    c. "Ask a neighbor to give the daily medications."
    d. "Write down the drugs that you have taken each day."

23. An 80-year-old client begins taking a tricyclic antidepressant. Which clinical manifestations suggest that she is experiencing side effects of this class of drug? (Select all that apply.)
    a. tachycardia
    b. bradycardia
    c. constipation
    d. hypotension
    e. urinary retention

24. In older adults, drug dosages are adjusted based on which factors? (Select all that apply.)
    a. laboratory test results
    b. amount of adipose tissue
    c. height
    d. health problems

25. Before administering drugs to older clients, what should the nurse know? (Select all that apply.)
    a. whether the drug is highly protein-bound
    b. the half-life of the drug
    c. the availability of the drug
    d. the serum levels of drugs with narrow therapeutic ranges

26. Which factors contribute to adverse reactions in older clients? (Select all that apply.)
    a. loss of protein-binding sites
    b. decline in hepatic first-pass metabolism
    c. prolonged half-life of the drug
    d. increase in hepatic first-pass metabolism

Case Study

Select the best answer.

M.Z., an octogenarian with few health issues, visits her health care provider for her annual check-up. During the health history, she complains of "trouble falling asleep and staying asleep and having to get up to go to the bathroom several times each night." M.Z. says her current medications are HydroDIURIL and Halcion. "I try to remember to take my meds, and sometimes I take an extra one, just in case I missed a dose," she says.

1. Which laboratory test would the nurse expect to be ordered to determine if M.Z. is having kidney problems?
   a. serum BUN and creatinine
   b. hemoglobin and hematocrit
   c. serum blood glucose levels
   d. serum troponin levels

2. The nurse is trying to help M.Z. decrease her sleep deprivation. What could M.Z. do to improve her ability to sleep? (Select all that apply.)
   a. Take her HydroDIURIL at night right before she goes to bed.
   b. Have a warm bath before she retires for the night.
   c. Avoid intake of caffeinated products after noon.
   d. Listen to soft music to decrease stress before bedtime.

3. The nurse is teaching M.Z. about her medications. Which statement by M.Z. indicates that she requires further education?
   a. "I should take my HydroDIURIL at bedtime so I won't have to get up so much to go to the bathroom."
   b. "I should put my medications in a daily or weekly pill box so that I can stay on schedule."
   c. "I need to report any side effects to my health care provider to prevent further problems from occurring."
   d. "I should write down when I take my medication so I don't take more than what is prescribed."

4. M.Z. is visiting her health care provider for her follow-up checkup. Which electrolyte alterations may be associated with her medications? (Select all that apply.)
   a. hypokalemia
   b. hypocalcemia
   c. hypernatremia
   d. hypomagnesemia

13 Medication Administration in Community Settings

Study Questions

Complete the following word search. Clues are given in questions 1-7. Circle your responses.

1. Medication administration in any community setting must be consistent with _____, _____, and _____ requirements.

2. Communication and tracking are required to _____ untoward responses and medication errors.

3. The five areas of suggested client teaching are _____, _____, _____, _____, and _____.

4. In all aspects of medication administration, client _____ is of primary concern.

5. Two necessary qualities related to the storage of medications are _____ containers; with _____ caps, as necessary.

6. As part of the cultural assessment, the nurse initially assesses the client's _____.

7. Nurses may demonstrate respect for cultural diversity by including _____ and _____ practices in the health care plan.

```
R C U L T U R A L C O N S I D E R A T I O N S J O A J V S V L Z
C E N Z E S B X A E F H R X U H S T E B S I D X E V S N E Y J R
G Q G W G W F E N O O L I V Z U Z X R I G L E U E O V S L U R Z
K V Q U T C S E L E Z E B K L I D K D A J I N Y Q I L U F H J T
S R I L L F H K I A Z E X J X O U E D U D N Y K Q D E X A N R O
G D X N N A L T K L P S M Q R F E E D K R I V J J B T C D Y C F
Q C L I D S T T K F E T O N U F L H C Y S Q T A E G T R M U O F
R L I E P I W O C H O B O X F E Z U P E C T H I X B N O I K E P
I L A E G V E B R W Y W L E B B G X Z U P H E G O X I F N U C G
U W S V M A W T B Y O X C A K X Z K T Q Z X M E G N P Z I J D U
R G R E U V L V I B F T L U N F K Z I U F X Z D M X A S S H X C
F E G J N T L B B J S L L E H O S M C G I B E I R U A L T C U J
S Z N E R X W O R G A R E C G C S H D Z A C X B F F W B R Y E O
I K B U N X H O I N R X J Z U F I R Z L J Y F M E W Z H A P R M
L W I E I E Q Y I S K O L V B L O N E A Y R E T Z Q V V T W J P
S X X D G D R G E F O H A G D C L M I P L I Y H V W G O I K Q C
B C V Q I U I A L T I E W S O N O W I I Q N X W E B Z I O F G S
T T P X U R Z B L J V O A I K H R B Q C K G D K C B K A N H H W
L H Y H O M W T R R A F L D D P R O F E S S I O N A L R R I F N
X B X B U F P D S Q E B O W V N L Z J W G W S F R E H T Y Q A V
```

Critical Thinking Exercises

Select the best response.

8. A client calls to find out how to discard expired medications. What is the nurse's best response?
    a. "Flush the medications down the toilet."
    b. "Crush the medications, put them in a plastic bag, and put the bag in the trash."
    c. "Crush the medications and wash them down the sink."
    d. "Mix the medications with used coffee grounds and put them in the trash."

9. The nurse is teaching a client about medications and appropriate diet during medication therapy. Which statement made by the client indicates a need for more education?
    a. "I can take all of my medications together first thing in the morning with breakfast."
    b. "When taking my MAO inhibitor, I should not eat any cheese products."
    c. "I should not take my pain medication while drinking any form of alcohol."
    d. "I will eat a banana every day while taking my potassium-wasting diuretic."

10. The nurse is teaching a client about medication side effects. What is the purpose of this teaching? (Select all that apply.)
    a. To help the client understand what to monitor when taking the medication.
    b. To assure the client that the side effects that may occur are expected.
    c. To inform the client what clinical manifestations should be reported to the health care provider.
    d. To help the client understand the importance of taking the medication.

NCLEX Review Questions

Select the best response.

11. Clients allergic to medications are advised to do which action?
    a. Wear medic-alert identification.
    b. Take extra vitamin C.
    c. Avoid use of penicillin.
    d. Have an annual CBC.

12. Administration of medication is ultimately regulated by which standard?
    a. guidelines of the agency
    b. state's nurse practice act
    c. ANA guidelines
    d. state nurses' association

13. A nurse at the work site may be responsible for identifying self-care centers for specific conditions. Which conditions are best suited for this level of service?
    a. abdominal pain and low-grade fever
    b. common cold and chest pain
    c. common cold and minor cuts
    d. headache and numbness in arm

14. What should be included in a complete prescription for a medication? (Select all that apply.)
    a. date
    b. drug
    c. dose
    d. frequency
    e. route
    f. health care provider signature
    g. number of refills
    h. generic, if available

15. Which commonly used over-the-counter preparations may not be compatible with prescription medications? (Select all that apply.)
    a. cough and cold preparations
    b. diet aids
    c. antacids
    d. fat-soluble vitamins

16. What should be included as part of dietary teaching related to medications? (Select all that apply.)

    a. drug-food interactions

    b. foods rich in vitamin C

    c. alcohol use

    d. foods to avoid

Case Study

Select the best answer.

The nurse is providing a new student orientation to parents before the start of the school year. As part of the orientation, the nurse is covering medication administration and what is required for the students to receive medications from the school nurse. The school at which the nurse works serves a very ethnically diverse population. The subsequent questions are specific to this situation.

1. The nurse is providing medications to 200 students. Which type(s) of medications are most frequently administered in the school setting? (Select all that apply.)

    a. asthma medications

    b. medications for ADHD

    c. OTC medications

    d. diabetes medications

2. The nurse is going to give medications to new students. What must the school nurse have to give medication to new students? (Select all that apply.)

    a. written permission from each child's parent or guardian to give the medication

    b. an individual pharmacy-labeled bottle for each child

    c. a medication record to record when the medications were given

    d. a request from each child for the medication every time it is administered

3. The nurse is assessing the safety of the medications kept at the school. What should the nurse assess to determine that safety of medications is maintained? (Select all that apply.)

    a. Policies and procedures must be in place prior to administering medications.

    b. Medications for students must be kept in a secure location with access limited to those giving the medication.

    c. The nurse should review the state's nurse practice act to ensure adherence to state law.

    d. The nurse should be sure to ask each child's age before documenting the medications.

14 The Role of the Nurse in Drug Research

Study Questions

Match the phrase in Column I to the applicable description in Column II.

Column I

_____ 1. Descriptive design
_____ 2. Quasi-experimental design
_____ 3. Intervening variables
_____ 4. Probability sampling
_____ 5. Crossover design
_____ 6. Matched pair design
_____ 7. Double and triple design
_____ 8. Independent variable
_____ 9. Control group
_____ 10. Experimental group
_____ 11. Dependent variable

Column II

a. Comparison of effectiveness of two antibiotics using two groups: clients receiving antibiotic A and clients receiving antibiotic B
b. Subjects randomly selected from the population
c. Subject is its own control
d. A chart review of hospitalized clients who received ritodrine at Evergreen Hospital in 1992
e. Preferred for drug research
f. Subjects matched on intervening variables and randomly assigned to experimental or control group
g. May include disease and state of severity, age, and weight
h. Participant receives treatment
i. The drug itself
j. Provides a baseline to measure the effects
k. Subjects' clinical reactions

Match the terms in Column I with the definitions in Column II.

Column I

_____ 12. Risk-to-benefit ratio
_____ 13. Respect for person
_____ 14. Beneficence
_____ 15. Justice
_____ 16. Informed consent
_____ 17. Truth-telling
_____ 18. Autonomy

Column II

a. Individual should be treated as capable of making decisions in his/her own best interest
b. Right of self-determination
c. Telling the whole truth, even bad news
d. The client has the right be to informed and make decisions without coercion
e. Weighing the risk versus the benefit to the client
f. All people should be treated fairly
g. Duty not to harm others

NCLEX Review Questions

Select the best response.

19. What is an integral component of respect for persons?
    a. risk
    b. beneficence
    c. autonomy
    d. justice

20. Which ethical principle can be defined as duty not to harm?
    a. risk
    b. beneficence
    c. autonomy
    d. justice

21. Which principle includes the objective allocation of social benefits and burdens?
    a. risk
    b. beneficence
    c. autonomy
    d. justice

22. Few potential drugs are actually used in clinical situations based on the findings of the research and development process. What is the potential for a drug to be used in a clinical trial?
    a. 1 in 1000
    b. 1 in 5000
    c. 1 in 10,000
    d. 1 in 20,000

23. What is the objective in determining the safe therapeutic dose and drug-related abnormal changes in animal organs?
    a. human clinical experimentation
    b. toxicity screening
    c. risk-to-benefit ratio
    d. peak levels

24. A multidisciplinary team ensures that data will answer the clinical questions in which phase of human experimentation?
    a. I
    b. II
    c. III
    d. IV

25. Long-term use of a drug is addressed in which phase of human experimentation?
    a. I
    b. II
    c. III
    d. IV

26. What is a standard for the many aspects of clinical trials?
    a. Declaration of Helsinki
    b. institutional review boards
    c. good clinical practice (GCP)
    d. self-determination

27. What is required in an experimental study design? (Select all that apply.)
    a. researcher controls treatment
    b. alternate treatment methods
    c. control groups
    d. random assignment

28. The nurse is working on a clinical drug trial. Which interventions are appropriate for the nurse to provide the client? (Select all that apply.)
    a. Obtain informed consent.
    b. Screen subjects.
    c. Adhere to protocols.
    d. Monitor selected parameters.
    e. Document data.
    f. Record subject's own evaluation.
    g. Evaluate significance of findings.

Case Study

Select the best answer.

The nurse is working with a drug company that is in stage II and moving to stage III in a double-blind clinical trial. The drug has been shown to have several minor side effects but has been approved to move to stage III.

1. Which statement made by the client indicates that he or she doesn't understand what occurs in a double-blind study?
    a. "I know the doctor knows that I am receiving the drug under study and not the control drug."
    b. "I know no-one knows which drug I am receiving, but I suspect it is the control drug."
    c. "We will find out which drug we received at the end of the study."
    d. "I know I can withdraw from this study at any time without penalty."

2. The study is just about ready to move to stage III. What could possibly delay or prevent it from moving to stage III? (Select all that apply.)
    a. A large number of participants have withdrawn from the study.
    b. No new side effects have been identified in the last several weeks.
    c. Several participants have been hospitalized with major side effects.
    d. Several participants have recently complained of experiencing new side effects.

15 Vitamin and Mineral Replacement

Study Questions

Match the letter of the fat- or water-soluble vitamins in Column II with the appropriate word or phrase in Column I.

Column I

____ 1. Vitamin A
____ 2. Vitamin B complex
____ 3. Vitamin C
____ 4. Vitamin D
____ 5. Vitamin E
____ 6. Vitamin K
____ 7. Toxic in excessive amounts
____ 8. Metabolized slowly
____ 9. Minimal protein binding
____ 10. Readily excreted in urine
____ 11. Slowly excreted in urine

Column II

a. Fat-soluble vitamins
b. Water-soluble vitamins

Match the letter of the common food sources in Column II with the appropriate vitamin in Column I.

Column I

____ 12. Vitamin A
____ 13. Vitamin B_{12}
____ 14. Vitamin C
____ 15. Vitamin D
____ 16. Vitamin E

Column II

a. Fermented cheese, egg yolk, milk
b. Wheat germ, egg yolk, liver
c. Fish, liver, egg yolk
d. Green and yellow vegetables
e. Tomatoes, pepper, citrus fruits
f. Whole grains and cereals
g. Milk and cream

NCLEX Review Questions

Select the best response.

17. Inappropriate indications for vitamin therapy include which of the following?
    a. feeling tired
    b. debilitating illness
    c. improvement of overall health
    d. a and c only

18. The USDA's Food Guide Pyramid recommends that fat be limited to what percentage of caloric intake?
    a. 10%
    b. 20%
    c. 30%
    d. 40%

19. Regulation of calcium and phosphorus metabolism and calcium absorption from the intestine is a major role of which of the following vitamins?
    a. A
    b. B$_{12}$
    c. C
    d. D

20. Synthesis of prothrombin and other clotting factors is a role of which of the following vitamins?
    a. E
    b. K
    c. A
    d. D

21. Protection of red blood cells from hemolysis is a role of which of the following vitamins?
    a. E
    b. K
    c. A
    d. D

22. There is a disruption in cellular division without which of the following acids?
    a. pyloric
    b. lactic
    c. folic
    d. gastric

23. Which of the following minerals is essential for regeneration of hemoglobin?
    a. copper
    b. selenium
    c. chromium
    d. iron

24. Sixty percent of iron is found in which component of red blood cells?
    a. hemoglobin
    b. hematocrit
    c. plasma
    d. blastocysts

25. Egg yolks, dried beans, and fruits are foods rich in what vitamin/mineral?
    a. vitamin C
    b. zinc
    c. iron
    d. vitamin D

26. Antacids have which of the following effects on iron absorption?
    a. decrease
    b. increase
    c. no change
    d. synergetic

27. The client is advised to drink a liquid iron preparation through a straw because it may do which of the following?
    a. cause bleeding gums
    b. discolor tooth enamel
    c. corrode tooth enamel
    d. cause esophageal varices

28. Vitamin A is essential for maintaining which body tissues? (Select all that apply.)
    a. skin
    b. hair
    c. ovaries
    d. eyes

29. Vitamin A is stored in the liver, kidneys, and fat. How is it excreted?

    a.   rapidly from the body

    b.   slowly from the body

    c.   only in the bile and feces

    d.   several hours after ingestion

30. A 15-year-old client is prescribed large doses of vitamin A as treatment for acne. Massive doses of vitamin A may be toxic; therefore, client teaching should include which actions? (Select all that apply.)

    a.   encouraging the client to contact the health care provider concerning drug dosing

    b.   informing the client that high doses of vitamin A could cause toxicity (hypervitaminosis A)

    c.   teaching the client not to exceed the recommended dietary allowance without health care provider approval

    d.   instructing the client that massive doses of vitamin A are needed for months to alleviate acne

31. Which vitamin would be considered less toxic than vitamin A?

    a.   vitamin K

    b.   vitamin D

    c.   vitamin E

    d.   vitamin C

32. Which of the following statements is true about zinc?

    a.   found in lamb, eggs, and leafy vegetables

    b.   to be taken 2 hours after antibiotic

    c.   adult RDA is 12-19 mg

    d.   all of the above

33. Chromium is thought to be helpful in control of what condition?

    a.   non–insulin-dependent diabetes

    b.   common cold

    c.   Raynaud's phenomenon

    d.   Alzheimer's disease

34. Which statement is true about copper?

    a.   Deficiency is corrected by iron supplements.

    b.   Deficiency is associated with Wilson's disease.

    c.   Found in shellfish, legumes, and cocoa.

    d.   All of the above.

35. Vitamin K is used to treat which condition? (Select all that apply.)

    a.   peripheral neuritis

    b.   oral anticoagulant overdose

    c.   hypoprothrombinemia or vitamin K deficiency

    d.   anemia

36. Vitamins are organic chemicals that are most necessary for which process? (Select all that apply.)

    a.   tissue healing

    b.   tissue growth

    c.   metabolic functions

    d.   eyesight

37. Vitamin intake should be increased in the presence of which condition? (Select all that apply.)

    a.   alcoholism

    b.   balanced diet

    c.   fad diets

    d.   breastfeeding

16 Fluid and Electrolyte Replacement

Study Questions

Match the electrolyte in Column I with the normal values in Column II.

Column I		Column II	
____ 1.	Magnesium	a.	95-108 mEq/L
____ 2.	Calcium	b.	135-145 mEq/L
____ 3.	Sodium	c.	1.7-2.6 mEq/L
____ 4.	Potassium	d.	1.5-2.5 mEq/L
____ 5.	Chloride	e.	3.5-5.3 mEq/L
____ 6.	Phosphorus	f.	4.5-5.5 mEq/L

Match the terms in Column II with the descriptions in Column I.

Column I		Column II	
____ 7.	Similar to plasma concentration	a.	Osmolality
____ 8.	Based on milliosmoles per kilogram of water	b.	Osmolarity
		c.	Iso-osmolar
____ 9.	Fluids contain fewer particles and more water	d.	Hypo-osmolar
		e.	Hyperosmolar
____ 10.	Fluids have a higher solute/particle concentration		

Match the electrolyte in Column II with the related drug in Column I (answers may be used more than once).

Column I		Column II	
____ 11.	Normal saline	a.	Potassium
____ 12.	Potassium chloride	b.	Sodium
____ 13.	Maalox	c.	Calcium
____ 14.	Epsom salt	d.	Magnesium
____ 15.	Calcium chloride		
____ 16.	Slow-K		

Critical Thinking Exercises

T.C. is receiving fluid and electrolytes. Questions 17-22 are related to this client.

17. The nurse has taught T.C. how to take his potassium. Which statement by T.C. indicates that he requires more education on taking this medication once he is discharged?
    a. "I can take this medication with a few sips of water."
    b. "I can take this medication with 6 ounces of water or more."
    c. "I can take this medication with meals."
    d. "I can take this medication with a large glass of juice."

18. T.C.'s condition changes, and his potassium level is less than 3.0 mEq/L. He is started on potassium chloride IV. What is the nurse's best action when preparing to give this medication?
    a. Prepare the syringe with the ordered amount medication to be given IV push.
    b. Push the potassium chloride into the IV fluid bag and keep it still before administration.
    c. Push the potassium chloride into the IV fluid bag and shake it vigorously before administration.
    d. Push the potassium chloride into the IV fluid bag and invert it several times before administration.

19. T.C. continues on his potassium therapy, and the skin around his IV becomes reddened and edematous. What is the nurse's best action when this condition is assessed?
    a. Flush the IV with sterile water and increase the rate of administration of the potassium.
    b. Flush the IV with normal saline and decrease the rate of administration of the potassium.
    c. Stop the IV fluids and determine if there is a backflow of blood in the IV.
    d. Discontinue the IV and restart it in another vein.

20. T.C.'s potassium level is improving, but his urine output has decreased to about 30 mL in 2 hours. What would the nurse expect to find when assessing this client?
    a. confusion
    b. abdominal distension
    c. tachycardia
    d. weakening muscle strength

21. It is determined that T.C. has become hyperkalemic. What would the nurse anticipate giving him?
    a. 10 mEq/L potassium mixed in 1000 mL IV
    b. 0.9% sodium/chloride IV
    c. a hyperosmolar IV fluid challenge
    d. sodium polystyrene sulfonate (Kayexalate) with sorbitol

22. T.C.'s potassium level has normalized, and his health care provider is prescribing potassium to take at home. What should be included in his discharge planning? (Select all that apply.)
    a. the signs and symptoms of both hyperkalemia and hypokalemia
    b. he will need to have his potassium levels checked regularly
    c. he will need to increase his intake of potassium-rich foods
    d. he should take his medication with food or a large glass of water

NCLEX Review Questions

Select the best response.

23. What is the normal range of serum osmolality?
    a. 175-195 mOsm/kg
    b. 280-295 mOsm/kg
    c. 375-395 mOsm/kg
    d. 475-495 mOsm/kg

24. How is serum osmolality calculated?
    a. doubling the serum sodium level
    b. halving the serum sodium level
    c. doubling the serum calcium level
    d. halving the serum calcium level

25. What is the term used to describe the body fluid when the serum osmolality is 285 mOsm/kg?
    a. hypo-osmolar
    b. iso-osmolar
    c. hyperosmolar
    d. neo-osmolar

26. An IV solution with an osmolality of 540 mOsm is considered to be what type of solution?
    a. hypotonic
    b. isotonic
    c. hypertonic
    d. neotonic

27. How is the majority of potassium excreted?
    a. through the liver
    b. through the kidneys
    c. through the lungs
    d. in the feces

28. When administering potassium orally, the nurse knows that it must be taken with at least how many ounces of water or juice?
    a. 2
    b. 4
    c. 6
    d. 8

29. The nurse is teaching a client about calcium absorption and includes in the health teaching that vitamin D is needed for calcium absorption. Where in the body is calcium absorbed?
    a. GI tract
    b. liver
    c. colon
    d. kidneys

30. Calcium is distributed intercellularly and intracellularly in what proportions?
    a. 25%; 75%
    b. 75%; 25%
    c. 50%; 50%
    d. 90%; 10%

31. Thiazide diuretics such as hydrochlorothiazide (HydroDIURIL) have what effect on the serum calcium level?
    a. decrease
    b. increase
    c. no change
    d. marked decrease

32. A client is receiving 2 L of IV fluids: 1000 mL (1 L) of D_5W and 1000 mL of $D_5/0.45\%$ NaCl ($D_5/\frac{1}{2}$ NS). What are the client's solutions classified as?
    a. colloids
    b. crystalloids
    c. lipids
    d. blood products

33. One liter (1000 mL) of 5% dextrose in ½ normal saline solution ($D_5/0.45\%$ NaCl) is what type of IV fluid?
    a. isotonic
    b. hypotonic
    c. hypertonic
    d. isohypotonic

34. A client has received a continuous D_5W infusion for the past several days. When this type of infusion is given for an extended period of time, what type of solution does it become?
    a. hypotonic
    b. hypertonic
    c. isotonic
    d. isohypertonic

35. What is the client's serum osmolality according to the following current laboratory values: serum sodium 140 mEq/L; BUN 15 mg/dl; blood glucose 110 mg/dl?
    a. 280 mOsm
    b. 285 mOsm
    c. 291 mOsm
    d. 296 mOsm

36. How is a serum osmolality of approximately 290 mOsm classified?
    a. iso-osmolar
    b. hypo-osmolar
    c. hyperosmolar
    d. isohyperosmolar

37. Which body component has a similar composition to lactated Ringer's IV solution?
    a. white blood cells
    b. plasma
    c. body tissue
    d. skin

38. A 43-year-old client is taking Slow-K. She is taking hydrochlorothiazide 50 mg daily to control her hypertension. The client's serum potassium level is 3.2 mEq/L. What clinical manifestations would the nurse expect to assess in this client?
    a. headache
    b. increased serum glucose
    c. bradycardia
    d. confusion

39. The nurse is giving a client Slow-K. What is the best way this should be given?
    a. when the client's stomach is empty
    b. at bedtime
    c. with 8 ounces of water
    d. 2 hours before meals

40. A client who is taking Slow-K complains of nausea, vomiting, and abdominal distention. These clinical manifestations are associated with which electrolyte imbalance?
    a. hyponatremia
    b. hypernatremia
    c. hyperkalemia
    d. hypokalemia

41. A client with a serum potassium level of 3.2 mEq/L asks why she has to take potassium. What reasons should the nurse give her for taking this medication? (Select all that apply.)
    a. "Your diuretic causes not only water and sodium to be excreted but also potassium."
    b. "Your serum potassium level is low, and Slow-K helps to prevent a potassium deficit."
    c. "Your health care provider should discontinue the potassium supplement after a week."
    d. "The potassium supplement should maintain a normal potassium level in your body while you are taking the diuretic (potassium-wasting)."

42. Which serum potassium levels indicate hyperkalemia?
    a. 5.9 mEq/L
    b. 4.6 mEq/L
    c. 3.8 mEq/L
    d. 2.9 mEq/L

43. A 65-year-old client's serum potassium level is 6.1 mEq/L. What clinical manifestations should the nurse expect to assess in this client? (Select all that apply.)
    a. abdominal cramps
    b. muscle weakness
    c. tachycardia and later bradycardia
    d. oliguria

44. Which drugs are used to treat hyperkalemia? (Select all that apply.)
    a. glucagon
    b. IV sodium bicarbonate, calcium gluconate
    c. insulin and glucose
    d. kayexalate and sorbitol

45. A 68-year-old client has a calcium deficit. Her serum calcium level is 3.6 mEq/L. What clinical manifestations should the nurse expect to assess in this client? (Select all that apply.)
    a. irritability
    b. tetany
    c. numbness of the fingers
    d. pathologic fractures

46. The health care provider orders calcium chloride in 5% dextrose and 0.45% sodium chloride (D$_5$/½ NS) for a client with a calcium deficit. What effect may saline solution have on calcium chloride?

    a. It may increase the effects of calcium; calcium should always be mixed with a saline solution.

    b. It has little or no effect on the calcium additive.

    c. Calcium additives should always be added to IV solutions containing sodium chloride.

    d. Sodium encourages calcium loss; calcium should not be mixed with a saline solution.

47. What is the best response by the nurse to an IV order of calcium chloride in 5% dextrose and 0.45% sodium chloride (D$_5$/½ NS)?

    a. Explain to the client that she should not accept this IV fluid.

    b. Suggest to the health care provider to change the IV order to 5% dextrose in water (D$_5$W) and explain why.

    c. Do nothing, because this solution would not have any effect on the calcium chloride additive.

    d. Report the health care provider to the chiefs of both nursing and medicine.

48. The nurse is teaching the client to eat foods rich in potassium. Which potassium-rich foods should the nurse recommend? (Select all that apply.)

    a. dry fruits

    b. bananas and prunes

    c. broccoli and peanut butter

    d. eggs and whole-grain breads

Case Study

Select the best answer.

A.F. is taken to the emergency department after an automobile accident. He is losing large amounts of blood. Vital signs are BP 100/60 mm Hg; pulse 112 beats/min; respiratory rate 32 breaths/min.

1. What is a priority action for the nurse when receiving this client?

    a. Ask the family members for a health history.

    b. Call the physician for assistance.

    c. Start an IV line to begin IV fluids.

    d. Listen to the client's lungs.

2. What is the advantage of using whole blood versus packed red blood cells (RBCs)?

    a. Whole blood provides both fluid volume and red blood cells.

    b. Whole blood provides more clotting factors than packed red blood cells

    c. Whole blood helps to prevent additional blood loss in clients with excessive bleeding.

    d. Whole blood provides less fluid volume and prevents fluid overload.

3. Which statement(s) best explain(s) the significance of A.F.'s vital signs? (Select all that apply.)

    a. The low blood pressure and heart rate demonstrate that he is in shock.

    b. The high respiratory rate demonstrates that not enough oxygen is getting to the tissues.

    c. The high heart rate is due to increased vasodilation with low blood pressure.

    d. The low blood pressure is due to fluid moving from the interstitium into the vasculature.

A.F. is admitted to the hospital after receiving 2 L of crystalloids and 2 units of whole blood. After receiving the IV fluids, his vital signs are BP 122/65 mm Hg; pulse 92 beats/min; respiratory rate 28 breaths/min. His urine output is 400 mL in 8 hours.

4. Which statement best explains why A.F.'s vital signs improved? (Select all that apply.)

    a. increased vascular fluid volume

    b. increased number of circulating red blood cells

    c. increased number of clotting factors

    d. decreased need for oxygen at the tissue level

During the next 23 hours, A.F. receives 3 L of D_5W, with 20 mEq of potassium chloride in 2 of the liters. His serum potassium level is 3.3 mEq/L.

5. What type of IV solution, if any, is missing with this 24-hour IV fluid order and why?

   a. Sodium is missing and it should be given to prevent water intoxication.

   b. Lactated Ringer's is missing and should be given to maintain osmolality.

   c. Nothing is missing as the client is receiving a dose of potassium chloride.

   d. Crystalloids are missing as they are better at long-term support of fluid volume.

6. What is the difference in the fluid osmolalities of the following crystalloids: D_5W, D_5/0.45% NaCl, and lactated Ringer's solution?

   a. D_5W and lactated Ringer's are isotonic and D_5/0.45% NaCl is hypotonic.

   b. D_5W and lactated Ringer's are hypotonic and D_5/0.45% NaCl is isotonic.

   c. D_5W and lactated Ringer's are isotonic and D_5/0.45% NaCl is hypertonic.

   d. D_5W and lactated Ringer's are hypertonic and D_5/0.45% NaCl is hypotonic.

7. What occurs when a client receives all hypertonic IV fluid?

   a. increased urine output from the increased vascular fluid volume

   b. decreased urine output as the body needs to conserve fluid volume

   c. the cells become dehydrated and the extra fluid volume is excreted

   d. the cells will absorb more fluid volume and urine output decreases

8. What is the purpose of giving this client the potassium chloride (KCl) in his IV?

   a. It prevents intracellular dehydration.

   b. It prevents increased urine output.

   c. It helps to reestablish normal potassium levels.

   d. It prevents decreased urine output.

9. What are priority nursing actions for A.F. related to his IV therapy? (Select all that apply.)

   a. Monitor his vital signs.

   b. Monitor for clinical manifestations of increased bleeding.

   c. Maintain the client on a liquid diet while undergoing IV therapy.

   d. Monitor intake and output to maintain appropriate fluid balance.

17 Nutritional Support

Study Questions

Crossword puzzle: Use the definitions to determine the correct terms.

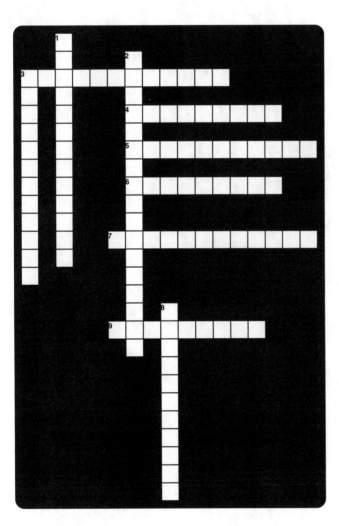

Across

3. May be caused by sudden interruption of TPN
4. Provides partially digested nutrients for feedings
5. May occur during changing of IV tubing when the Valsalva maneuver is not used (2 words)
6. May occur if poor technique is used during IV insertion
7. Accidental puncture of the pleural cavity
9. Supplements prescribed for clients who have normal or near-normal gastrointestinal (GI) function

Down

1. May occur as a result of the hypertonic dextrose solution when TPN is initiated
2. Another name for total parenteral nutrition
3. Fluid shift from cellular to vascular spaces because of hypertonic solutions
8. Occurs when the catheter perforates the vein, releasing solution into the chest

10. Label the routes for enteral feedings.

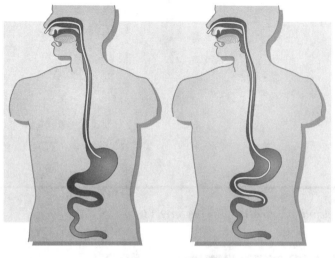

a. _____   b. _____

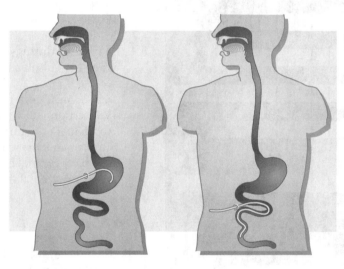

c. _____   d. _____

Match the terms in Column I with the descriptions in Column II.

Column I

____ 11. Bolus
____ 12. Intermittent
____ 13. Continuous
____ 14. Cyclic

Column II

a. Feeding given every 3-6 hours for 30-60 minutes by gravity infusion
b. Feeding given continuously into the small intestine
c. Feeding infused over 8-16 hours per day
d. 250-400 mL given at one time, used for ambulatory clients

NCLEX Review Questions

Select the best response.

15. The client has diabetes mellitus. Which enteral formulas would you expect to be prescribed?
    a. Glucerna
    b. Respalor
    c. Nepro
    d. NutriHep

16. The client has COPD. Which enteral formula would you expect this client to receive?
    a. Glucerna
    b. Respalor
    c. Nepro
    d. NutriHep

17. Which type of solution can be used for nutritional support?
    a. 5% dextrose in water (D_5W)
    b. 0.9% sodium chloride (normal saline)
    c. lactated Ringer's
    d. Ensure

18. Ensure and Sustacal are examples of which type of solutions?
    a. blenderized solutions
    b. polymeric, lactose-free solutions
    c. polymeric, milk-based solutions
    d. elemental or monomeric solutions

19. What type of enteral feeding is administered over 30-60 minutes by drip or pump infusion?
    a. bolus
    b. intermittent
    c. gravity
    d. continuous

20. The client is receiving TPN. What is the most appropriate method for TPN to be given?
    a. orally
    b. via a peripheral vein
    c. via a central venous line
    d. via a subcutaneous line

21. What is the average percentage of dextrose in TPN?
    a. 5%
    b. 10%
    c. 25%
    d. 50%

22. Continuous feedings into the small intestine are commonly infused at which rate per hour?
    a. 25-50 mL
    b. 50-125 mL
    c. 100-175 mL
    d. 150-200 mL

23. What is the most appropriate nursing action to manage diarrhea associated with enteral feedings?
    a. changing the enteral solution
    b. decreasing the rate of infusion
    c. diluting the solution
    d. all of the above

24. The nurse is measuring residual volume in a client receiving tube feedings. A residual volume greater than what percentage of previous feeding indicates delayed gastric emptying?
    a. 30
    b. 40
    c. 50
    d. 60

25. What are the best reasons enteral feeding should be used before TPN? (Select all that apply.)
    a. It is less costly.
    b. It poses less risk of infection.
    c. It maintains GI integrity.
    d. There is less risk of aspiration.

26. Which complications are associated with use of TPN? (Select all that apply.)
    a. pneumothorax
    b. aspiration
    c. air embolism
    d. infection

27. Sequence the steps of transitional parenteral to enteral feeding: _____

    a. Stop parenteral feeding when about 75% of nutritional needs are met via enteral nutrition.

    b. Introduce small amount of enteral feeding at a slow rate of 25-40 mL/hr.

    c. Reduce parenteral feeding by appropriate amount.

    d. Determine GI tolerance.

    e. Increase amount of enteral feeding q8-12h.

28. What can be done by the nurse to prevent aspiration in a client receiving tube feeding? (Select all that apply.)

    a. Place the client in high Fowler's position.

    b. Decrease the infusion rate if the client is receiving continuous infusion feeding.

    c. Check for residual before administering a feeding.

    d. Monitor I & O for this client.

29. A client has just had a central catheter line inserted for TPN administration. He was doing well, but now complains of shortness of breath, sharp chest pain, and has decreased breath sounds. What should the nurse suspect may be occurring? (Select all that apply.)

    a. hyperglycemia

    b. pneumothorax

    c. hemothorax

    d. hydrothorax

18 Adrenergic Agonists and Adrenergic Blockers

Study Questions

Match the terms in Column I with the definition in Column II.

Column I

____ 1. Alpha blocker

____ 2. Beta blocker

____ 3. Selectivity

____ 4. Sympathomimetic

____ 5. Sympatholytic

Column II

a. Same as alpha blockers

b. Has a greater affinity for certain receptors

c. Helpful in decreasing symptoms of benign prostatic hypertrophy (BPH)

d. Propranolol hydrochloride

e. Mimics stimulation of the sympathetic nervous system

Complete the following word search. Clues are given in questions 6-16. Circle your responses.

```
S Y M P A T H O L Y T I C S B M A
Y F K H M A S T H M A S B K L I D
S H F D R E G I T I N E T L H N R
P T N O I S N E T O P Y H G Z I E
G I M C Z F M A G T V F K L L P N
C F G P L Q B O N S I M M X C R E
L Q Z K R L G E O Y P N R S J E R
A N T A G O N I S T S A G Q M S G
F G A J V R E G E H H H E U Q S I
F V Q A K Y Q U I B F R I C P R C
A G B E T A B L O C K E R S H G N
```

6. Adrenergic receptors are located on the cells of _____ muscle.

7. Urinary retention may occur with high doses of _____ drugs.

8. Nasal sprays should be used with the client (sitting up / lying down). (Circle correct answer.)

9. Sympathomimetics (do / do not) pass into the breast milk. (Circle correct answer.)

10. Adrenergic blockers are the same as _____.

11. The antidote for IV infiltration of alpha- and beta-adrenergic drugs such as norepinephrine and dopamine is _____.

12. The alpha blocker that may cause impotence or a decrease in libido is _____.

13. Mood changes such as depression and suicidal tendencies are possible when taking which type of adrenergic blocker? _____

14. Abruptly stopping a beta blocker can cause rebound _____.

15. Nonselective beta blockers such as Inderal are contraindicated in clients with _____ and _____.

16. What is most likely to occur if a client is taking an adrenergic agonist with an adrenergic blocker? _____

Match the letter of the receptor in Column II with the associated adrenergic response in Column I.

Column I

____ 17.   Increases gastrointestinal relaxation

____ 18.   Increases force of heart contraction

____ 19.   Dilates pupils

____ 20.   Decreases salivary secretions

____ 21.   Inhibits release of norepinephrine

____ 22.   Dilates bronchioles

____ 23.   Increases heart rate

____ 24.   Promotes uterine relaxation

____ 25.   Dilates blood vessels

Column II

a.   Alpha$_1$

b.   Alpha$_2$

c.   Beta$_1$

d.   Beta$_2$

NCLEX Review Questions

Select the best response.

26.   Isoproterenol (Isuprel) may be taken by clients with asthma. What does this drug cause in order to improve a client's breathing condition?

a.   decreased heart rate

b.   bronchodilation

c.   increased urinary output

d.   increased state of alertness

27.   When isoproterenol stimulates beta$_1$ receptors, what would the nurse assess?

a.   increased heart rate

b.   bronchospasm

c.   acute heart block

d.   nasal congestion

28.   A client taking isoproterenol for asthma is experiencing tachycardia and tremors. What is occurring in this client?

a.   side effects of the adrenergic drugs

b.   normal responses to the adrenergic drugs

c.   allergic reaction to the medication

d.   synergistic medication reactions

29.   The nurse is administering a client's adrenergic medication with food. What is the purpose of administering this medication with food?

a.   decrease incidence of diarrhea

b.   decrease incidence of nausea and vomiting

c.   decrease incidence of gastric bleeding

d.   decrease incidence of constipation

30.   Over-the-counter drugs for cold symptoms have sympathetic properties and are contraindicated in clients diagnosed with which disease process?

a.   hypertension

b.   diabetes mellitus

c.   coronary artery disease

d.   all of the above

31.   Which adrenergic drug used to treat acute hypotension does not decrease renal function?

a.   epinephrine

b.   norepinephrine bitartrate

c.   metaraminol bitartrate

d.   dopamine hydrochloride

32. For a client with asthma, beta$_2$-adrenergic drugs are more desirable than those that have beta$_1$ and beta$_2$ properties. What would be an advantage of a giving a beta$_2$ (selective) adrenergic agonist?

    a. increases heart rate

    b. increases blood pressure

    c. dilates bronchial tubes

    d. increases urine output

33. A 64-year-old client is receiving methyldopa (Aldomet) for dysrhythmias. What should the nurse assess in this client to determine if he is experiencing a common side effect of methyldopa?

    a. constipation

    b. decreased heart rate

    c. excessive saliva

    d. hypertension

34. The nurse is preparing to give medication. The medication record reads that the client should take Minipress 25 mg PO once daily. What is the nurse's best action?

    a. Give the client the medication after identifying the client.

    b. Hold the medication and contact the physician for a dosage within the correct range.

    c. Give the medication and request a new order when you see the client's physician.

    d. Take the client's blood pressure and then give the medication.

35. Which statement(s) by a client taking doxazosin mesylate (Cardura) would indicate that he understands his teaching plan? (Select all that apply.)

    a. "I need to monitor my blood glucose level because this medication will block some hypoglycemic symptoms."

    b. "I need to change positions slowly to avoid orthostatic hypotension."

    c. "I need to increase my daily fluid intake to match my urine output."

    d. "I should contact my physician if I experience dizziness."

36. Which beta blocker is used to decrease blood pressure and pulse (heart) rate in asthmatic clients with little effect on bronchial tubes?

    a. propranolol hydrochloride

    b. nadolol

    c. pindolol

    d. atenolol

37. Which clinical manifestations are common side effects/adverse effects of albuterol (Proventil)? (Select all that apply.)

    a. tremors

    b. dizziness

    c. somnolence

    d. bradycardia

    e. palpitations

Case Study

Select the best answer.

K.S. is taking propranolol (Inderal) 40 mg t.i.d. for angina pectoris and cardiac dysrhythmias. During the nursing assessment, the nurse records that the client stated, "I'm troubled at times with asthma." Vital signs are BP 136/84 mm Hg; pulse 88 beats/min; respiratory rate 24 breaths/min.

1. K.S.'s blood pressure is elevated. What should concern the nurse about this dosage level?

    a. The daily dose may be too high as the heart rate is too high.

    b. The daily dose may be too low as the blood pressure is too high.

    c. The daily dose is OK; increased blood pressure is a side effect.

    d. The daily dose is too high as the blood pressure is too high.

2. What should concern the nurse about K.S. taking propranolol and his difficulty with asthma? (Select all that apply.)

    a. The difficulty he has with asthma may be related to his taking propranolol.

    b. The propranolol has no impact on his asthma.

    c. The physician should be informed that he is experiencing asthma symptoms.

    d. The physician should increase the asthma medication that K.S. is taking.

3. Which action should the nurse take before giving a beta blocker?

   a. Determine serum glucose level.

   b. Determine heart rate.

   c. Determine urine output.

   d. Determine respiratory rate.

4. The nurse is teaching K.S. about side effects that may be experienced when using propranolol over a long period. Which statement indicates that K.S. understands the teaching? (Select all that apply.)

   a. "I will take my pulse daily before taking the medication."

   b. "I will notify my physician if I experience decreased libido."

   c. "I will change positions slowly so I don't pass out."

   d. "I can take double the medication dose if I miss a dose."

5. When teaching K.S. about his medication, the nurse tells him that he should inform his health care provider if he takes OTC medication. What statement(s) by KS indicate(s) that he requires more teaching? (Select all that apply.)

   a. "I should call my doctor before taking any new OTC."

   b. "I can take NSAIDs for a headache without any major impact."

   c. "I should take only cold medications but no other OTC medications."

   d. "I can take any OTC as long as I monitor my blood pressure."

6. Which beta blocker could K.S. take that might cause fewer side effects? (Select all that apply.)

   a. metoprolol

   b. atenolol

   c. acebutolol

   d. reserpine

19 Cholinergic Agonists and Anticholinergics

Study Questions

Match the term in Column I with the definition in Column II.

Column I

_____ 1. Acetylcholine
_____ 2. Anticholinergic
_____ 3. Cholinergic
_____ 4. Cholinesterase
_____ 5. Muscarinic receptor
_____ 6. Nicotinic receptor
_____ 7. Parasympathomimetic
_____ 8. Anticholinesterase

Column II

a. Stimulates smooth muscle and slow heart rate

b. Impacts skeletal muscles

c. Stimulates muscarinic receptors

d. Types of drugs that stimulate the parasympathetic system

e. Blocks the action of acetylcholine

f. Mimics cholinergic actions

g. Blocks the breakdown of acetylcholine

h. Causes the breakdown of acetylcholine

NCLEX Review Questions

Select the best response.

9. Which receptor stimulates smooth muscle and slows the heart rate?
   a. nicotinic
   b. muscarinic
   c. acetylcholine
   d. sympathomimetic

10. Which cholinergic drug is used primarily to increase urination?
   a. bethanechol chloride (Urecholine)
   b. metoclopramide hydrochloride (Reglan)
   c. edrophonium chloride (Tensilon)
   d. neostigmine (Prostigmin)

11. Anticholinesterases are used to produce which type of pupillary changes?
   a. dilation
   b. constriction
   c. nonresponsiveness
   d. dilation and constriction (one pupil dilated and one constricted)

12. The client has glaucoma and is prescribed an anticholinergic drug. What is the nurse's priority action?
   a. Give the medication as ordered after identifying the client.
   b. Give half of the normal dose because the client has glaucoma.
   c. Hold the dose and contact the physician about the client's diagnosis of glaucoma.
   d. Hold the medication until after the client has taken eye drops for glaucoma.

13. Bethanechol is what type of medication?
    a. cholinergic agonist
    b. anticholinergic
    c. cholinesterase inhibitor
    d. sympatholytic

14. How does bethanechol work in the body?
    a. It stimulates nicotinic receptors.
    b. It stimulates muscarinic receptors.
    c. It inhibits muscarinic receptors.
    d. It inhibits nicotinic receptors.

15. How does bethanechol correct a client's clinical problem of urinary retention?
    a. It promotes contraction of the bladder.
    b. It inhibits bladder contraction.
    c. It stimulates kidney secretion.
    d. It decreases bladder tone.

16. How does the body tissue respond to large doses of cholinergic drugs? (Select all that apply.)
    a. increased bronchial secretions
    b. decreased salivation
    c. urinary retention
    d. decreased blood pressure

17. A client taking bethanechol is experiencing decreased urinary output. What is the nurse's priority action?
    a. Encourage the client to increase fluid intake to increase his output.
    b. Catheterize the client to drain the bladder and measure output.
    c. Notify the physician as it may be related to the client's medications.
    d. Encourage the client to try to relax when urinating.

18. A client who takes bethanechol is experiencing flushing, sweating, nausea, and abdominal cramps. What is the nurse's best action?
    a. Prepare to give the client IV atropine sulfate.
    b. Document the client's clinical manifestations.
    c. Increase the client's fluid intake.
    d. Give the client a laxative.

19. Which drug treats myasthenia gravis by increasing muscle strength?
    a. bethanechol (Urecholine)
    b. pilocarpine (Pilocar)
    c. neostigmine bromide (Prostigmin)
    d. edrophonium chloride (Tensilon)

20. For which situations is atropine frequently prescribed? (Select all that apply.)
    a. as a preoperative medication
    b. as an antispasmodic
    c. to treat bradycardia
    d. to treat urinary retention

21. Which client should not receive any atropine-like drugs?
    a. A 50-year-old with parkinsonism
    b. A 35-year-old with a peptic ulcer
    c. A 60-year-old with glaucoma
    d. A 55-year-old with cirrhosis

22. A 70-year-old client is admitted for evaluation of peptic ulcers. She is taking propantheline (Pro-Banthine) three times a day. The nurse is teaching this client about her medications. The priority teaching point is that the client should eat which types of foods?
    a. those high in fiber
    b. those high in protein
    c. those low in fat
    d. those low in salt

23. Which information is important to include in the teaching plan for a 70-year-old client who is admitted for evaluation of peptic ulcers and who is taking propantheline (Pro-Banthine) three times a day? (Select all that apply.)
    a. Avoid alcohol.
    b. Use artificial tears.
    c. Decrease fluid intake.
    d. Avoid constipation.

24. Anticholinergic drugs are contraindicated in clients with which disease process?
    a. coronary artery disease
    b. diabetes
    c. gastrointestinal obstruction
    d. heart block

25. A specific group of anticholinergics may be prescribed in the early treatment of which neuromuscular disorders?
    a. myasthenia gravis
    b. parkinsonism
    c. multiple sclerosis
    d. muscular dystrophy

26. Which drug is used to treat an overdose of organophosphate pesticides that causes paralysis?
    a. neostigmine
    b. edrophonium chloride
    c. pralidoxime chloride
    d. tacrine hydrochloride

27. What advice should the nurse give the client taking anticholinergic drugs?
    a. Increase intake of vitamins A and C.
    b. Increase intake of fluids and foods high in fiber.
    c. Increase caffeine intake.
    d. Avoid organic meats.

28. Which clinical manifestations are effects of anticholinergics? (Select all that apply.)
    a. constrict pupils
    b. increase heart rate
    c. decrease salivation
    d. increase GI motility
    e. decrease muscle rigidity
    f. relax bladder detrusor muscle

29. Which clinical manifestations would the nurse possibly assess in a client experiencing side effects/adverse effects of atropine? (Select all that apply.)
    a. diarrhea
    b. flushing
    c. headache
    d. dry mouth
    e. blurred vision
    f. urinary frequency

Case Study

Select the best answer.

Q.T. has been prescribed bethanechol for urinary retention. She is also taking propranolol for high blood pressure.

1. What should the nurse monitor closely in this client? (Select all that apply.)
    a. heart rate
    b. dietary intake
    c. fluid intake
    d. blood pressure

2. Q.T. informs the nurse that she was diagnosed with asthma several years ago and since she started on bethanechol her asthma attacks have become more frequent. What is the nurse's best action?
    a. Encourage Q.T. to continue to take the bethanechol as it decreased her urinary frequency.
    b. Ask Q.T. what she is using to treat her asthma and the exacerbations.
    c. Notify her physician about this information given the medication she is taking.
    d. Encourage Q.T. to continue to monitor her asthma attacks and severity of the attacks.

3. The nurse is teaching Q.T. how to take her medications. Which statement by Q.T. indicates she requires more teaching? (Select all that apply.)
    a. "I should take the medication at the same time with my other medications."
    b. "I should increase my fluid intake while taking this medication."
    c. "I am so glad I can take this medication with my breakfast."
    d. "I will notify my health care provider if I experience any urinary retention."

Q.T. fell down at home and is now back in the hospital, scheduled for a hip replacement. She is receiving atropine preoperatively.

4. Which clinical manifestation should the nurse be concerned about following administration of atropine?

   a. tachycardia

   b. hypothermia

   c. increased pain

   d. increased urine output

5. While doing the postoperative assessment, the nurse notes that Q.T. has decreased bowel sounds. What should the nurse suspect may be occurring in this client?

   a. constipation

   b. paralytic ileus

   c. diarrhea

   d. decreased urinary output

6. Q.T. is being discharged from the hospital. What should the nurse tell her to decrease the potential for constipation? (Select all that apply.)

   a. Increase fiber in her diet.

   b. Increase fluid intake.

   c. Increase exercise as allowed.

   d. Increase calcium intake.

20 Central Nervous System Stimulants

Study Questions

Crossword puzzle: Use the definitions to determine the correct terms.

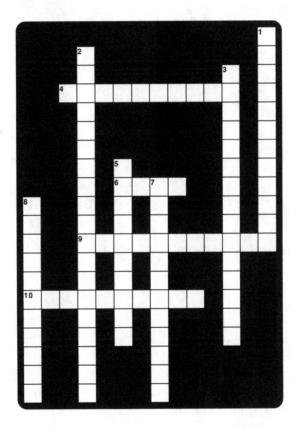

Across

4. Larger doses needed to reproduce the initial response
6. Attention-deficit hyperactivity disorder
9. Used to treat obesity
10. Used to stimulate respirations

Down

1. Cause euphoria and alertness
2. FDA required its removal from OTC weight loss drugs
3. Used to correct attention-deficit hyperactivity disorder
5. Falling asleep during normal activities
7. Hypermovement
8. Used to treat narcolepsy

NCLEX Review Questions

Select the best response.

11. The client is prescribed a CNS stimulant. Which conditions have these medications been approved to treat? (Select all that apply.)

    a. narcolepsy

    b. ADHD

    c. obesity

    d. anorexia

12. The nurse is caring for a client who takes a CNS stimulant. What are priority nursing implications in caring for this client? (Select all that apply.)

    a. Monitor the client's heart rate and blood pressure.

    b. Administer 6-8 hours before sleep.

    c. Taper the medication when discontinuing.

    d. Report significant changes in urine output.

13. What are priority teaching considerations for a client taking CNS stimulants? (Select all that apply.)

    a. Client must take the medication before meals.

    b. Alcohol and caffeine-containing foods should be avoided.

    c. Client must report any weight gain.

    d. Nervousness and tremors may occur.

    e. Client must avoid hazardous equipment when experiencing tremors.

14. Which drug group acts on the brain stem and medulla to stimulate respiration?

    a. triptan

    b. analeptic

    c. anorexiant

    d. amphetamine

15. What are other terms used for clients with ADHD?

    a. minimal brain dysfunction

    b. hyperkinesis

    c. hyperkinetic syndrome

    d. all of the above

16. A 16-year-old client is receiving methylphenidate (Ritalin) for treatment of ADHD. Which common side effects should the client be informed may occur? (Select all that apply.)

    a. euphoria and alertness

    b. hypertension

    c. irritability

    d. orthostatic hypotension

17. To maintain the half-life of Ritalin, how often should this medication be given?

    a. daily

    b. 1-3 times per day

    c. every 3 hours

    d. every 12 hours

18. A client who takes Ritalin for treatment of ADHD develops CNS toxicity. What is the goal of treatment?

    a. decreasing urine pH

    b. increasing urine pH

    c. decreasing fluids

    d. increasing fluids

19. What is the best time for the nurse to administer an amphetamine?

    a. at bedtime

    b. 1-2 hours before sleep

    c. with meals

    d. 6-8 hours before sleep

20. What is an adverse finding in clients with long-term use of amphetamines?

    a. diarrhea

    b. cardiac dysrhythmias

    c. urinary retention

    d. rash

21. A client is 11 years old and is taking anorexiants. What should be included in health teaching to this client?

    a. that children under 12 should not take anorexiants

    b. the need to monitor dose

    c. that the drug should be taken at regular mealtimes

    d. that the drug should be taken with limited fluid

22. Which anorexiant has a high potential for abuse?

    a. phentermine (Adipex-P)

    b. doxapram (Dopram)

    c. benzphetamine (Didrex)

    d. naratriptan (Amerge)

23. Which statement is true of Ritalin? (Select all that apply.)

    a. It may increase hypertensive crisis with monoamine oxidase inhibitors.

    b. It may increase effects of oral anticoagulants.

    c. It may alter effects of insulin.

    d. It may cause hyperglycemia.

24. If CNS toxicity from amphetamines is suspected, what aids in the excretion of the drug?

    a. increasing urine pH

    b. decreasing urine pH

    c. increasing fluids

    d. using diuretics

25. In which clients are CNS stimulants contraindicated?

    a. heart disease and renal disease

    b. heart disease and liver disease

    c. heart disease and hyperthyroidism

    d. all of the above

26. Caffeine is used to treat which conditions in newborns? (Select all that apply.)

    a. apnea

    b. narcolepsy

    c. respiratory distress

    d. hyperactive disorder

27. What are side effects/adverse reactions of methylphenidate? (Select all that apply.)

    a. diarrhea

    b. weight gain

    c. bradycardia

    d. hypotension

    e. restlessness

Case Study

Select the best answer.

There is a new school nurse at Countryside Elementary, which has 1000 students. The nurse notes that more than 100 students come to the nurse's office "around midday" to take their medications for ADHD. The majority of them take pemoline and the rest take methylphenidate.

1. What is the most appropriate time to take these medications?

    a. with meals

    b. before meals

    c. at bedtime

    d. first thing in the morning

2. What are the priority nursing implications in giving this medication as a school nurse? (Select all that apply.)

    a. Schedule the medication to be given before lunch.

    b. Monitor the children's blood pressure before giving the medication.

    c. Maintain student confidentiality concerning the medication being taken.

    d. Make sure there is enough room for the number of children taking medications.

3. What priority nursing assessment is important to monitor in these students? (Select all that apply.)

    a. measurement of height, weight, and growth

    b. monitoring of blood pressure

    c. daily blood glucose measurements

    d. use of daily caffeine

4. What laboratory tests should the nurse expect to monitor in these students? (Select all that apply.)
   a. CBC
   b. WBC with differential
   c. platelet count
   d. Hgb and Hct

5. What information concerning these medications should be taught to these students? (Select all that apply.)
   a. Chew sugarless gum to relieve dry mouth.
   b. Avoid taking OTC medications that contain caffeine.
   c. The importance of eating three nutritional meals if experiencing anorexia.
   d. Monitor blood levels of the medication monthly.

6. The school nurse starts a support group for parents and teachers of these children. What are priorities for this group? (Select all that apply.)
   a. opportunity to discuss feelings and ask questions
   b. discussion of the need for appropriate counseling along with pharmacological interventions
   c. discussion of the fact that long-term use of ADHD drugs may lead to drug abuse
   d. education on the lack of side effects seen with clients taking this medication

21 Central Nervous System Depressants

Study Questions

Crossword puzzle: Use the definitions to determine the correct terms.

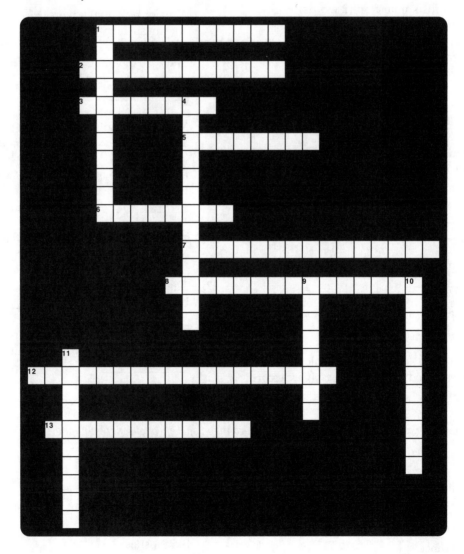

Across

1. Given at the lower end of the spinal column to block the perineal area (2 words)
2. The first anesthetic (2 words)
3. Residual drowsiness resulting in impaired reaction time
5. Inability to fall asleep

6. Herb that should not be taken with barbiturates (2 words)
7. Increase the action of the neurotransmitter GABA
8. Used to block pain at the site while consciousness is maintained (2 words)
12. Combination of drugs used in general anesthesia (2 words)
13. Should be restricted to short-term (2 weeks or less)

Down

1. Penetration of the anesthetic into the subarachnoid membrane (2 words)
4. Placement of a local anesthetic in the outer covering of the spinal cord (2 words)
9. Mildest form of central nervous system (CNS) depression
10. Placed near the sacrum (2 words)
11. First benzodiazepine introduced

Complete the following.

14. The broad classification of CNS depressants includes the following seven groups: _____, _____, _____, _____, _____, _____, and _____.

15. The two phases of sleep are _____ and _____.

16. The mildest form of CNS depression is _____.

17. Anesthesia (may / may not) be achieved with high doses of sedative-hypnotics. (Circle correct answer.)

18. Thiopental is used in general anesthesia as a(n) _____ anesthetic.

19. General anesthesia depresses the _____ system, alleviates _____, and causes a loss of _____.

20. An operation is performed during the _____ stage of anesthesia. The other three stages are _____, _____, and _____.

21. Bupivacaine and tetracaine are drugs commonly used for _____ anesthesia.

22. A major potential adverse effect of spinal anesthesia is _____.

23. The type of spinal anesthesia frequently used for clients in labor is a(n) _____ _____.

24. Muscle relaxants (are / are not) part of balanced anesthesia. (Circle correct answer.)

25. Drugs used to induce sleep in those who have difficulty getting to sleep are _____-acting barbiturates.

26. A popular non-benzodiazepine for the treatment of insomnia is _____.

27. The drug of choice for the management of benzodiazepine overdose is _____.

28. Local anesthetics are divided into two groups: _____ and _____.

Match the letter of the description in Column II with the common side effect of sedative-hypnotics in Column I.

Column I

_____ 29. Hangover
_____ 30. REM rebound
_____ 31. Dependence
_____ 32. Tolerance
_____ 33. Respiratory depression
_____ 34. Hypersensitivity

Column II

a. Need to increase dosage to get desired effect
b. Suppression of respiratory center in the medulla
c. Skin rashes
d. Residual drowsiness
e. Results in withdrawal symptoms
f. Vivid dreams and nightmares

NCLEX Review Questions

Select the best response.

35. Because of a high incidence of sleep disorders, what is the most frequently prescribed type of drug?
    a. triptans
    b. analeptics
    c. anesthetics
    d. sedative-hypnotics

36. Which drugs are frequently prescribed to control seizures?
    a. ultra-short–acting barbiturates
    b. short-acting barbiturates
    c. intermediate-acting barbiturates
    d. long-acting barbiturates

37. A 48-year-old client returns to the unit after surgery; she has had spinal anesthesia. What is/are the best action(s) for the nurse to take to decrease the possibility of a spinal headache?
    a. Position the client in high-Fowler's position.
    b. Position the client flat in bed.
    c. Increase fluid intake.
    d. b and c

38. What is the reasoning for putting a client in a specific position after spinal anesthesia?
    a. to decrease leakage of spinal fluid
    b. to increase leakage of spinal fluid
    c. has no relation to leakage of spinal fluid
    d. to maintain the body in good alignment

39. On the night of postoperative day 4, a client who had spinal anesthesia requests a sleeping pill. Which barbiturate may be used when the client has difficulty falling asleep and nonpharmacologic measures have not been effective?
    a. secobarbital
    b. amobarbital
    c. butabarbital
    d. aprobarbital

40. Which type of anesthesia frequently is administered using lidocaine? (Select all that apply.)
    a. spinal anesthesia
    b. local anesthesia
    c. intravenous anesthesia
    d. general anesthesia

41. What are the primary ingredients in OTC sleep medications?
    a. barbiturates
    b. benzodiazepines
    c. tranquilizers
    d. antihistamines

42. Which drug(s) is/are considered safer than barbiturates in older clients?
    a. estazolam (ProSom)
    b. temazepam (Restoril)
    c. triazolam (Halcion)
    d. all of the above

43. The advantage(s) of balanced anesthesia include(s) which?
    a. slow induction of anesthesia
    b. reduction of drugs to maintain desired state of anesthesia
    c. maximum adverse effects postoperatively
    d. all of the above

44. Local anesthesia is indicated for which procedures? (Select all that apply.)
    a. dental procedures
    b. diagnostic procedures
    c. suturing a skin laceration
    d. long-duration surgery at a localized area
    e. blocking nerves above spinal anesthetic insertion

45. Balanced anesthesia is comprised of which? (Select all that apply.)
    a. inhaled gas
    b. muscle relaxant
    c. long-acting barbiturate
    d. hypnotic the night before
    e. narcotic analgesic and anticholinergic about 1 hour preoperatively

46.   Which are possible complications of spinal anesthesia? (Select all that apply.)

   a.   headache

   b.   drowsiness

   c.   hypotension

   d.   dysrhythmias

   e.   respiratory distress

Case Study

Select the best answer.

B.Z. visits the clinic complaining of "trouble sleeping." He states, "I'm afraid to take anything because I may sleep through the alarm clock I set for work."

1.   What questions should the nurse ask B.Z. to determine his sleep patterns? (Select all that apply.)

   a.   "Do you have a usual time at which you go to bed?"

   b.   "Do you take naps during the day and if so, for how long?"

   c.   "How much caffeine do you ingest on a daily basis?"

   d.   "What medications are you currently taking?"

   e.   "How much fluid do you drink within the 3 hours prior to going to sleep?"

2.   B.Z.'s physician ordered secobarbital for sleep, and B.Z. has now taken this medication for 1 month. What is the best action by the nurse?

   a.   Continue to give the medication as ordered at bedtime.

   b.   Request a dosage increase as he has been taking this drug a long time.

   c.   Question the order given that this client has been taking this drug for at least 1 month.

   d.   Ask the client how well the medication is working and his total hours of sleep nightly.

3.   B.Z. is being discharged with a sleep medication for long-term use. Which medication would the nurse expect to be ordered for this client?

   a.   phenobarbital

   b.   butabarbital

   c.   quazepam

   d.   lidocaine

4.   What priority information should the nurse include in the health teaching for this client? (Select all that apply.)

   a.   methods for inducing sleep without using medications

   b.   information on side effects of the medications

   c.   instructions to void prior to taking the sleep medication

   d.   instructions to skip a dose every other night to improve the drug's effectiveness

22 Anticonvulsants

Study Questions

Crossword puzzle: Use the definitions to determine the correct terms.

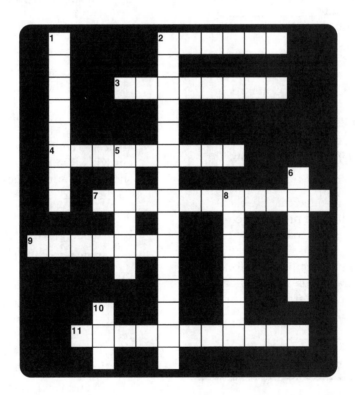

Across
2. Head drop, loss of posture, and sudden loss of muscle tone
3. Absence seizure (2 words)
4. Isolated clonic contraction or jerks lasting 3 to 10 seconds
7. Involuntary paroxysmal muscular contractions
9. Seizure that involves one hemisphere of the brain
11. Drugs that have a negative impact on the fetus

Down
1. Tonic-clonic seizure (2 words)
2. Drugs used for epileptic seizures
5. Dysrhythmic muscle contraction seizure
6. Absence of oxygen to the brain
8. Results from abnormal electric discharges from the cerebral neurons
10. Useful in diagnosing epilepsy

Complete the following.

12. Epilepsy occurs in approximately _____% of the population.

13. To diagnose epilepsy, results of a(n) _____ are useful.

14. Fifty percent of all epilepsy is considered to be primary or _____.

15. The international classification of seizures describes the two categories of seizures as _____ and _____.

16. Anticonvulsant drugs suppress abnormal electrical impulses, thus _____ the seizure, but they (do/do not) eliminate the cause. (Circle correct answer.)

17. Anticonvulsants (are/are not) used for all types of seizures. (Circle correct answer.)

18. The first anticonvulsant used to treat seizures was _____, discovered in 1938, and today is the most commonly used drug for this condition.

19. It is strongly recommended that the client check with the health care provider before taking _____ preparations.

20. Administration of phenytoin via the (oral/ intramuscular/intravenous) route is not recommended because of its erratic absorption rate. (Circle correct answer.)

NCLEX Review Questions

Select the best response.

21. The client has not responded to other anticonvulsant drug therapy. Which drug would expect to be prescribed for this client?
    a. diazepam
    b. valproic acid
    c. ethosuximide
    d. carbamazepine

22. The client has just found out she is pregnant and is in need of seizure medications. Which medication has been shown to be teratogenic and should not be given to a pregnant client?
    a. Phenytoin
    b. Valproic acid
    c. Anticonvulsants
    d. Trimethadione

23. The client is receiving phenytoin and asks how this medication works in the body. What is the nurse's best response?
    a. "It inhibits the enzyme that destroys GABA."
    b. "It suppress the entry of sodium into the cell."
    c. "We are not sure how it works, but it suppresses seizures."
    d. "It increases the amount of calcium that enters the cell."

24. A 24-year-old who has a seizure disorder is going to start taking phenytoin, the drug of choice, to control her seizure activity. The client will initially receive IV phenytoin. What should the nurse check before giving this medication?
    a. urine output
    b. blood glucose levels
    c. patency of the client's IV
    d. dietary intake

25. A client's initial order is to receive phenytoin for a seizure disorder. The nurse is getting ready to administer the next dose and notices that the medication is mixed with a dextrose solution. What is the nurse's best action?
    a. Administer the medication after flushing the IV to assure patency.
    b. Administer the medication but decrease the rate of infusion to prevent a reaction.
    c. Send the medication back to the pharmacy and request the drug be mixed in a saline solution.
    d. Contact the physician and request that the medication be changed to an oral dose.

26. A client is receiving phenytoin intravenously for a seizure disorder. After several days of IV medication, the nurse notices that the client's IV insertion site is red and swollen. What is the best action by the nurse?
    a. Discontinue the medication and request that the client be changed to an oral dose.
    b. Continue the medication infusion and monitor the IV site more frequently.
    c. Flush the IV with normal saline and continue the current infusion.
    d. Discontinue this IV infusion, restart the IV in another site and restart the infusion.

27. A client who has been receiving phenytoin intravenously for a seizure disorder has been changed to an oral medication. Which order for oral administration should the nurse question?
    a. 100 mg, PO, daily
    b. 100 mg, PO, t.i.d.
    c. 100 mg, PO, b.i.d.
    d. All of the above

28. A client who is to begin taking oral phenytoin for a seizure disorder asks how long she will need these medications. What is the nurse's best response to this question?
    a. "You will need to take this medication for a lifetime."
    b. "This medication should taken until you are seizure-free."
    c. "Unfortunately, seizures are unpredictable, and therefore so is the drug regimen."
    d. "For a short period of time, as seizure disorders are cured by medications."

29. When a client is taking phenytion for a seizure disorder, serum phenytoin levels should be monitored to determine if the blood serum level is within the therapeutic range, thus avoiding toxic levels. Which result is within the therapeutic range?
    a. 5 mcg/mL
    b. 12 mcg/mL
    c. 23 mcg/mL
    d. 42 mcg/mL

30. A client is receiving anticonvulsant medication and many other medications. Which type of drug(s) should the nurse question before administration? (Select all that apply.)
    a. digoxin
    b. antineoplastics
    c. sulfonamides
    d. laxatives

31. In the event that a client taking anticonvulsant medication experiences a seizure, what information should be included in the nurse's documentation? (Select all that apply.)
    a. type of movements
    b. time the movements started and ended
    c. ability to stop the movements
    d. progression of movements

32. A client who has been receiving phenytoin for a seizure disorder will be discharged in a couple of days. The nurse is preparing for discharge teaching. What information about side effects of this medication should the client receive?
    a. The client may have a permanent brown discoloration of her urine.
    b. The client should brush her teeth with a firm toothbrush.
    c. The client may experience nosebleeds and a sore throat.
    d. The client may experience orthostatic hypotension.

33. The nurse is conducting an admission assessment for a client who has been taking phenytoin for 20 years. The client has not reported any seizure activity while taking the maintenance dose. What would the nurse expect to see if this client is experiencing a common side effect of the drug?
    a. gingival hyperplasia
    b. polyuria
    c. weight gain
    d. irritability

34. As a result of a client's long-term use of phenytoin, which laboratory test would the nurse want ordered for the client?
    a.   serum potassium (K)
    b.   serum BUN and creatinine
    c.   platelet count
    d.   serum blood glucose

35. The client is diagnosed with status epilepticus. Which medication would the nurse expect to be prescribed?
    a.   diazepam
    b.   primidone
    c.   acetazolamide
    d.   valproic acid

36. Which statement(s) is/are true about seizures and anticonvulsant use during pregnancy? (Select all that apply.)
    a.   Seizures increase 25% in epileptic women.
    b.   Many anticonvulsants have teratogenic properties.
    c.   Anticonvulsant use increases loss of folic acid.
    d.   Anticonvulsants increase the effects of vitamin K.
    e.   Valproic acid causes major malformations in 40-80% of fetuses.

37. The nurse assesses the client for side effects of phenytoin. What clinical manifestations might the nurse see? (Select all that apply.)
    a.   nausea
    b.   vomiting
    c.   diarrhea
    d.   headache
    e.   nystagmus
    f.   gingival hyperplasia

38. What should be included in the health teaching plan for the client taking phenytoin? (Select all that apply.)
    a.   Restrict fluids while taking phenytoin.
    b.   Urine may be a harmless pink or reddish brown color.
    c.   Alcoholic beverages are not recommended.
    d.   The drug may have a teratogenic effect on a fetus.
    e.   Avoid aspirin while taking phenytoin.

Case Study

Select the best answer.

M.B. is a 44-year-old attorney who has been taking phenytoin for epilepsy for more than 25 years. Review of her records indicates she has missed several of her regularly scheduled appointments. The nurse discusses this with M.B., and her response is, "I know all about the disease and the drugs."

1. M.B.'s drug level is 8 mcg/mL. What should concern the nurse about this level?
    a.   Nothing, it is within normal limits
    b.   It is too low.
    c.   It is too high.
    d.   It is OK as she is not experiencing side effects.

2. M.B.'s medication has been changed to ethotoin. What disadvantage of this medication could be problematic for this client?
    a.   This medication has more side effects than phenytoin.
    b.   This medication has to be taken more frequently than phenytoin.
    c.   Use of this medication has to be monitored more closely than phenytoin.
    d.   This medication will cause temporary discoloration of the skin.

3. M.B. does not like taking ethotoin, so the physician put her back on phenytoin. She has been reporting gastric upset and her physician has put her on cimetidine. What should the nurse be concerned about with this combination of medications?

    a. The effectiveness of phenytoin will be decreased.

    b. The drug levels of cimetidine will rise to toxic levels.

    c. The actions of phenytoin will be increased.

    d. The effectiveness of cimetidine will be decreased.

4. M.B. has become perimenopausal, and she informs the nurse that she is taking evening primrose, an OTC herbal supplement. What should concern the nurse about M.B. taking evening primrose?

    a. The evening primrose will not be effective when taking it with phenytoin.

    b. The phenytoin dosage will need to be decreased.

    c. The phenytoin dosage will need to be increased.

    d. This combination should not concern the nurse.

23 Drugs for Neurologic Disorders: Parkinsonism and Alzheimer's Disease

Study Questions

Match the term in Column I with the definition in Column II.

Column I

_____ 1. Acetylcholinesterase inhibitor

_____ 2. Dopamine agonist

_____ 3. Dystonic movement

_____ 4. Bradykinesia

_____ 5. Pseudoparkinsonism

Column II

a. Stimulates dopamine receptors

b. Adverse reaction to antipsychotic drugs

c. Permits more acetylcholine in the neuron receptors

d. Involuntary abnormal movement

e. Slowed movements

Complete the following.

6. The two neurotransmitters within the neurons of the striatum of the brain that have opposing effects are _____ and _____.

7. Which of the neurotransmitters is deficient in parkinsonism? _____

8. The drug prescribed to treat parkinsonism by replacing the neurotransmitter is _____.

9. The substance that inhibits the enzyme dopa decarboxylase and allows more levodopa to reach the brain is _____.

10. An example of an acetylcholinesterase inhibitor is _____.

11. Acetylcholinesterase inhibitors _____ transmission at the cholinergic synapses, both peripheral and central.

12. The drug _____ prolongs action of levodopa and can decrease "on-off" fluctuations in clients with parkinsonism.

13. Entacapone (Comtan) is the newest FDA-approved COMT inhibitor that does not affect _____ function.

14. FDA-approved anticholinergic drugs are _____ and _____.

NCLEX Review Questions

Select the best response.

15. The nurse is giving a 51-year-old client with parkinsonism his carbidopa-levodopa. Which order should the nurse question before administering the drug?
    a. Carbidopa 5 mg/levodopa 200 mg b.i.d.
    b. Carbidopa 25 mg/levodopa 150 mg b.i.d.
    c. Carbidopa 25 mg/levodopa 250 mg t.i.d.
    d. Carbidopa 10 mg/levodopa 100 mg q.i.d.

16. A 51-year-old client with parkinsonism has been taking carbidopa-levodopa for 2 years. What clinical manifestations would the nurse observe if this client is experiencing side effects?
    a. headache
    b. hyperglycemia
    c. fever
    d. orthostatic hypotension

17. The nurse is teaching a client with parkinsonism about the carbidopa-levodopa he takes. Which statement by the client indicates the need for more teaching? (Select all that apply.)
    a. "This medication may increase abnormal movements."
    b. "My urine will darken with exposure to air."
    c. "I need to take vitamin B$_6$ with this medication."
    d. "I need to take this medication before meals."

18. The nurse should recommend that a client with parkinsonism who takes carbidopa-levodopa avoid which foods?
    a. leafy green and yellow vegetables
    b. beans and cereals
    c. cheese and milk
    d. citrus fruits

19. A client with parkinsonism who takes carbidopa-levodopa has been prescribed a medication for his depression. Which order should the nurse question before administering the new drug?
    a. MAOI antidepressant
    b. atypical antidepressant
    c. SSRI antidepressant
    d. tricyclic antidepressant

20. A client with parkinsonism who takes carbidopa-levodopa needs medication for depression. The client's physician adds the medication entacapone to the client's drug regimen. What would the nurse expect to occur with the carbidopa-levodopa dosage?
    a. There should be no change in the medication dosage.
    b. Both carbidopa and levodopa dosages should be decreased.
    c. The levodopa dosage should decrease.
    d. The carbidopa dosage should be decreased.

21. The nurse is teaching a client about an appropriate diet while taking carbidopa-levodopa. Which foods should this client be taught to avoid? (Select all that apply.)
    a. most cereals
    b. lima beans
    c. kidney beans
    d. chicken
    e. seafood

22. What common side effects of acetylcholinesterase inhibitors are assessed in clients taking this medication? (Select all that apply.)
    a. rhinitis
    b. depression
    c. constipation
    d. weight gain
    e. increased appetite

23. Anticholinergics are contraindicated for which clients? (Select all that apply.)
    a. 60-year-old with shingles
    b. 45-year-old with glaucoma
    c. 77-year-old with GI obstruction
    d. 65-year-old with urinary frequency
    e. 71-year-old with prostatic hypertrophy

24. A client has been taking tacrine for 2 months. Which vital sign finding specific to a client taking this medication should concern the nurse?
    a. pulse of 51 beats/min
    b. pulse of 92 beats/min
    c. blood pressure of 120/80 mm Hg
    d. blood pressure of 100/70 mm Hg

25. A client's wandering and hostility levels have increased. What should concern the nurse in this client who is taking tacrine?
    a. The client is taking too high of a daily dosage to maintain mental status.
    b. The client requires more medication to maintain mental status.
    c. The medication is not working as effectively as it could be.
    d. The medication is no longer able to control the client's mental deterioration.

Case Study

Select the best answer.

D.G., 76 years old, was diagnosed as having parkinsonism 6 years ago, for which he took levodopa 750 mg t.i.d. Because of side effects, levodopa was discontinued and carbidopa-levodopa was started.

1. The nurse needs to assess D.G. Which classic clinical manifestations should the nurse expect to assess? (Select all that apply.)
    a. bradykinesia
    b. rigidity
    c. tremors
    d. blurred vision

2. D.G.'s spouse said he is beginning to have some side effects from the medication. Which clinical manifestations might the nurse assess that are related to D.G.'s medication regimen? (Select all that apply.)
    a. frequent headaches
    b. psychosis
    c. vomiting
    d. increased blood pressure

3. D.G. is being changed from levodopa to carbidopa-levodopa and wants to know how this medication is going to be more effective. What is the nurse's best response?
    a. "This medication will increase the amount of serotonin released in the brain, thus increasing muscle tone."
    b. "This medication will allow more dopamine to be broken down, thus decreasing muscle spasms."
    c. "This medication will increase the amount of dopamine to reach the brain, thus decreasing movement symptoms."
    d. "This medication decreases the amount of dopamine in the periphery, thus increasing muscle tone."

4. D.G. is also taking other medications. Which medication, when given with carbidopa-levodopa, should the nurse question before administering?
    a. digoxin
    b. antacid
    c. MAOI
    d. antihypertensive

5. D.G. is being discharged on carbidopa-levodopa. Which information should be a priority to include in the teaching for this client? (Select all that apply.)
    a. The client may take this medication with food if experiencing GI upset.
    b. The client's perspiration may become dark and may stain clothing.
    c. The client will have to monitor blood pressure weekly and report any increases.
    d. The client should not abruptly stop the medication without contacting the health care provider.

24 Drugs for Neuromuscular Disorders: Myasthenia Gravis, Multiple Sclerosis, and Muscle Spasms

Study Questions

Crossword puzzle: Use the definitions to determine the correct terms.

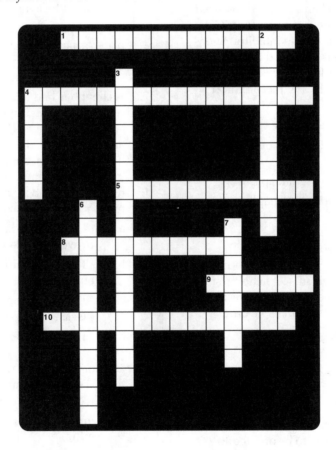

Across

1. Myasthenia gravis (MG) clients lack this neurotransmitter
4. Generalized muscular weakness of the client with MG (2 words)
5. Drug used to diagnose MG
8. Paralysis of one side of the body
9. Drooping eyelid
10. Involuntary muscle twitching

Down

2. First acetylcholinesterase inhibitor used to control MG
3. An acute exacerbation of MG symptoms (2 words)
4. Abnormal pupil constriction
6. Multiple sclerosis (MS) forms plaques on this area of the nerve (2 words)
7. Drug most effective in reducing spasticity in clients with MS

NCLEX Review Questions

Select the best response.

11. A 62-year-old client is receiving treatment for MG with an acetylcholinesterase inhibitor. The nurse is assessing the client. What clinical manifestations would be noted to determine if the medication is working?
    a. experiencing the side effect of GI upset
    b. miosis
    c. increased salivation
    d. maintenance of muscle strength

12. The nurse observes changes in a 62-year-old client who is receiving treatment for MG with an acetylcholinesterase inhibitor. She is drooling, and she has increased tearing and sweating. What should concern the nurse about the client's exhibiting these clinical manifestations?
    a. She is having cholinergic crisis.
    b. She is in the early stages of myasthenic crisis.
    c. She is having a vascular spasm.
    d. She is experiencing an anaphylactic reaction.

13. What emergency medication should the nurse administer to a client who is receiving treatment for MG with an acetylcholinesterase inhibitor to relieve clinical manifestations such as drooling, tearing, and sweating?
    a. edrophonium
    b. atropine
    c. Valium
    d. pyridostigmine

14. MS is difficult to diagnose. Which study should the nurse expect to be ordered to diagnose MS and identify new lesions?
    a. magnetic resonance imaging (MRI)
    b. computed tomography (CT)
    c. x-ray
    d. angiography

15. What are the actions of adrenocorticotropic hormone (ACTH) in clients with MS?
    a. increase blood flow
    b. increase exacerbations
    c. increase demyelinating axons
    d. decrease the acute inflammatory process

16. A client was given 80 units of ACTH in 500 mL of D_5W per day for 5 days. Which medication when ordered by the physician should the nurse question before administering it to the client?
    a. histamine$_2$ blockers
    b. beta blockers
    c. cephalosporins
    d. certain nonsteroidal antiinflammatory drugs (NSAIDs)

17. A client has had MS for several years, during which he has had many remissions and exacerbations. He has been prescribed Imuran and Betaseron. The client wants to know how the new medications (biologic response modifiers and immunosuppressants) will help his current physical state. What is the nurse's best response?
    a. "They will reduce spasticity and improve muscular movement."
    b. "They will help to form new neurons and axons."
    c. "They will stop the progression of this disease."
    d. "They will improve muscle strength."

18. A client had an acute attack of MS. Which drug(s) should the nurse be prepared to administer? (Select all that apply.)
    a. immunosuppressant (cyclophosphamide)
    b. ACTH
    c. glucocorticoid (prednisone)
    d. 6α-methylprednisolone

19. A client with MS is experiencing muscle spasms. How will centrally acting muscle relaxants improve his status?
    a. They can decrease pain and do not affect range of motion.
    b. They can decrease pain and increase range of motion.
    c. They can increase range of motion and do not affect pain.
    d. They can decrease pain and decrease range of motion.

20. The nurse is assessing a client who is taking carisoprodol. Which assessed clinical manifestations would indicate the client is experiencing side effects? (Select all that apply.)
    a. nausea
    b. insomnia
    c. weakness
    d. bradycardia
    e. hypertension

21. The nurse is administering medications to her clients. Which medication order should the nurse question before administration?
    a. meprobamate for a 33-year-old with muscle trauma
    b. dantrolene sodium for a 50-year-old with muscle spasms
    c. edrophonium for a 30-year-old who is undergoing diagnostic testing for MG
    d. diazepam for a 60-year-old who also has glaucoma

Case Study

Select the best answer.

G.D., 21 years old, has muscle spasms following a spinal cord injury. He is receiving carisoprodol (Soma) to relax his muscles, antacids, insulin, and an inhaler. He also has been diagnosed with asthma and type I diabetes.

1. The nurse is reviewing G.D.'s medications and health history. What should concern the nurse about G.D. taking carisoprodol?
   a. It will cause hyperglycemia.
   b. It can cause hypoglycemia.
   c. It can increase asthma attacks.
   d. It causes stomach irritation.

2. G.D. states that he has been depressed since his injury and sometimes drinks too much alcohol when taking the Soma. What is a priority concern for the nurse with this combination?
   a. It can cause severe muscle relaxation.
   b. Alcohol and Soma cannot be taken together as one blocks the actions of the other.
   c. It can cause an increase in muscle spasms.
   d. It can increase CNS depression.

3. The nurse is passing out 2 PM medications for several people, including G.D. Which client should receive medication first?
   a. 25-year-old with MG taking neostigmine bromide
   b. G.D., who is receiving insulin for a blood glucose level of 160 mg/dl
   c. 30-year-old with MG taking ambenonium
   d. 40-year-old with a broken leg requesting pain medication

4. Which medication, if ordered for G.D., should be questioned by the nurse?
   a. antihistamine
   b. antacid
   c. NSAID
   d. proton-pump inhibitor

5. G.D. is being discharged. What information is a priority to be included in his discharge teaching? (Select all that apply.)
   a. Avoid use of alcohol and CNS depressants.
   b. Do not abruptly stop taking the muscle relaxant.
   c. Follow up with the health care provider for required lab tests.
   d. Avoid eating beans and cereals.

25 Antiinflammatory Drugs

Study Questions

Match the term in Column I with the definition in Column II.

Column I

_____ 1. Salicylates
_____ 2. Para-chlorobenzoic acid
_____ 3. Ketorolac
_____ 4. Fenamates
_____ 5. Oxicams
_____ 6. Gold
_____ 7. Immunomodulators
_____ 8. Colchicine
_____ 9. Allopurinol

Column II

a. Disrupts the inflammatory process and delays disease progression
b. Most frequently used DMARD
c. Indicated for long-term arthritic conditions
d. One of the first NSAIDs introduced
e. Oldest antiinflammatory agent
f. The first injectable NSAID
g. The first drug used to treat gout
h. Drug of choice for clients with chronic tophaceous gout
i. Potent NSAIDs used for acute and chronic arthritic conditions

Complete the following.

10. Inflammation is a response to tissue _____ and _____.

11. The five cardinal signs of inflammation are _____, _____, _____, _____, and _____.

12. Leukocyte infiltration of the inflamed tissue occurs during the _____ phase of inflammation.

13. The half-life of each NSAID (does/does not) differ greatly. (Circle correct answer.)

14. When using NSAIDs for inflammation, the dosage is generally _____ than for pain relief.

15. The half-life of corticosteroids is greater than _____ hours.

NCLEX Review Questions

Select the best response.

16. What occurs during the vascular phase of inflammation?
    a. vasoconstriction and fluid influx to the interstitial space
    b. vasodilation with increased capillary permeability
    c. leukocyte and protein infiltration to inflamed tissue
    d. vasoconstriction with leukocyte infiltration to inflamed tissue

17. The client who is taking NSAIDs complains of heartburn. What should concern the nurse about this symptom?

    a. Nothing, it is a known side effect of NSAIDs.

    b. This indicates the client should be taken off NSAIDs.

    c. This indicates the client's dosage is too high.

    d. This indicates the client's dosage is too low.

18. The client asks how the NSAID he just took works. What is the nurse's best response?

    a. "It enhances the body's inflammatory process."

    b. "It inhibits the synthesis of prostaglandins."

    c. "It inhibits phagocytic activity."

    d. "It decrease the response of red and white blood cells."

19. The client is taking large doses of aspirin for an arthritic condition. Which of the following should concern the nurse? (Select all that apply.)

    a. Tinnitus is a common symptom of early toxicity.

    b. The half-life of aspirin in large doses is approximately 2-20 hours.

    c. Aspirin can lower blood sugar in clients with diabetes, causing hypoglycemia.

    d. Aspirin not taken at mealtime or with food can increase GI distress.

20. A father presents to the emergency department with his 4-year-old son. The father explains that his son had a temperature and that he gave him baby aspirin to decrease his fever, but it has not worked. What should concern the nurse about a 4-year-old receiving aspirin?

    a. Aspirin has the potential to cause GI bleeding in children.

    b. Aspirin has the potential to cause ringing in the ears in children.

    c. Aspirin has the potential to cause hyperglycemia in children.

    d. Aspirin has the potential to cause Reye's syndrome in children.

21. A 25-year-old client with asthma has been prescribed aspirin for arthritis. What should concern you about this client taking aspirin?

    a. Aspirin can cause severe headaches.

    b. Aspirin can cause osteoarthritis.

    c. Aspirin can cause bronchospasms.

    d. Aspirin can cause hyperglycemia.

22. Ibuprofen (Motrin, Advil, Nuprin) is a frequently taken antiinflammatory, analgesic, and antipyretic agent. What is a positive aspect of this drug in relation to other NSAIDs?

    a. It causes less GI upset.

    b. It can be taken between meals with water.

    c. It has a long half-life of 20 to 30 hours.

    d. It has no potential side effects.

23. Which statement by a client would indicate a need for further education on ibuprofen?

    a. "This medication will cause less GI upset than the other NSAID I was taking."

    b. "I will be glad to decrease how much I drink daily."

    c. "I can take this 4 times a day without going over the approved limit."

    d. "I know I might experience diarrhea while using this medication."

24. Piroxicam (Feldene) is an NSAID. What advantage does it have over other NSAIDs?

    a. well-tolerated

    b. low incidence of toxic problems

    c. long half-life

    d. fast-acting

25. What information should the nurse provide to an individual taking NSAIDs? (Select all that apply.)

    a. The client should report epigastric distress.

    b. Alcohol can be taken with NSAIDs.

    c. The client should observe for tarry stools, bleeding gums, and bruising if taking NSAIDs for an extended time.

    d. Those clients with a heavy menstrual flow should take NSAIDs 1 to 2 days before menstruation and not during heavy flow.

26. What characteristics are associated with celecoxib (Celebrex)? (Select all that apply.)
    a. It is not to be used for cardiac precautions like aspirin.
    b. It is to be avoided during the third trimester of pregnancy.
    c. It relieves pain and inflammation without causing GI distress.
    d. It is not to be used by persons with hyperglycemia.

27. Clients receiving gold (a DMARD) therapy for advanced arthritic conditions may receive a corticosteroid as part of the early multiple-dosage regimen. The client may ask about the reason for the combination of a steroid and a DMARD. What would be the nurse's best response?
    a. "The health care provider usually combines these drugs."
    b. "The combination of drugs improves the outcome."
    c. "The gold takes time to achieve its effects; the steroid assists immediately in the alleviation of arthritic symptoms."
    d. "The combination of drugs causes an absence of symptoms."

28. By which action does colchicine relieve the symptoms of gout?
    a. inhibition of the migration of leukocytes to the inflamed area
    b. inhibition of the final steps of uric acid biosynthesis
    c. blocking reabsorption of uric acid excretion
    d. reabsorbing uric acid from distal tubules of the kidney

29. Uricosuric agents such as probenecid (Benemid) are used in the treatment of gout. What does this medication promote?
    a. retention of urate crystals in the body
    b. uric acid excretion via the kidney
    c. reabsorption of urates from the kidney
    d. uric acid excretion via the sweat glands

30. What would the nurse assess in an individual experiencing side effects from Benemid?
    a. sore gums and headache
    b. flushed skin and oliguria
    c. constipation and edema
    d. blurred vision and urinary retention

31. A client is taking corticosteroids for an arthritic condition. What information should the nurse include in a health teaching plan? (Select all that apply.)
    a. Corticosteroids are used to control arthritic flare-ups in severe cases.
    b. Corticosteroids have a short half-life and are taken several times a day.
    c. Corticosteroid dosage must be tapered when discontinuing therapy.
    d. Corticosteroid drugs may not be effective when given as monotherapy.

32. When discontinuing steroid therapy, the dosage should be tapered over a period of how many days?
    a. 1 to 3
    b. 4 to 6
    c. 5 to 10
    d. more than 10

33. Which statements are true regarding ketorolac? (Select all that apply.)
    a. It can be administered orally.
    b. It has an efficacy equal to morphine.
    c. It can be administered intramuscularly.
    d. It can be administered intravenously.
    e. It may be given only for 5 days or less.
    f. It has a usual adult dose of 15 mg IM q6h.

34. A client should receive what information concerning gold therapy? (Select all that apply.)
    a. Desired clinical effect may take 3 to 4 months.
    b. Adherence to scheduled lab tests is essential.
    c. Meticulous dental hygiene is required.
    d. Measures to control constipation are needed.
    e. Metallic taste or pruritus should be reported to the health care provider.

35. The nurse is planning teaching related to antigout drugs. Which information should be included? (Select all that apply.)
   a. Take large doses of vitamin C.
   b. Increase fluid intake.
   c. Avoid alcohol and caffeine.
   d. Avoid foods high in purine.
   e. Take medication with food.

Case Study

Select the best answer.

M.B., 37 years old, comes to the clinic for treatment of an inflammatory condition. She reports taking 975 mg of aspirin q4h for the past week.

1. M.B.'s serum level for aspirin is 33 ng/dl. What should concern the nurse about the drug blood level?
   a. It is below the therapeutic range.
   b. It is within the therapeutic range.
   c. It is at a mildly toxic level.
   d. It is at highly toxic levels.

2. M.B.'s health care provider places her on potassium supplements. She does not like to take medications and asks the nurse why she now has to take potassium. What is the nurse's best response?
   a. "You should speak with your health care provider because she ordered the medication."
   b. "Someone your age should be taking potassium to help your heart."
   c. "You need potassium to decrease the GI distress caused by the aspirin."
   d. "Aspirin can decrease serum potassium levels."

3. M.B. is talking about her medication and wants to know if she should take her medication next week because she is having a tooth pulled. What is the nurse's best response?
   a. "You can continue to take your medication without difficulty before this dental work."
   b. "You should discontinue the medication now so you won't have problems during the procedure next week."
   c. "You should contact your dentist before this appointment to determine what should be done."
   d. "Your health care provider will need to put you on a different medication before this procedure."

4. M.B. also complains of loss of appetite and stomach pains and wonders, "Is there something else is wrong with me?" What is the nurse's best response?
   a. "These are normal problems experienced in individuals taking aspirin."
   b. "There might be; we need to contact your health care provider."
   c. "I don't think anything is wrong with you. You should not worry so much."
   d. "I will discontinue the aspirin until we can find out what else is going on with you."

5. M.B. wants to know if there are other things that she should be concerned about while taking aspirin. What other clinical manifestations should the nurse discuss with the client? (Select all that apply.)
   a. ringing in the ears
   b. drowsiness
   c. dizziness
   d. headache

6. The nurse is planning discharge teaching for M.B. What information should be included in her teaching plan? (Select all that apply.)
   a. Take medication with meals to decrease stomach upset.
   b. Avoid intake of alcohol.
   c. Keep medication out of the reach of children.
   d. Increase intake of fluids.

26 Nonopioid and Opioid Analgesics

Study Questions

Crossword puzzle: Use the definitions to determine the correct terms.

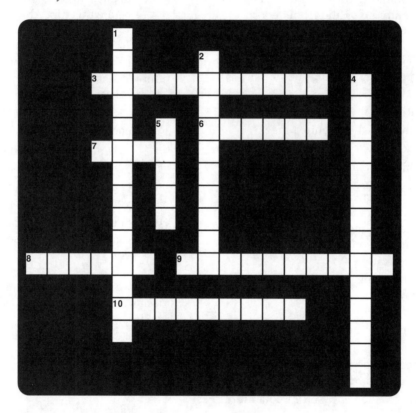

Across
3. Sensory pain receptors
6. Drug type for deep pain
7. This type of drug should not be given with meperidine
8. Drug type for somatic pain
9. Type of drugs prescribed for pain
10. Drug type for chronic pain

Down
1. NSAIDs inhibit synthesis of this
2. NSAID that has an analgesic effect
4. Most serious result of an overdose of Tylenol
5. Type of infection in which aspirin should not be given

Complete the following.

11. Opioids act primarily on the _____
     and nonopioid analgesics act on the
     _____ at the pain receptor sites.

12. In addition to suppressing pain impulses,
     opioids also suppress _____ and
     _____.

13. In addition to pain relief, many opioids have
     _____ and _____ effects.

14. Opioids are contraindicated for use in clients
     with _____ and _____.

15. The client taking meperidine reports
     blurred vision. The nurse knows this is a(n)
     _____ and would report this find-
     ing to the _____.

16. Pentazocine, an opioid agonist-antagonist,
     is classified as a Schedule _____
     drug.

NCLEX Review Questions

Select the best response.

17. A 53-year-old client has just returned to the
     unit from the OR for the placement of a pin
     to stabilize her fractured hip. For the first 48
     hours postoperatively, meperidine (Demerol)
     is ordered for pain control. During the time
     the client is taking meperidine, frequent
     monitoring of what is required?
     a. urine output
     b. temperature
     c. pulse
     d. blood pressure

18. The nurse assesses for toxic effects of meperi-
     dine. What would the nurse expect to find if
     the client is experiencing toxic effects?
     a. tachycardia
     b. constipation
     c. urinary retention
     d. constricted pupils

19. Which nursing assessment would be *least*
     important when monitoring a client who is
     receiving meperidine?
     a. fluid intake
     b. bowel sounds
     c. urinary output
     d. vital signs

20. What should the nurse include in a teaching
     plan for a client who is taking meperidine
     for pain control after surgery? (Select all that
     apply.)
     a. instruction not to use alcohol and cen-
         tral nervous system (CNS) depressants
         while taking meperidine
     b. instruction to report side effects
     c. information on how to prevent consti-
         pation
     d. information on orthostatic hypotension

21. Which factor is most relevant to the relief of
     chronic pain?
     a. administration of drugs at client's re-
         quest
     b. use of injectable drugs
     c. opioid analgesics
     d. use of drugs with long half-lives

22. What is the opioid antagonist used to treat an
     overdose of a morphine-like substance?
     a. pentazocine (Talwin)
     b. ibuprofen (Motrin)
     c. naloxone (Narcan)
     d. probenecid (Benemid)

23. Mixed opioid agonist-antagonists were
     developed in hopes of decreasing which
     problem?
     a. pain
     b. renal failure
     c. opioid abuse
     d. respiratory depression

24. Withdrawal symptoms usually occur how
     many hours after the last opioid dose?
     a. 6 to 12
     b. 24 to 48
     c. 48 to 72
     d. 72 to 96

25. Methadone treatment programs can be effective in helping the opioid-addicted person withdraw. Which is the recommended maintenance dose of methadone?
    a. 100-150 mg/day
    b. 15-120 mg/day
    c. 10-35 mg/day
    d. 2-10 mg/day

26. What is a benefit of methadone over other opioids?
    a. reduced dependency
    b. shorter half-life
    c. daily dosing
    d. both a and c

27. Older clients frequently require a reduction in opioid dosage to avoid severe side effects. What changes occur that require a reduction in opioid dosage? (Select all that apply.)
    a. decreased excretion of drug
    b. decreased metabolism of drug
    c. polypharmacy
    d. increased fluid volume

28. The 70-year-old client is 12 hours post-surgery and is reporting severe discomfort. The physician has ordered Demerol for relief of pain. What should concern the nurse about giving this medication to the client?
    a. Nothing; Demerol works well to relieve pain in older clients.
    b. Demerol tends to be more toxic in older clients.
    c. Not enough time has passed since surgery for the client to be experiencing pain.
    d. The dosage should be cut in half given that this is a recently postoperative client.

29. It may be difficult to assess pain in children. What should the nurse do to be more successful in assessing pain in children? (Select all that apply.)
    a. use age-appropriate communication skills
    b. use the "ouch scale"
    c. discuss the child's response with parents
    d. ask the parents if the child is in pain

30. The nurse is reading the client's medication administration record and notes that she is taking acetaminophen. Which type of drug or drugs should the client not receive when taking this drug?
    a. cholestyramine
    b. beta-blockers
    c. antibiotics
    d. diuretics

31. The nurse is concerned that the client is experiencing side effects of opioid analgesics/agonists. What might the nurse assess if this client is experiencing side effects? (Select all that apply.)
    a. sedation
    b. constipation
    c. hypertension
    d. urinary frequency
    e. nausea and vomiting
    f. respiratory depression

32. The client is taking morphine for pain after a procedure. He has asked for pain medication. This will be his fourth dose of morphine. The nurse goes to his room to administer the drug. His respiratory rate is 12. What is the best action by the nurse?
    a. Give the medication and contact the client's health care provider about his pain.
    b. Give the medication and contact the client's health care provider about his respiratory rate.
    c. Hold the medication and contact the client's health care provider about his pain.
    d. Hold the medication and contact the client's health care provider about his respiratory rate.

33. The client is taking morphine for her postoperative pain. What should the nurse assess in this client to determine if she is experiencing side effects of this medication?
    a. headaches
    b. increased blood pressure
    c. increased coughing
    d. urinary retention

34. What statement by a client taking morphine for pain indicates a need for more teaching?

   a. "I need to monitor my respiratory rate before taking this medication."

   b. "I may need to take a laxative with this medication to prevent constipation."

   c. "Having a few beers on the weekends will help me to relax."

   d. "I should increase the fiber in my diet while taking this medication."

35. The client is taking morphine and reports she is having dizzy spells when she changes position. What is the nurse's best response to this concern?

   a. "Don't worry about it; this will change after you have been taking the medication for a period of time."

   b. "You should move slowly when changing positions and it will decrease the incidence of this."

   c. "You will not experience that once you discontinue the medication."

   d. "We need to change you to another medication; this is a toxic side effect."

36. The nurse is working in the postanesthesia care unit, and the client has received morphine for pain and subsequently is breathing at a rate of less than 8 breaths/minute. What medication should the nurse give to increase this client's respiratory rate?

   a. Robinul

   b. romazicon

   c. naloxone

   d. meperidine

Case Study

Select the best answer.

E.K., 55 years old, is brought to the emergency department complaining of severe chest pain of 30 minutes' duration that began after a tense business meeting and was unrelieved by nitroglycerin. The nurse does a thorough assessment. The health care provider's orders include morphine sulfate 10 mg IV push for the severe pain.

1. The nurse has administered the 10 mg of morphine IV. What is a priority to assess in this client? (Select all that apply.)

   a. blood pressure

   b. blood glucose level

   c. urinary output

   d. respiratory rate

2. E.K. says, as the nurse is giving the medication, that she takes kava kava daily and took it this morning. Given this combination, what should the nurse monitor in this client?

   a. increased respiratory rate

   b. increased sleepiness

   c. decreased pain relief

   d. decreased heart rate

3. E.K.'s chest discomfort is relieved, and she is transferred to the ICU on morphine for pain. What should the nurse continue to monitor in this client? (Select all that apply.)

   a. blood pressure

   b. blood glucose levels

   c. urinary output

   d. respiratory rate

Three hours later, E.K. is resting more comfortably in high-Fowler's position and complains, "I'm not able to pass my water." The nurse notes that her blood pressure has dropped to 120/40 mm Hg. Laboratory test results are pending.

4. What, if anything, should concern the nurse about the blood pressure finding?

   a. Nothing; this is a normal response to morphine.

   b. Nothing, because the client is sitting up, the diastolic reading will be low.

   c. Nothing, because the systolic reading is within an appropriate range.

   d. Nothing, because the client is speaking without slurring.

5. Given that the client is not able to "pass water," what is the first action that should be taken by the nurse?

   a. Notify the physician.

   b. Assess for bladder distention.

   c. Catheterize the client.

   d. Check the client's blood pressure.

6. The nurse takes E.K. to the bathroom, and she is able to void but complains of being light-headed and dizzy when standing up. She wants to know why this is happening. What is the nurse's best response?

    a. "Your heart rate is too low and we need to get you back to bed quickly."

    b. "Your blood pressure drops when changing positions; we need to move slowly."

    c. "Your blood pressure has increased, and we need to get you to bed quickly."

    d. "Your blood glucose must be low; we need to check it immediately."

7. E.K.'s lab results show that she is experiencing noncardiac pain. Her physician has changed her order to oral morphine. What priority teaching information should be given to this client? (Select all that apply.)

    a. Do not continue to take your kava kava until approved by your physician.

    b. Be sure to monitor your bowel movements as this medication can cause constipation.

    c. You will need to monitor your blood glucose level while on this medication.

    d. Do not drink any alcohol when taking this medication.

8. E.K. knows that this medication is addictive. She wants to know how long she can take it without becoming addicted. What is the nurse's best response?

    a. "Each individual is different. Make sure you take the medication as needed to relieve pain."

    b. "You won't be on this medication long enough to become addicted."

    c. "Each individual is different. As long as you don't take it more than 1 month you should be OK."

    d. "You should speak to your physician about taking a different medication."

9. The nurse is reviewing discharge teaching with E.K. What statement(s) by her indicate she has an understanding of her pain medications? (Select all that apply.)

    a. "I will start eating more fruits and vegetables."

    b. "I will not take my kava kava until directed by my physician."

    c. "I will move quickly when changing positions so that my blood pressure will stay OK."

    d. "I will not drink alcohol while taking this medication. Even a small drink can cause problems."

27 Antipsychotics and Anxiolytics

Study Questions

Match the term in Column I to the corresponding statement in Column II.

Column I

_____ 1. Acute dystonia
_____ 2. Akathisia
_____ 3. Anxiolytics
_____ 4. Neuroleptic
_____ 5. Psychosis
_____ 6. Schizophrenia
_____ 7. Tardive dyskinesia
_____ 8. Pseudoparkinsonism

Column II

a. Losing contact with reality
b. Extrapyramidal reaction to antipsychotics
c. Muscle tremors, rigidity, shuffling gait
d. Restlessness, inability to sit still, foot-tapping
e. Spasms of tongue, face, neck, and back
f. Used to treat anxiety and insomnia
g. Drug that modifies psychotic behavior
h. Chronic psychotic disorder

Complete the following.

9. Antipsychotic drugs were developed to improve the _____ and _____ of clients with psychotic symptoms resulting from an imbalance in the neurotransmitter _____.

10. Typical antipsychotics are subdivided into phenothiazines and nonphenothiazines. Nonphenothiazines are divided into four classes: _____, _____, _____, and _____.

11. The most common side effect of all antipsychotics is _____.

12. Antipsychotics may lead to side effects that include _____ and _____.

13. Phenothiazines (increase / decrease) the seizure threshold; adjustment of anticonvulsants may be required. (Circle correct answer.)

14. Anxiolytics (are / are not) usually given for secondary anxiety. (Circle correct answer.)

15. Long-term use of anxiolytics is not recommended because _____ may develop within a short time.

16. The action of anxiolytics resembles that of _____, not antipsychotics.

Match the following drugs in Column I with their drug classification in Column II.

Column I

_____ 17.   clozapine (Clozaril)

_____ 18.   chlorpromazine (Thorazine)

_____ 19.   fluphenazine (Prolixin)

_____ 20.   droperidol (Inapsine)

_____ 21.   haloperidol (Haldol)

_____ 22.   risperidone (Risperdal)

Column II

a.   Phenothiazines

b.   Nonphenothiazines

c.   Atypical antipsychotics

NCLEX Review Questions

Select the best response.

23.   Antipsychotic drugs are useful in the management of what types of illness?

    a.   anxiety and neurosis

    b.   psychotic illnesses

    c.   depression and lifting of mood

    d.   psychosomatic disorders

24.   The client has been prescribed an antipsychotics and would like to know when it will take effect. What is the best answer?

    a.   24 hours

    b.   3 days

    c.   1 week

    d.   3-6 weeks

25.   Client education for use of these drugs is important. What information should be included in education about antipsychotic drugs?

    a.   A therapeutic response to the medication is expected in a few days.

    b.   The drug should be taken as prescribed and the health care provider consulted before discontinuing use.

    c.   Taking alcohol or barbiturates with the drug is acceptable.

    d.   A rapid change in position from supine to standing may cause vertigo.

26.   Typical or traditional antipsychotics may cause extrapyramidal symptoms (EPS) or pseudoparkinsonism. Which symptom is an EPS?

    a.   intentional tremors

    b.   shuffling gait

    c.   downward eye movement

    d.   loss of hearing

27.   Clients taking high-potency typical antipsychotics may develop adverse extrapyramidal reactions. What is one type of these abnormal reactions?

    a.   paralysis of the extremities

    b.   akathisia

    c.   disorientation

    d.   talking excessively

28.   What is the most severe adverse extrapyramidal reaction?

    a.   acute dystonia

    b.   akathisia

    c.   tardive dyskinesia

    d.   pseudoparkinsonism

29.   Which agent would the nurse expect to give to decrease EPS?

    a.   benztropine (Cogentin) and trihexyphenidyl (Artane)

    b.   atropine and bethanechol (Urecholine)

    c.   doxepin (Sinequan) and nortriptyline (Aventyl)

    d.   diazepam (Valium) and alprazolam (Xanax)

30. Phenothiazines are grouped into three categories based on their side effects. In which group is fluphenazine (Prolixin) found?
    a. aliphatic phenothiazine
    b. piperazine phenothiazine
    c. piperidine phenothiazine
    d. thioxanthene

31. What is a common side effect of fluphenazine (Prolixin)?
    a. bradycardia
    b. EPS
    c. oliguria
    d. diarrhea

32. A 72-year-old client is taking fluphenazine (Prolixin) for schizophrenia. In reviewing his medication dosage, the nurse notes that it is the normal dose for an adult. What should concern the nurse about this amount of medication prescribed?
    a. Nothing; the client is an adult and should receive the normal dosage.
    b. The client's dose should be 10% less than an adult dose.
    c. The client's dose should be 25-50% less than an adult dose.
    d. The client should not take this medication because he is older than 70 years.

33. A client presents to the emergency department with an overdose of fluphenazine. What is the priority action by the nurse?
    a. administration of activated charcoal
    b. starting an intravenous line
    c. administration of cholinergics
    d. administration of beta-adrenergic blockers

34. Haloperidol (Haldol) is frequently used as an antipsychotic. What should the nurse know about this medication when giving it as an antipsychotic?
    a. It has a sedative effect on agitated, combative persons.
    b. It is the drug of choice for older clients with liver disease.
    c. It will not cause EPS.
    d. It can be used by clients with narrow-angle glaucoma.

35. The client is taking Haldol 5 mg t.i.d. and complains of nearly falling down when he gets out of bed. What is this client experiencing?
    a. anticholinergic reaction
    b. tardive dyskinesia
    c. orthostatic hypotension
    d. tachycardia

36. What is the drug category for atypical antipsychotics?
    a. phenothiazines
    b. serotonin/dopamine antagonists
    c. butyrophenones
    d. thioxanthenes

37. The atypical antipsychotics, marketed in the United States since 1990, have a weak affinity for the D_2 receptors. As such, what type of EPS does the client experience?
    a. an increase in EPS
    b. fewer EPS
    c. an absence of EPS
    d. no effect on EPS

38. Atypical antipsychotics have a stronger affinity to which receptors?
    a. D_1 receptors
    b. D_2 receptors; they block serotonin receptors
    c. D_3 receptors
    d. D_4 receptors; they block serotonin receptors

39. Serotonin antagonists, atypical antipsychotics, are effective for treating which type of schizophrenia?

    a. positive symptoms

    b. negative symptoms

    c. both positive and negative symptoms

    d. anxiety

40. The anxiolytic alprazolam (Xanax) is from which drug group?

    a. antihistamines

    b. azapirones

    c. benzodiazepines

    d. propanediol

41. Dependency can occur when taking benzodiazepines over extended periods. When these medications are abruptly withdrawn, what might the nurse assess in this client?

    a. gastrointestinal discomfort

    b. drowsiness

    c. increased thirst

    d. irritability and nervousness

42. Valium is classified as which type of drug?

    a. phenothiazine

    b. benzodiazepine

    c. antihistamine

    d. serotonin antagonist

43. A client asks what "b.i.d." means. What is the best response?

    a. "Once a day."

    b. "Twice a day."

    c. "Three times a day."

    d. "Four times a day."

44. The nurse is teaching a client how to take his Valium. What should he avoid when taking Valium?

    a. Vitamins, because they increase the effects of Valium to toxic levels.

    b. Antacids, because they increase serum Valium levels.

    c. Alcohol, because it can cause CNS depression and respiratory distress.

    d. An antihypertensive agent, because the client's blood pressure could be increased.

45. Which patient(s) should not be taking fluphenazine? (Select all that apply.)

    a. 53-year-old with blood dyscrasias

    b. 35-year-old with hepatic dysfunction

    c. 62-year-old neuromuscular pain

    d. 47-year-old with subcortical brain damage

    e. 32-year-old with narrow-angle glaucoma

46. Lorazepam is an anxiolytic drug; however, it may be prescribed for other clinical problems. For which other conditions may it be prescribed? (Select all that apply.)

    a. anxiety

    b. status epilepticus

    c. preoperative sedation

    d. manage schizophrenia

    e. depression and delusions

Case Study

Select the best answer.

Clozapine (Clozaril) was the first atypical antipsychotic to be effective in treating clients with severe schizophrenia. B.B. had been taking mesoridazine besylate (Serentil), which was ineffective in treating his withdrawal behavior and his lack of interest in himself and his surroundings. B.B. has been prescribed clozapine (Clozaril) 50 mg per day for the initial dose. If tolerated, the dosage will increase to 100 mg, t.i.d.

1.   B.B. wants to know why he is being changed from mesoridazine to clozapine. What is the nurse's best response?

   a.   "Clozapine has less severe side effects."

   b.   "Clozapine works better on the symptoms you're experiencing."

   c.   "Clozapine requires less frequent monitoring."

   d.   "Clozapine has less drug-to-drug interactions."

2.   What is the most severe side effect of clozapine?

   a.   photosensitivity

   b.   sudden death

   c.   agranulocytosis

   d.   liver failure

3.   The nurse is teaching B.B. about his follow-up care. Which lab values should be monitored in this client?

   a.   Hct and Hgb

   b.   liver enzymes

   c.   troponin levels

   d.   WBCs

4.   Which statement by B.B. during his teaching should concern the nurse and indicate that he requires more education?

   a.   "I will continue to drink two glasses of red wine every day for their health benefits."

   b.   "I need to have my doctor check my antihypertensive medication."

   c.   "I will continue with my normal exercise routine."

   d.   "I won't have to change my diet in order to take this medication."

28 Antidepressants and Mood Stabilizers

Study Questions

Complete the following word search. Clues are given in questions 1-7. Circle your responses.

```
T C S R V R N M J R D M J A H J H
R I Y Y V X R S A N O D J J Y E B
A N O D U O I A N N O Y N J Y V O
P I M J L R W L L D I K Q P B I I
L K F X S J G Q M O H C T W V T F
N M D S K W V O B N P I L W O C B
M A G W I G D V D L Q I T X K A U
J O T R I C Y C L I C S B U J E K
Y I Z Y M P F R F J A K P H C R V
Q S Q M U H G O U I D O F U C C X
L S T N A S S E R P E D I T N A Q
```

1. Swing-type moods
2. Abbreviation for selective serotonin reuptake inhibitors
3. Abbreviation for monoamine oxidase inhibitors
4. A sense of euphoria
5. Group of drugs used to treat depression
6. Depression that has a sudden onset
7. Block the uptake of norepinephrine and serotonin in the brain

Match the drugs in Column I with their drug classification in Column II.

Column I

____ 8. mirtazapine (Remeron)
____ 9. reboxetine (Vestra)
____ 10. citalopram (Celexa)
____ 11. amitriptyline (Elavil)
____ 12. tranylcypromine (Parnate)
____ 13. paroxetine (Paxil)

Column II

a. Atypical antidepressants
b. Selective serotonin reuptake inhibitors (SSRIs)
c. Monoamine oxidase inhibitors (MAOIs)
d. Tricyclic antidepressants (TCAs)

Crossword puzzle: Use the definitions to determine the correct terms.

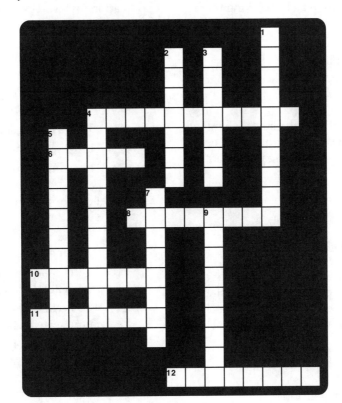

Across

4. Herbal supplement used for depression (3 words)
6. Depression that involves loss of interest in work and home
8. Depression that occurs with a sudden onset following an event
10. Depression that involves swings between two moods
11. Best time to take a TCA
12. Avoid foods with _____ when taking an MAOI

Down

1. First TCAs produced
2. First drug to treat bipolar affective disorder
3. Supplement when taken with MAOIs may lead to manic episodes
4. May cause serotonin syndrome when taken with an SSRI (3 words)
5. TCA used to treat enuresis
7. Herbal supplement that interferes with effects of fluoxetine
9. Clinical response to TCAs takes _____ weeks (3 words)

NCLEX Review Questions

Select the best response.

14. Which is the drug of choice for treatment of enuresis in children?
    a. fluvoxamine (Luvox)
    b. sertraline (Zoloft)
    c. citalopram (Celexa)
    d. imipramine (Tofranil)

15. A client is taking an MAOI for chronic anxiety and fear. The client begins taking phenelzine (Nardil). What is the schedule for the nurse to administer this medication?
    a. once daily
    b. 2-3 times daily
    c. every 4 hours
    d. every other day

16. An order for which type of medication should be questioned in a client taking phenelzine?
    a. NSAID
    b. birth control pills
    c. cold medications with phenylephrine
    d. antacids

17. Assessment is essential with clients taking MAOIs. Which indicator is a priority assessment for the nurse when caring for a client taking phenelzine?
    a. blood pressure
    b. pulse
    c. urine output
    d. hemoglobin levels

18. The nurse is conducting an assessment of a client who is taking phenelzine. Which finding should be of concern to the nurse specific to the client's medications? (Select all that apply.)
    a. headache
    b. sleepiness
    c. orthostatic hypotension
    d. tachycardia

19. If a client were to ingest drugs and/or foods that interact with phenelzine, which change might the nurse assess?
    a. anaphylaxis
    b. orthostatic hypotension
    c. hypertensive crisis
    d. hallucinations

20. A client taking phenelzine is having difficulty selecting foods from his menu. Which foods should he be instructed to avoid?
    a. cheese, chocolate, and raisins
    b. sausage, beer, and whole-grain breads
    c. yogurt, eggs, and bananas
    d. spinach, liver, and milk

21. A client with depression tells you that he would prefer to take herbal supplements rather than prescription medications. What could you recommend for this client?
    a. ephedra and garlic
    b. St. John's wort and ginkgo
    c. feverfew and ginger
    d. garlic and goldenseal

22. The nurse is conducting a preoperative medication review. The client tells the nurse that she takes herbal supplements for depression. The nurse tells the client which medications/supplements she can take, and when. How long before surgery should the client stop taking herbal products?
    a. 24 hours before surgery
    b. 5 days before surgery
    c. 1 to 2 weeks before surgery
    d. 1 month before surgery

23. What are the advantages of SSRIs over TCAs?
    a. SSRIs cause less sedation and fewer hypotensive effects.
    b. SSRIs cause less hypotension and fewer circulatory changes.
    c. SSRIs cause less GI distress and fewer hypotensive effects.
    d. SSRIs cause less sexual dysfunction and moderate sedation.

24. What nursing interventions should be implemented for an acutely manic client who is taking lithium? (Select all that apply.)
    a. Blood levels are drawn monthly to ensure a blood level between 0.5-1.5 mEq/L.
    b. Understanding that the drug is most effective in the depressive phase.
    c. Monitoring for thirst, weight gain, and increased urination.
    d. Emphasizing the importance of taking the medication as ordered.

25. Which specific nursing interventions should be included in monitoring an acutely manic client who is taking lithium? (Select all that apply.)
    a. daily weight
    b. serum lithium level
    c. daily ECG
    d. intake and output

26. What is the recommended daily intake of fluid for an acutely manic client who is taking lithium?

   a. 500 mL

   b. 2000 mL

   c. 3000 mL

   d. 4000 mL

27. After taking lithium carbonate 1200 mg/day for 5 days, the acutely manic client remains agitated and hyperactive. The plasma level is 0.8 mEq/L, and the client complains of feeling slowed down and having increased thirst. What do you suspect is occurring?

   a. The client is still manic, with serious signs of toxicity.

   b. The client is toxic.

   c. The client is still manic, without serious signs of toxicity.

   d. The client is a nonresponder.

28. The nurse is teaching an acutely manic client who is taking lithium about his medication. Which statement by the client indicates a need for more education?

   a. "If I stop taking my medication, the depressive symptoms will reappear."

   b. "I should avoid caffeine products that may aggravate the manic phase."

   c. "I should take my medication with food."

   d. "I should wear or carry an ID tag indicating the drug I take."

29. The nurse is teaching a client who has been prescribed phenelzine (Nardil). Which types of drugs/foods should the patient be taught to avoid? (Select all that apply.)

   a. beer

   b. pork

   c. cheese

   d. citrus fruits

   e. many cold medications

30. Your client is taking fluoxetine (Prozac). About which potential side effects should this client be taught? (Select all that apply.)

   a. tremors

   b. seizures

   c. insomnia

   d. headache

   e. dysrhythmias

Case Study

Select the best answer.

R.C., a 65-year-old executive with the local newspaper company, has recently moved to the area. She says that she is taking Prozac 80 mg at night because of insomnia, lack of energy, and grief at the death of her daughter in a motor vehicle accident 2 months ago. The nurse conducts a thorough nursing assessment.

1. What should concern the nurse about the medication R.C. is taking?

   a. Nothing; it is within the normal dosage range.

   b. It is too low a dose, and R.C.'s physician should be contacted.

   c. It is too high a dose, and R.C.'s physician should be contacted.

   d. The medication should be given in doses throughout the day, not just at night.

2. The nurse is conducting an initial assessment of R.C. Which assessment indicators should the nurse be sure to evaluate? (Select all that apply.)

   a. history of depression

   b. coping behaviors

   c. vital signs

   d. drug history

   e. urine output

3. R.C. said she was started on Prozac a few days ago. She wants to know when she should see clinical effects of the medication. What is the nurse's best response?

   a. "You should already be seeing effects from the medication."

   b. "You won't see effects for at least 2 weeks."

   c. "You will begin to see effects from the medication in 3 weeks."

   d. "You will begin to see effects of the medication in 4 weeks."

4. R.C. will be discharged today. What community resources should the nurse recommend to her? (Select all that apply.)

   a. grief support

   b. peer counseling programs

   c. AA meetings

   d. mental health support groups

5. What information should be included in R.C.'s discharge instructions? (Select all that apply.)

   a. Take medication as prescribed.

   b. Avoid use of alcohol.

   c. Take the medication with food.

   d. Do not abruptly stop taking the medication.

   e. Avoid sun exposure when taking the medication.

29 Penicillins and Cephalosporins

Study Questions

Crossword puzzle: Use the definitions to determine the correct terms.

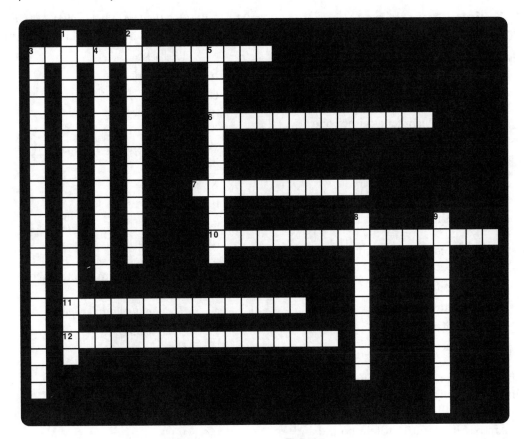

Across

3. Resistance to antibacterial drugs that have similar actions (2 words)
6. Drugs that inhibit the growth of bacteria
7. The first penicillinase-resistant penicillin
10. Caused by prior exposure to antibacterial (2 words)
11. Antibody proteins such as IgG and IgM
12. Bacterial resistance that may occur naturally (2 words)

Down

1. Infections acquired when in a health care facility (2 words)
2. Toxicity of drugs in the kidneys
3. Should be checked before administration of antibiotics (3 words)
4. Occurrence of a secondary infection when the flora of the body are disturbed
5. Substances that inhibit bacterial growth or kill bacteria
8. Introduced during World War II
9. Drugs that kill bacteria

Match the antibiotic in Column I to its category in Column II.

Column I

___ 13. Penicillin G

___ 14. Amoxicillin

___ 15. Oxacillin

___ 16. Carbenicillin indanyl

___ 17. Ancef

___ 18. Cefaclor

___ 19. Cefdinir

___ 20. Cefepime

Column II

a. First generation

b. Second generation

c. Third generation

d. Fourth generation

e. Basic penicillin

f. Penicillinase-resistant penicillins

g. Broad-spectrum penicillin

h. Extended-spectrum penicillins

NCLEX Review Questions

Select the best response.

21. There are several drugs with similar actions, such as penicillins and cephalosporins. What can result when a client takes either one of these medications?

    a. cross-resistance

    b. inherent resistance

    c. nosocomial infections

    d. bacteriostatic effect

22. What condition can occur when the normal flora are disturbed during antibiotic therapy?

    a. organ toxicity

    b. superinfection

    c. hypersensitivity

    d. allergic reaction

23. Which statements are true about the pharmacokinetics of penicillin derivatives amoxicillin and dicloxacillin? (Select all that apply.)

    a. Amoxicillin is 20% protein-bound and dicloxacillin is about 95% protein-bound.

    b. Both drugs have short half-lives.

    c. Amoxicillin is excreted in the urine and dicloxacillin is excreted in bile and urine.

    d. Both drugs are absorbed well from the GI tract.

24. Allergic effects occur in what percentage of persons receiving penicillin compounds?

    a. 1% to 4%

    b. 5% to 10%

    c. 11% to 15%

    d. more than 15%

25. What should a client taking cephalosporins be taught to avoid?

    a. alcohol

    b. anticonvulsants

    c. antacids

    d. antihypertensives

26. Aztreonam (Azactam) is effective against which bacteria?

    a. *Haemophilus influenzae*

    b. *Escherichia coli*

    c. *Proteus* spp.

    d. *Pseudomonas* spp.

27. What happens when probenecid is administered with cefazolin (Ancef) or cefamandole (Mandol)?

    a. Hypersensitivity is common.

    b. Glucosuria occurs.

    c. Drug action is decreased.

    d. Drug action is increased.

28. A 40-year-old client is suffering from an *E. coli* infection. She is unable to swallow pills, so an oral suspension of cephalexin (Keflex) 250 mg is ordered. How should the nurse expect this medication to be scheduled for administration?
    a. q2h
    b. q4h
    c. q6h
    d. q12h

29. What is the usual dose of Keflex?
    a. 250-500 mg q6h
    b. 250 mg-1 g q6h
    c. 1-2 g q6h
    d. 2-3 g q6h

30. Available:

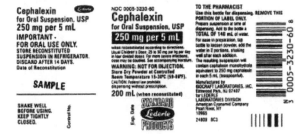

    How many mL of this drug should a client receive receive per dose, and per 24 hours, if receiving the usual dose?
    a. 5 mL/20 mL
    b. 10 mL/20 mL
    c. 5 mL/15 mL
    d. 10 mL/15 mL

31. Which drugs/foods are known to change the action of Keflex?
    a. laxatives
    b. antacids
    c. alcohol
    d. uricosurics

32. What should be included in a health teaching plan for a client taking Keflex? (Select all that apply.)
    a. taking total amount of prescribed antibiotic
    b. resting
    c. finishing antibiotics from a previous prescription
    d. being alert for signs and symptoms of superinfection

33. Which drug may a client use as a substitute for penicillin?
    a. erythromycin
    b. amoxicillin
    c. cephalosporin
    d. tetracycline

34. When given together, broad-spectrum penicillins may decrease the effectiveness of which type of medications?
    a. antacids
    b. oral contraceptives
    c. anticonvulsants
    d. cholinergics

35. Quinupristin/dalfopristin (Synercid) is marketed for IV use against life-threatening infection caused by which bacteria?
    a. vancomycin-resistant *Enterococcus faecium*
    b. *Streptococcus* spp.
    c. *Escherichia coli*
    d. *Proteus mirabilis*

36. The nurse is assessing a client taking a cephalosporin. Which assessment findings are recognized as side effects of the medication? (Select all that apply.)
    a. nausea
    b. vomiting
    c. tinnitus
    d. diarrhea
    e. itching

37. Which specific nursing interventions should be done for a client taking ceftazidime (Fortaz)? (Select all that apply.)
    a. taking culture for culture and sensitivity
    b. administering IV dose over 20 minutes every day
    c. assessing for allergic reaction
    d. monitoring urinary output
    e. restricting fluids

38. Which client must be monitored carefully if receiving carbenicillin indanyl?
    a. 34-year-old with diabetes
    b. 50-year-old with Parkinson's disease
    c. 58-year-old with heart failure
    d. 70-year-old with Alzheimer's disease

39. A client is taking penicillin G. When is the best time for the client to take the medications?
    a. with meals
    b. 1 hour before or 2 hours after meals
    c. at bedtime
    d. upon arising in the morning

40. The client is taking high doses of penicillin G sodium/potassium. What should be monitored in this client?
    a. Hgb and Hct
    b. blood glucose levels
    c. sodium and potassium levels
    d. urine output

41. The nurse is caring for a client who has been prescribed cefpodoxime. When is the best time for the client to take this medication?
    a. with meals
    b. 1 hour before meals
    c. 2 hours after meals
    d. at bedtime

Case Study

Select the best answer.

J.L., 25 years old, is hospitalized for treatment of a severe penicillin G–resistant *Staphylococcus aureus* infection. He is receiving nafcillin parenterally.

1. J.L. requests to take the medication orally. What is the nurse's best response to this request?
    a. "Okay, I will contact the physician and determine if she will change the order."
    b. "We can't give you the medication orally, as it is metabolized too quickly."
    c. "This method of administration is the best because gastric juices decrease its absorption."
    d. "This method of administration is the best because the pill is large and difficult to swallow."

2. Available:

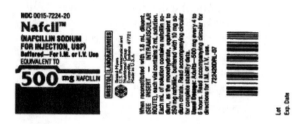

How many mL are required to administer 500 mg IM of the drug?
    a. 1 mL
    b. 2 mL
    c. 3 mL
    d. 4 mL

3. The nurse is assessing J.L. for potential superinfection. What would the nurse expect to see if this client has a superinfection? (Select all that apply.)
    a. stomatitis
    b. genital itching
    c. discoloration of urine
    d. constipation

4. The nurse is monitoring J.L., and he starts having difficulty breathing, wheezing, palpitations, and hives. What should the nurse administer to this client?
    a. a different antibiotic
    b. digoxin
    c. epinephrine
    d. prednisone

5. What nursing interventions should be included in a plan of care for J.L.? (Select all that apply.)
    a. Monitor for allergic reactions.
    b. Monitor client's temperature.
    c. Dilute antibiotic for IV infusion.
    d. Encourage greater than 2500 mL fluid intake.

30 Macrolides, Tetracyclines, Aminoglycosides, and Fluoroquinolones

Study Questions

Match the drug in Column I with the category in Column II.

Column I

_____ 1. Amikacin
_____ 2. Clindamycin
_____ 3. Tigecycline
_____ 4. Erythromycin
_____ 5. Telithromycin
_____ 6. Zithromax
_____ 7. Doxycycline
_____ 8. Ciprofloxacin
_____ 9. Streptomycin
_____ 10. Demeclocycline
_____ 11. Daptomycin

Column II

a. Macrolides
b. Lincosamides
c. Ketolides
d. Lipopeptide
e. Tetracyclines
f. Glycylcyclines
g. Aminoglycosides
h. Fluoroquinolones

Crossword puzzle: Use the definitions to determine the correct terms.

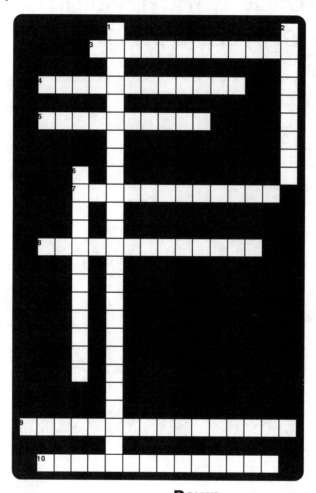

Across

3. First tetracycline
4. First macrolide
5. Works against drug-resistant *Staphylococcus aureus*
7. Given to those who have penicillin allergies
8. Single IM drug for treatment of gonorrhea
9. Azithromycin works through this action on bacteria (2 words)
10. Synthetic analogue of the tetracyclines

Down

1. Adverse reactions to vancomycin (2 words)
2. Antibiotics related to macrolides
6. Action of fluoroquinolones on bacteria

NCLEX Review Questions

Select the best response.

12. Which fluoroquinolone order should the nurse question?
    a. levofloxacin 500 mg IV q day
    b. ofloxacin 300 mg IV q day
    c. gatifloxacin 400 mg IV q day
    d. norfloxacin 400 mg PO b.i.d.

13. What is the usual dose of tetracycline?
    a. 250 to 500 mg q6h
    b. 250 to 500 mg q4h
    c. 500 mg to 1 g q4h
    d. 1 to 2 g q4h

14. Which laboratory test is influenced by tetracycline?

    a. blood urea nitrogen

    b. serum calcium level

    c. prothrombin time

    d. white blood cell count

15. The nurse is teaching a client how to take tetracycline. For best results, how should this medication be administered?

    a. with meals

    b. with extra fluids

    c. on an empty stomach

    d. one-half hour after meals

16. What should the nurse include in teaching for a client taking tetracycline for a respiratory tract infection? (Select all that apply.)

    a. Outdated tetracycline breaks down into toxic byproducts and must be discarded.

    b. Observe for superinfection.

    c. Avoid tetracycline during pregnancy.

    d. Anticipate urinary urgency.

17. The nurse assesses a client who is taking gentamicin (Garamycin). What assessment findings should be cause for concern? (Select all that apply.)

    a. nausea

    b. ototoxicity

    c. constipation

    d. photosensitivity

    e. thrombocytopenia

18. Which drugs and/or food if ordered for a client taking tetracycline should the nurse question? (Select all that apply.)

    a. iron

    b. antacids

    c. warfarin

    d. milk products

    e. beta blockers

19. Which specific nursing interventions should be implemented for a 34-year-old woman taking tetracycline? (Select all that apply.)

    a. restricting fluids

    b. storing the drug away from light

    c. monitoring laboratory test results

    d. obtaining a specimen for culture and sensitivity

    e. advising the client to use additional contraceptives when taking this drug

20. The client is taking gentamicin for a postsurgical infection, and the nurse needs to draw a trough level. The client takes the medication at 9:00 AM and at 9:00 PM. When is the correct time to draw a drug trough level?

    a. 10:00 AM

    b. 8:50 PM

    c. 1:00 PM

    d. 7:30 PM

21. The trough level that the nurse drew for a client taking gentamicin is 3.5 mcg/mL. What is the best action by the nurse?

    a. Administer the medication at the correct time.

    b. Hold the medication and contact the physician.

    c. Repeat the trough level after the next dose of medication.

    d. Give the client Benadryl to decrease the risk of a reaction.

22. A client tells the nurse that she has developed a vaginal discharge since she began taking gentamicin. What does the nurse suspect is occurring?

    a. The client has been exposed to other infectious agents since her admission to the hospital.

    b. The client is experiencing a reaction to the medication.

    c. The client is experiencing a superinfection.

    d. The client is experiencing a drug-to-drug interaction.

23. The nurse is doing a morning assessment on a 65-year-old client taking gentamicin, and the client states that her ears have been ringing all night. What should concern the nurse about this assessment finding?

    a. The noise in the hospital is causing hearing problems.

    b. The tinnitus is a negative side effect of gentamicin.

    c. The tinnitus is a mild side effect of gentamicin.

    d. The tinnitus is common in senior citizens.

24. The nurse is noting the intake and output on a 65-year-old client taking gentamicin and sees that the client's urine output has decreased to 500 mL/day. What is the best action by the nurse?

    a. Increase the client's oral intake.

    b. Increase the client's IV rate.

    c. Contact the physician.

    d. Document this in her chart.

25. What should the nurse routinely monitor for a 65-year-old client taking gentamicin? (Select all that apply.)

    a. heart rate and blood pressure

    b. urine output, noting clarity of urine

    c. oral and IV intake

    d. serum BUN and creatinine

Case Study

Select the best answer.

A.B., a 24-year-old woman, comes to the health care provider complaining of a productive cough, fever, and flu-like symptoms. Ciprofloxacin (Cipro) is prescribed.

1. Should the order for ciprofloxacin for A.B. concern the nurse?

    a. No, this drug is an appropriate medication for the client's illness.

    b. Yes, this drug does not work on respiratory infections.

    c. Yes, this drug should not be given to women of childbearing age.

    d. No, this drug will relieve the flu-like symptoms.

2. What specific nursing assessments are indicated for this client? (Select all that apply.)

    a. vital signs

    b. intake and output

    c. other medications taken by the client

    d. blood glucose levels

3. Which assessment findings should the nurse be concerned about when this drug is used?

    a. The client has a history of hypertension.

    b. The client has a history of a seizure disorder.

    c. The client's mother had breast cancer.

    d. The client's father has multiple allergies to medications.

4. What laboratory tests require monitoring?

    a. serum BUN and creatinine

    b. Hct and Hgb

    c. blood glucose levels

    d. platelet count

5. A.B. requires medication information. What information is a priority to include in the teaching? (Select all that apply.)

    a. Avoid caffeine.

    b. Use a sunblock.

    c. Don't take with antacids.

    d. Monitor for hearing changes.

31 Sulfonamides

Study Questions

Complete the following word search. Clues are given in questions 1-8. Circle your responses.

```
W J Q I O K D N F A B U L H N R Q
W D P E N I C I L L I N O K R H K
B L R Y E D R M C P S D D O V P A
L K C O V N V E E A U L G Y Q N M
M C R C C E R M V F C L J M E C T
P A A N Y Y I U A I F I U S Q X Y
V X B J D S S C D C L F L S K K E
E Q A R G I N C R E A S E O N W S
B Q A R E N O T L Q V U Z D F D L
Y N C I T A T S O I R E T C A B E
R T R I M E T H O P R I M C J C F
```

1. Sulfonamides inhibit bacterial synthesis of
   _____.

2. Clinical use of sulfonamides has decreased because of the availability and effectiveness of _____.

3. The new antibacterial drug that has a synergistic effect with sulfonamides is
   _____.

4. Sulfonamides (are/are not) effective against viruses and fungi. (Circle correct answer.)

5. Anaphylaxis (is/is not) common with the use of sulfonamides. (Circle correct answer.)

6. Sulfonamide drugs are metabolized in the _____ and excreted by the
   _____.

7. Sulfonamides are (bacteriostatic/bactericidal). (Circle correct answer.)

8. The use of warfarin with sulfonamides (increases/decreases) the anticoagulant effect. (Circle correct answer.)

Match the drug in Column I with its duration of action in Column II.

Column I

____ 9. Sulfisoxazole

____ 10. Sulfamethoxazole

____ 11. Sulfasalazine

____ 12. Sulfadiazine

____ 13. Sulfamethizole

Column II

a. Short-acting

b. Intermediate-acting

NCLEX Review Questions

Select the best response.

14. Which sulfonamide derivative may be used for the treatment of second- and third-degree burns?
    a.   sulfamethizole (Sulfasol)
    b.   sulfasalazine (Azulfidine)
    c.   sulfacetamide sodium (Isopto Cet-amide)
    d.   sulfadiazine (Silvadene)

15. Which drug may be used to treat seborrheic dermatitis?
    a.   sulfacetamide sodium (Isopto Cet-amide)
    b.   mafenide acetate (Sulfamylon)
    c.   sulfisoxazole (Gantrisin)
    d.   sulfadiazine (Microsulfon)

16. What is the usual adult dose of Septra?
    a.   160 mg TMP/800 mg SMZ q6h
    b.   160 mg TMP/800 mg SMZ q12h
    c.   40 mg TMP/60 mg SMZ q6h
    d.   40 mg TMP/60 mg SMZ q12h

17. The nurse is preparing to give a 45-year-old client admitted for treatment of a severe urinary tract infection Septra (trimethoprim/sulfamethoxazole) and digoxin. The nurse finds the following available:

    Septra tablets: each scored tablet contains 80 mg of trimethoprim and 400 mg of sulfamethoxazole.

    How many tablets should the client take for each dose and per 24 hours?
    a.   1 and 2
    b.   2 and 4
    c.   2 only
    d.   4 and 6

18. What interventions should the nurse implement in a 45-year-old client admitted for treatment of a severe urinary tract infection who is receiving Septra and digoxin? (Select all that apply.)
    a.   Administer medications and extra fluids.
    b.   Monitor urinary output.
    c.   Observe for allergic response.
    d.   Encourage the client to stop smoking.

19. What occurs with displacement of the sulfonamides from the protein-binding sites?
    a.   increased levels of free drug in the blood
    b.   decreased levels of free drug in the blood
    c.   no change in free drug levels in the blood
    d.   synergistic effect of the drug

20. Which possible side effects/adverse reactions of trimethoprim/sulfamethoxazole should the nurse advise the client about? (Select all that apply.)
    a.   anorexia
    b.   constipation
    c.   crystalluria
    d.   photosensitivity
    e.   decreased WBCs and platelets

21. Which statements are true regarding sulfonamides? (Select all that apply.)
    a.   They are considered safe in newborns.
    b.   They increase anticoagulant effect of warfarin.
    c.   Stevens-Johnson syndrome is an adverse reaction.
    d.   They may lead to decreased serum creatinine levels.
    e.   They increase hypoglycemic effect with sulfonylureas.

Case Study

Select the best answer.

Y.M., a 24-year-old man, presents to the emergency department with complaints of "pain when I go to the bathroom." Gantrisin is prescribed.

1. What nursing interventions should be implemented when giving Y.M. this medication? (Select all that apply.)
    a. The medication should be taken with a full glass of water.
    b. The nurse should use two methods of identification before giving the medication.
    c. The nurse should monitor the client's fluid intake and output.
    d. The nurse should monitor for a superinfection.

2. Y.M. does not drink very much and wants to know why he has to drink a full glass of water when taking this medication. What is the nurse's best response?
    a. "You need this much water to make sure the pills end up in your stomach."
    b. "You need this much to make sure that you have a normal output."
    c. "Drinking that much water helps to decrease the incidence of crystalluria."
    d. "Drinking that much water helps to decrease the incidence of constipation."

3. What information should Y.M. receive related to the prescribed medication? (Select all that apply.)
    a. "Make sure you take the medication with water and drink several full glasses of water throughout the day."
    b. "Observe for a sore throat and purpura, which may indicate a potential reaction to the medication."
    c. "Observe for mouth ulcers, a furry black tongue, and anal or genital discharge."
    d. "Observe for increased number of hard stools per day."

32 Antituberculars, Antifungals, Peptides, and Metronidazole

Study Questions

Crossword puzzle: Use the definitions to determine the correct terms.

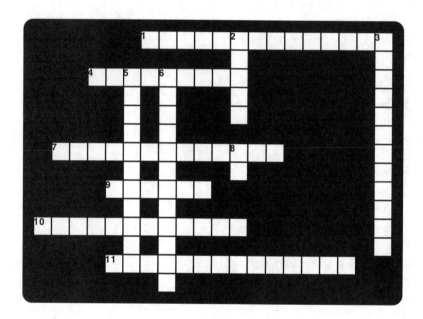

Across

1. Type of drugs that are more effective and less toxic than other drugs (3 words)
4. Drug of choice to prevent disseminated *Mycobacterium avium* complex
7. Drug of choice for severe systemic fungal infections (2 words)
9. One body area where fungi are normal flora
10. Polymyxins are effective on this type of bacteria (2 words)
11. Liver toxicity

Down

2. Target area for systemic fungal infections
3. First drug prescribed for tuberculosis
5. Common oral antifungal
6. Action of polymyxins
8. Preferred route for administration of polymyxins

Match the drug in Column I with its type in Column II.

Column I	Column II
____ 12. Ethambutol	a. First-line drug
____ 13. Pyrazinamide	b. Second-line drug
____ 14. Capreomycin	
____ 15. Isoniazid	
____ 16. Streptomycin	
____ 17. Aminosalicylate	
____ 18. Ethionamide	
____ 19. Amikacin	
____ 20. Rifapentine	

NCLEX Review Questions

Select the best response.

21. Which outcome is a serious adverse effect of isoniazid?

   a.   ototoxicity

   b.   crystalluria

   c.   palpitations

   d.   hepatotoxicity

22. Which person should not receive prophylactic treatment for tuberculosis?

   a.   46-year-old with alcoholism

   b.   65-year-old with parkinsonism

   c.   57-year-old concurrently taking warfarin

   d.   29-year-old concurrently taking theophylline

23. Your patient has just started taking rifapentine (Priftin). How often should this medication be given?

   a.   twice a week

   b.   three times a week

   c.   five times a week

   d.   daily

24. Your patient is taking capreomycin (Capastat). Which vitamin should be given to this patient to avoid peripheral neuropathy?

   a.   vitamin D

   b.   vitamin B$_6$

   c.   vitamin E

   d.   vitamin K

25. Which herbal supplement when taken with ketoconazole may cause hepatotoxicity?

   a.   St. John's wort

   b.   ginkgo biloba

   c.   echinacea

   d.   kava kava

26. During the admission interview, which information should the nurse seek to obtain from a 69-year-old client taking isoniazid (INH)? (Select all that apply.)

   a.   history of TB

   b.   last PPD, chest x-ray, and results

   c.   drug allergies

   d.   blood glucose level

27. What is usual dose of INH for active treatment of TB?

   a.   1-4 mg/kg/day, max 300 mg daily

   b.   5-10 mg/kg/day, max 300 mg daily

   c.   11-15 mg/kg/day, max 300 mg daily

   d.   16-20 mg/kg/day, max 300 mg daily

28. When a client is taking INH, frequent monitoring of which lab result should be a nursing priority?

   a.   liver enzymes

   b.   WBCs

   c.   creatinine

   d.   BUN

29. Which drugs/foods should a client taking INH be taught to avoid?

    a. laxatives

    b. cheese

    c. antacids

    d. digoxin

30. What is priority health teaching for a client taking INH? (Select all that apply.)

    a. Possible need to take vitamin B$_6$ to avoid peripheral neuritis.

    b. Need to increase fluid intake and avoid alcohol.

    c. That urine and saliva may be red-orange.

    d. That weight should be monitored daily.

31. How should rifapentine be taken to decrease the incidence of resistance?

    a. It should be taken daily.

    b. It should be taken once a week.

    c. It should be taken with another antitubercular drug.

    d. It should be taken only with a productive cough.

32. A client is receiving amphotericin B for histoplasmosis. What is the routine method of administration?

    a. rectally

    b. topically

    c. intramuscularly

    d. intravenously

33. What is the usual dose of amphotericin B?

    a. 0.25-1 mg/kg/day

    b. 1-2 mg/kg/day

    c. 2-3 mg/kg/day

    d. 3-4 mg/kg/day

34. A client is receiving amphotericin B for histoplasmosis. What is a priority frequent monitoring that should be done by the nurse?

    a. WBCs

    b. BUN

    c. platelets

    d. eosinophils

35. What is priority information that should be part of the health teaching plan for a client receiving amphotericin B for histoplasmosis? (Select all that apply.)

    a. Avoid operating hazardous equipment.

    b. Report weakness.

    c. Obtain lab testing as ordered.

    d. Consume no alcohol.

36. Metronidazole is primarily used for treatment of disorders caused by organisms in which area of the body?

    a. respiratory tract

    b. urinary tract

    c. GI tract

    d. peripheral nervous system

37. In combination with other agents, metronidazole is commonly used to treat *Helicobacter pylori* associated with which alteration?

    a. peptic ulcers

    b. urinary retention

    c. adenomas

    d. gastroesophageal reflux disease (GERD)

38. Which alteration in a client taking metronidazole should be an area of concern to the nurse? (Select all that apply.)

    a. toothache

    b. photophobia

    c. abdominal cramps and diarrhea

    d. headache and depression

39. Available:

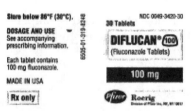 

The client's prescription is for a maintenance dose of fluconazole (Diflucan), 150 mg/day. How many tablets should the client take per dose?

    a. 1 tablet

    b. 1.5 tablets

    c. 2 tablets

    d. 2.5 tablets

40. Which laboratory value(s) or vital sign(s) must be frequently monitored for the client taking fluconazole? (Select all that apply.)
    a. AST
    b. ALT
    c. BUN
    d. pulse
    e. blood pressure

41. Which side effects might the nurse observe in a client taking peptides? (Select all that apply.)
    a. dizziness
    b. hypertension
    c. neurotoxicity
    d. nephrotoxicity
    e. tingling/numbness of the extremities

42. What change should the nurse be alert for in a client taking amphotericin B? (Select all that apply.)
    a. flushing
    b. hypotension
    c. hypertension
    d. hypokalemia
    e. thrombophlebitis

Case Study

Select the best answer.

C.J., 22 years old, has presented to the clinic complaining of "white spots in my mouth." She has been taking multiple antibiotics during the past month for a severe lower respiratory tract infection. Mycostatin is ordered, 250,000 units oral swish and swallow, q.i.d.

Available:

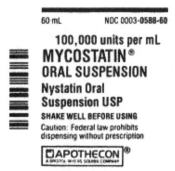

1. What questions should the nurse ask C.J.? (Select all that apply.)
    a. Do you have a vaginal discharge?
    b. Do you have anal itching?
    c. Did you take your antibiotics today?
    d. Have you treated these with any OTC medication?

2. What is the most likely cause of these "white spots"?
    a. a virus
    b. superinfection
    c. cross-contamination
    d. side effects of her medications

3. What is the most likely causative organism?
    a. gram-positive bacteria
    b. aspergillosis
    c. candida
    d. mucomycosis

4. What are specific instructions related to the correct administration of this drug? (Select all that apply.)
    a. C.J. should swish the medication around her mouth.
    b. C.J. should spit out the medication after swishing it around her mouth.
    c. C.J. should swallow the medication after swishing it around her mouth.
    d. C.J. should rinse out her mouth thoroughly after swishing the medication around in her mouth.

5. What is priority information that C.J. should know when taking this medication? (Select all that apply.)
    a. Adherence to the drug regimen is important for its effectiveness.
    b. She should be sure to follow up with lab tests.
    c. She should avoid drinking alcohol when taking this medication.
    d. She should be sure to monitor for constipation.

33 Antivirals, Antimalarials, and Anthelmintics

Study Questions

Complete the following word search. Clues are given in questions 1-6. Circle your responses.

```
E D I R O L H C O R D Y H U V O J
C Y T O M E G A L O V I R U S Z W
R T M C H E N I D A T N A M I R R
V A R I C E L L A F R E L K N C M
I G I X E L P M I S S E P R E H S
S K L S O H D A G C A X N X G U D
Z O G R N R X D T V R E T A G G D
U J R E W O L S A I S R P Q L D T
T B H R U X T O X I C I T Y R A R
X R E P L I C A T I O N T I T M O
B W H E R P E S Z O S T E R M O F
```

1. Antiviral drugs prevent _____ of the virus.

2. AZT (is / is not) the only FDA-approved antiviral drug for treating persons with AIDS. (Circle correct answer.)

3. Antiviral drug development has been (slower / faster) than antibacterial drug development in part because of _____ of some antivirals. (Circle correct answer.)

4. A new drug to treat influenza A is _____. When a client is taking this drug, two organ functions that require monitoring are _____ and _____.

5. The drug vidarabine, introduced as an antineoplastic for the treatment of leukemia, is now known to have effects against which four organisms? _____, _____, _____, and _____.

6. Amantadine hydrochloride (Symmetrel) and rimantadine hydrochloride (Flumadine) were used to treat _____ influenza.

164 Copyright © 2012, 2009, 2006, 2003, 2000, 1997, 1993 by Saunders, an imprint of Elsevier Inc. All rights reserved.

Match the term in Column I with the appropriate definition in Column II.

Column I	Column II
____ 7. Tissue phase	a. Prevention
____ 8. Erythrocyte phase	b. Worm infestation
____ 9. Prophylaxis	c. Invasion of the body
____ 10. Helminthiasis	d. Infections in an immunocompromised client
____ 11. Opportunistic infection	e. Invasion of the blood cells

NCLEX Review Questions

Select the best response.

12. What is a serious adverse effect of ganciclovir (Cytovene), which is used for treatment of cytomegalovirus?
    a. ototoxicity
    b. granulocytosis
    c. thrombocytopenia
    d. electrocardiogram changes

13. Which is the most common site for helminthiasis?
    a. liver
    b. blood
    c. intestines
    d. urinary tract

14. A 17-year-old client is receiving treatment for herpes simplex 1. Acyclovir sodium 200 mg q2h is prescribed.

Available:

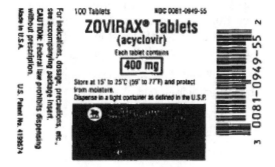

How many tablets should the client take at each dose?
    a. ½ tablet
    b. 1 tablet
    c. 1½ tablets
    d. 2 tablets

15. Acyclovir is effective against the herpes virus. What was it first introduced as?
    a. an antiviral
    b. an antineoplastic
    c. an antimalarial
    d. an antidepressant

16. The nurse is preparing to give a client acyclovir. Which medication seen on the MAR should concern the nurse?
    a. primaquine
    b. amantadine
    c. probenecid
    d. flucytosine

17. Which drugs are effective in combating herpes simplex viruses (HSV-1, HSV-2)? (Select all that apply.)
    a. famciclovir (Famvir)
    b. ganciclovir sodium
    c. valacyclovir (Valtrex)
    d. penciclovir (Denavir)

18. The client is taking ganciclovir. What baseline values should be obtained before administering this drug? (Select all that apply.)
    a. vital signs
    b. blood glucose levels
    c. serum creatinine and BUN
    d. bilirubin

19. What is the causative factor of malaria?

   a.   a fungus

   b.   a virus

   c.   bacteria

   d.   protozoa

20. The client has chloroquine-resistant malaria. What is the drug of choice for this type of malaria?

   a.   a combination of antimalarials

   b.   quinidine

   c.   Aralen

   d.   primaquine

21. Which lab values are affected by chloroquine usage? (Select all that apply.)

   a.   BUN

   b.   RBCs

   c.   hemoglobin

   d.   hematocrit

22. The client taking is taking chloroquine. What changes may occur as a result of taking this drug? (Select all that apply.)

   a.   blurred vision

   b.   headaches

   c.   pruritus

   d.   nausea and vomiting

23. Which nursing interventions should be part of care provided to a client undergoing antimalarial drug therapy?

   a.   monitoring urinary output and liver function

   b.   assessing hearing; drugs may be ototoxic

   c.   assessing for visual changes; chloroquine may cause retinopathy

   d.   monitoring blood glucose levels

24. What is the recommended schedule for taking chloroquine in preparation for a visit to a country infested with malaria?

   a.   during the visit

   b.   during the visit and after the visit

   c.   before the visit and during the visit

   d.   before, during, and after the visit

25. Which assessment information is a priority for individuals undergoing treatment with anthelmintics? (Select all that apply.)

   a.   history of food intake

   b.   collection of stool specimen

   c.   determining if other household members have the same signs and symptoms

   d.   frequency of infestation

26. Which drug is commonly used in the treatment of giant roundworms and pinworms?

   a.   bithionol (Actamer)

   b.   pyrantel pamoate (Antiminth)

   c.   mebendazole (Vermox)

   d.   oxamniquine (Vansil)

27. Long-term therapy with anthelmintics is required with which drugs? (Select all that apply.)

   a.   niclosamide

   b.   mebendazole

   c.   piperazine

   d.   thiabendazole

28. What is priority information that should be included in client teaching for anthelmintics? (Select all that apply.)

   a.   the importance of washing hands after toileting and before eating

   b.   the importance of showering rather than bathing

   c.   the importance of changing towels, underwear, and bedclothes daily

   d.   the fact that migraine headaches may occur with this type of drug

29. When teaching the client taking acyclovir (Zovirax) about the side effects/adverse reactions that are associated with this drug, what is priority information for the nurse to include? (Select all that apply.)

   a.   nausea

   b.   headache

   c.   lethargy

   d.   decreased BUN

   e.   increased AST

30. Chloroquine (Aralen) increases the effects of which drugs? (Select all that apply.)

    a. digoxin

    b. antacids

    c. anticoagulants

    d. anticonvulsants

    e. neuromuscular blockers

31. Which neurologic problems are associated with the use of anthelmintics? (Select all that apply.)

    a. dizziness

    b. headache

    c. weakness

    d. drowsiness

    e. urinary retention

Case Study

Select the best answer.

K.B., age 35 years, is being treated for HSV-1 with acyclovir (Zovirax). He is taking 550 mg t.i.d.

1. What should concern the nurse about this level of dosage?

    a. Nothing; it is within the regularly prescribed range.

    b. It is too low and should be changed.

    c. It is higher than the normal amount/dosage prescribed.

    d. It is at a toxic level.

2. What baseline assessment information should the nurse obtain before starting this medication? (Select all that apply.)

    a. history of renal or hepatic disease

    b. vital signs

    c. complete blood count

    d. regularity of bowel movements

3. Which laboratory value should concern the nurse when caring for K.B.? (Select all that apply.)

    a. decreased white blood cells

    b. low platelet count

    c. high Hgb and Hct

    d. high blood glucose level

4. What adverse reactions should the nurse teach K.B. to report to the health care provider? (Select all that apply.)

    a. decreased urine output

    b. dizziness and/or confusion

    c. constipation

    d. urticaria

5. What priority instructions should the nurse provide to K.B. concerning oral care?

    a. The client should brush his teeth twice a day.

    b. The client should brush his teeth several times during the day.

    c. The client should use glycerin swabs to maintain adequate oral moisture.

    d. The client should rinse his mouth out after eating rather than brush his teeth.

34 Drugs for Urinary Tract Disorders

Study Questions

Crossword puzzle: Use the definitions to determine the correct terms.

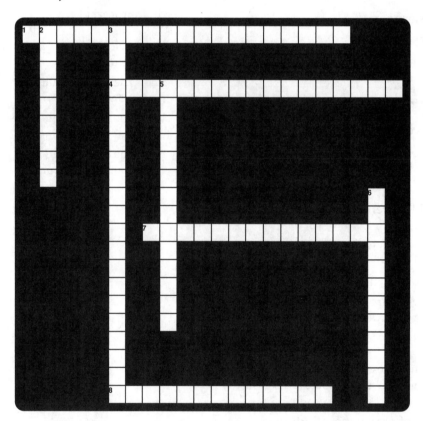

Across
1. Upper UTI (2 words)
4. Agents that increase muscle tone of urinary muscles (2 words)
7. Drugs that inhibit the growth of bacteria
8. Lower UTI (2 words)

Down
2. Juice that decreases urine pH
3. Resistant to nitrofurantoin (2 words)
5. Stains teeth
6. Drug that kills bacteria

NCLEX Review Questions

Select the best response.

9. What may occur when methenamine is given with sulfonamides?
   a. bleeding
   b. crystalluria
   c. chest pain
   d. intestinal distention

10. Which substances can be taken to decrease urine pH? (Select all that apply.)
    a. ammonium chloride
    b. cranberry juice
    c. potassium chloride
    d. ascorbic acid

11. Which is the correct dosage for long-term use of nalidixic acid?
    a. 1 g daily
    b. 1 g b.i.d.
    c. 1 g t.i.d.
    d. 1 g q.i.d.

12. The nurse is planning health teaching for a 53-year-old client receiving nalidixic acid for a chronic urinary tract infection. What priority information should be included? (Select all that apply.)
    a. Urine may turn orange.
    b. Protection against photosensitivity is necessary when taking this medication.
    c. Increase fluid intake.
    d. Avoid operating hazardous machinery.

13. Which are urinary antiseptic drug-drug interactions? (Select all that apply.)
    a. Nalidixic acid increases effects of warfarin.
    b. Antacids increase nitrofurantoin absorption.
    c. Antiseptics cause false-positive Clinitest results.
    d. Sodium bicarbonate inhibits action of methenamine.

14. Clients taking nitrofurantoin should report which alterations to the health care provider?
    a. chest pain
    b. fever
    c. cough
    d. leg pain

15. Which alteration is an adverse effect from nitrofurantoin?
    a. superinfection
    b. peripheral neuropathy
    c. anorexia
    d. drowsiness

16. For which alterations should the nurse expect to see urinary analgesics prescribed? (Select all that apply.)
    a. burning sensation
    b. frequency
    c. urgency
    d. retention

17. Which drug is a commonly prescribed urinary analgesic?
    a. phenazopyridine hydrochloride (Pyridium)
    b. trimethoprim (Trimpex)
    c. flavoxate (Urispas)
    d. bethanechol (Urecholine)

18. What are priority nursing interventions when administering urinary analgesics? (Select all that apply.)
    a. administering the drug with food or with milk
    b. instructing that chewable tablets must be chewed, never swallowed whole
    c. observing the client for any side effects
    d. monitoring the client's blood pressure

19. Which drug is commonly used to treat urinary tract spasms?
    a. trimethoprim (Trimpex)
    b. phenazopyridine hydrochloride (Pyridium)
    c. flavoxate (Urispas)
    d. bethanechol (Urecholine)

20. The client has overactive bladder. If she also has narrow-angle glaucoma, which drug should not be prescribed?

    a. tolterodine tartrate (Detrol)

    b. bethanechol chloride (Urecholine)

    c. flavoxate hydrochloride (Urispas)

    d. phenazopyridine hydrochloride (Pyridium)

21. Which drugs are considered to be urinary antiseptics? (Select all that apply.)

    a. aztreonam

    b. phenothiazide

    c. methenamine

    d. quinolones

    e. nitrofurantoin

22. What priority assessment information should the nurse obtain if the client is taking a fluoroquinolone? (Select all that apply.)

    a. headache and rash

    b. syncope and visual disturbance

    c. chest pain and fever

    d. peripheral neuritis

    e. photosensitivity

23. Clients taking bethanechol should report which alteration(s) to the health care provider? (Select all that apply.)

    a. abdominal discomfort

    b. headache

    c. increased salivation

    d. urgency

    e. abdominal cramps

Case Study

Select the best answer.

J.B., 11 years old, is taking a urinary antispasmodic for treatment of an injury to his urinary tract that is causing spasms of the smooth muscle. Ditropan 5 mg, t.i.d., has been prescribed.

1. What is the drug classification of Ditropan?

    a. antimuscarinic

    b. anticholinergic

    c. urinary antispasmodic

    d. urinary analgesic

2. What priority nursing interventions should be implemented when caring for J.B.? (Select all that apply.)

    a. Monitor urine output.

    b. Use two methods of identification before administering the medication.

    c. Encourage the client to decrease his fluid intake.

    d. Limit J.B.'s activity.

3. What side effects should be mentioned in J.B.'s health teaching? (Select all that apply.)

    a. drowsiness

    b. headache

    c. dry mouth

    d. blurred vision

4. For individuals with which conditions should Ditropan be avoided? (Select all that apply.)

    a. glaucoma

    b. GI obstruction

    c. urinary tract obstruction

    d. renal failure

35 HIV- and AIDS-Related Drugs

Study Questions

Crossword puzzle: Use the definitions to determine the correct terms.

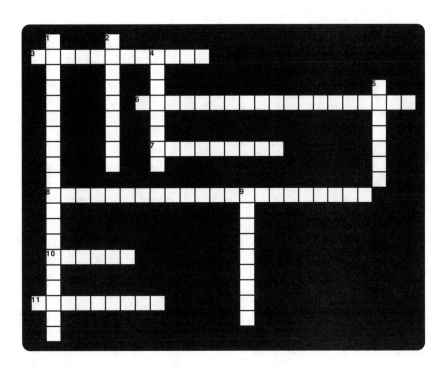

Across

3. Immunity that involves many leukocyte actions, reactions (2 words)
6. Inhibit synthesis of HIV by blocking growth of its DNA strand (2 words)
7. The first-choice drug within the NNRTI class
8. Bind to the center of reverse transcriptase and directly inhibit its production (2 words)
10. Genetically determined immunity
11. A test to measure the status of a person's immune system (2 words)

Down

1. Phase 2 of the HIV replication cycle (2 words)
2. The only nucleotide analogue
4. Immunity that every person's body makes or receives
5. Phase 6 of HIV replication cycle
9. Ability to carry out the therapeutic plan

Match the descriptors in Column I with the class of agents in Column II.

Column I

____ 12.   Block protease

____ 13.   Act by inhibiting HIV reverse transcriptase

____ 14.   Suppress virions in infected cell populations

____ 15.   Infection of new cells

Column II

a.   Nucleoside analogues

b.   Nonnucleoside analogues

c.   Protease inhibitors

NCLEX Review Questions

Select the best response.

16.   What finding is a leading AIDS indicator?
   a.   *Pneumocystis carinii* pneumonia
   b.   CD4 counts of less than 200 cells/mm^3
   c.   Kaposi's sarcoma
   d.   *Mycobacterium avium* complex

17.   What are the potential benefits of early initiation of antiretroviral therapy in the asymptomatic HIV-infected client? (Select all that apply.)
   a.   control of viral replication
   b.   decreased risk of drug toxicity
   c.   earlier development of drug resistance
   d.   prevention of progressive immunodeficiency

18.   What are potential risks of early initiation of antiretroviral therapy in clients with asymptomatic HIV infection? (Select all that apply.)
   a.   unknown long-term toxicity
   b.   reduction in quality of life from adverse effects
   c.   earlier development of drug resistance
   d.   decreased risk of selection of resistant virus

19.   What is the goal of combination antiretroviral therapy?
   a.   increase the CD4 count, decrease the viral load, and have the client clinically well
   b.   decrease the viral load and decrease the CD4 count
   c.   replace the memory cells within the immune system
   d.   decrease the CD4 count and increase the viral load

20.   The decision to treat asymptomatic individuals with detectable HIV RNA in plasma should include which information?
   a.   client's age and support
   b.   amount of time since diagnosis
   c.   client's willingness to accept therapy
   d.   probability of adherence to therapy

21.   What is the goal of combination therapy (HAART)?
   a.   It targets enzymes in the HIV lifecycle.
   b.   It offers a cure to AIDS-defined clients.
   c.   It offers a cure to pediatric patients.
   d.   It provides prophylaxis/treatment of major secondary infections.

22.   When did zidovudine receive FDA approval?
   a.   1987
   b.   1991
   c.   1994
   d.   1996

23. How frequently is zidovudine generally scheduled to be taken?
    a. daily
    b. q12h
    c. q4-6h
    d. q1-3h

24. Which is the usual adult dose of zidovudine?
    a. 300 mg b.i.d.
    b. 200 mg q12h
    c. 300 mg daily
    d. 1.5 mg/kg q3h

25. During the time that a client is taking zidovudine, frequent monitoring of which laboratory value is required? (Select all that apply.)
    a. CBC
    b. renal function
    c. hepatic function
    d. urine sedimentation rate

26. The nurse is assessing a client taking zidovudine. What should the nurse expect to see if the client is experiencing side effects? (Select all that apply.)
    a. numbness and pain in lower extremities
    b. headache
    c. seizures
    d. difficulty swallowing

27. In what year did efavirenz receive FDA approval?
    a. 2000
    b. 1998
    c. 1996
    d. 1994

28. Efavirenz is generally initially scheduled to be taken at which intervals?
    a. 14-day lead-in, one 600 mg tablet daily, then one 600 mg tablet twice a day in combination with other antiretroviral agents
    b. 600 mg q12h
    c. 600 mg q8h
    d. 600 mg q24h

29. During the time that a client is taking efavirenz, periodic monitoring of which laboratory values is required?
    a. CBC and platelets
    b. hepatic function
    c. renal function
    d. AST levels

30. What should the nurse assess in a client taking efavirenz if he appears to be experiencing side effects? (Select all that apply.)
    a. CNS effects
    b. diarrhea
    c. difficulty swallowing
    d. rash

31. A client is being discharged on efavirenz. What priority teaching information should be given to this client? (Select all that apply.)
    a. "Don't take St. John's wort with this drug as it will decrease its effectiveness."
    b. "Avoid alcohol while taking this drug."
    c. "This drug can cause convulsions and possibly liver failure."
    d. "Be sure to drink 2500 mL of fluid a day."

32. During which year did lopinavir receive FDA approval?
    a. 1998
    b. 1999
    c. 2000
    d. 2001

33. At what intervals is lopinavir generally scheduled to be taken?
    a. daily
    b. twice a day
    c. three times a day
    d. four times a day

34. What is the usual adult dose of lopinavir?
    a. 600 mg twice a day
    b. 800 mg/day in 2 divided doses
    c. 1200 mg/day
    d. 400 mg q8h

35. What laboratory values are priorities for the nurse to monitor in a patient taking lopinavir? (Select all that apply.)

    a. liver function

    b. triglycerides

    c. cholesterol

    d. blood glucose

36. The client is being discharged on lopinavir. What priority teaching information should this client receive? (Select all that apply.)

    a. "You cannot take St. John's wort while taking this drug."

    b. "You should take this medication with food."

    c. "You will need to learn to measure your blood glucose level."

    d. "You may experience an allergic reaction and should contact your health care provider if this occurs."

37. What is the first choice of drugs for prophylaxis for PCP?

    a. dapsone 50 mg PO b.i.d.

    b. atovaquone 750 mg PO b.i.d.

    c. Bactrim DS 1 tablet PO daily

    d. aerosolized pentamidine by mouth

38. In the pregnant client, zidovudine monotherapy is begun at how many weeks of gestation?

    a. 6

    b. 10

    c. 12

    d. 14

39. What is the dose of prophylactic zidovudine for the pregnant client?

    a. 100 mg five times a day

    b. 300 mg two times a day

    c. 200 mg three times a day

    d. 200 mg five times a day

40. What side effects would the nurse expect to see in a client taking lopinavir? (Select all that apply.)

    a. vomiting

    b. urinary retention

    c. diarrhea

    d. nausea

41. Which nursing interventions may help to increase adherence to the therapeutic regimen? (Select all that apply.)

    a. pill organizers

    b. pill counting

    c. timers/beepers

    d. scheduled pill holidays

Case Study

Select the best answer.

The nurse is caring for T.L., who has recently been diagnosed with AIDS. He is on a HAART regimen. T.L. is concerned about taking so many medications and about his ability to pay for his medications. He also has been asking questions about the drugs' side effects.

1. T.L. has been concerned about taking so many medications. What is the nurse's best response?

    a. "This is the best combination of drugs you can receive."

    b. "This combination of drugs will decrease your viral load without affecting the CD4 cells."

    c. "This combination of drugs will decrease the RNA HIV levels load and increase your CD4 cells."

    d. "This combination of drugs does not lead to drug resistance."

2. The nurse is teaching T.L. about his medications. T.L. complains that he has experienced a lot of nausea and diarrhea since starting the medications. What is the nurse's best response?

    a. "This lasts for quite a while; you will need to drink lots of fluid so you don't get dehydrated."

    b. "This will only last for a few weeks at the beginning of therapy."

    c. "You will need to take medications to decrease the nausea and diarrhea while you take this medication."

    d. "You will get used to the nausea so you won't notice it as much in a few weeks."

3. One of T.L.'s drugs is ritonavir. What is priority teaching information related to this drug? (Select all that apply.)

    a. This medication may cause cardiovascular problems, so T.L. may have to make some lifestyle changes.

    b. The GI effects can be irritating. If they get intolerable, T.L. should contact his health care provider rather than stopping the drugs.

    c. This medication has lots of drug-to-drug interactions. T.L. must check with his health care provider before taking any new medications.

    d. Adherence to the drug therapy regimen is important in decreasing the viral load and maintaining health status.

4. What are the nursing interventions that the nurse should perform for T.L.? (Select all that apply.)

    a. Monitor lab values.

    b. Monitor nutritional status.

    c. Provide emotional support.

    d. Monitor fluid intake.

36 Vaccines

Study Questions

Crossword puzzle: Use the definitions to determine the correct terms.

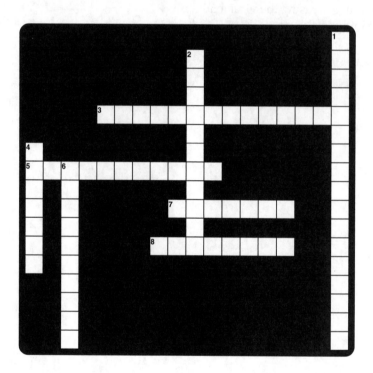

Across
3. Acquisition of detectable levels of antibodies in the bloodstream
5. A potentially life-threatening reaction
7. Transient immunity
8. Bacterium or virus that invades the body

Down
1. Weakened microorganisms (2 words)
2. Vaccines that involve the insertion of some of the genetic material
4. A small amount of antigen that stimulates an immune response
6. Also called immunoglobulins

NCLEX Review Questions

Select the best response.

9. What are vaccines made from the inactivated disease-causing substances produced by some microorganisms?

    a. toxoids

    b. recombinant subunit vaccines

    c. conjugate vaccines

    d. attenuated vaccines

10. In which situations is acquired passive immunity important? (Select all that apply.)

    a. when time does not permit active vaccination alone

    b. when the exposed individual is at high risk for complications of the disease

    c. in newborns

    d. when a person suffers from an immune system deficiency that renders that person unable to produce an effective immune response

11. What is the process in which antibodies are received by an individual, used for protection against a particular pathogen, and acquired from another source?

    a. active immunity

    b. most childhood immunizations

    c. toxoids

    d. passive immunity

12. What occurs when there is an acquisition of detectable levels of antibodies in the bloodstream?

    a. passive immunity

    b. acquired natural immunity

    c. immunization

    d. seroconversion

13. What do most vaccines do in the body?

    a. Stimulate an immune response.

    b. Cause an allergic reaction.

    c. Are perceived by the body as antibodies.

    d. Produce mild disease.

14. What is the type of immunity that usually persists for the remainder of the individual's life?

    a. humoral

    b. passive natural

    c. active natural

    d. passive acquired

15. When is a child's first vaccine usually administered?

    a. at age 6 months

    b. at age 2 months

    c. at birth

    d. at age 4 months

16. What is rubella also known as?

    a. smallpox

    b. German measles

    c. hard measles

    d. rubeola

17. Susceptible individuals age 13 years or older receive two doses of varicella vaccine spaced how long apart?

    a. at least 4 weeks

    b. 3 months

    c. 6 months

    d. 1 month

18. In the event of an adverse reaction to a vaccine, to whom should a health care provider report the details?

    a. to his or her immediate supervisor

    b. to the Vaccine Adverse Events Reporting System

    c. to the vaccine manufacturer

    d. to the Centers for Disease Control and Prevention (CDC)

19. Which vaccines are administered to adults age 65 years and older?

    a. Td, pneumococcal (PPV), influenza, zoster

    b. human papillomavirus (HPV), Td, influenza, pneumococcal (PPV)

    c. rotavirus, Td, influenza

    d. Tdap, pneumococcal (PPV), influenza, zoster

20. Which type of immunity is conferred by the tetanus-diphtheria (Td) vaccine?
    a. active
    b. passive
    c. natural
    d. inactive

21. Which immunizations are examples of live, attenuated vaccines?
    a. measles-mumps-rubella (MMR) and *Haemophilus influenzae* type B (Hib)
    b. varicella and Td
    c. MMR and varicella
    d. influenza and hepatitis B

22. What are the clinical manifestations of influenza?
    a. vomiting and diarrhea
    b. abdominal pain and cough
    c. fever and diarrhea
    d. fever, myalgias, and cough

23. A physically and medically neglected 15-month-old child has recently been placed in foster care. The foster parents present with this child today for immunization update. They have no idea what, if any, vaccines the child has previously received. What immunizations would the nurse would most likely administer?
    a. no vaccines because it is assumed the child is up-to-date
    b. DTaP #4, Hib #4, and MMR #1
    c. DTaP, Hib, hepatitis A, hepatitis B, MMR, IPV, pneumococcal (PCV), and varicella
    d. DTaP, Hib, hepatitis B, and MMR; have the child return in 2 weeks for hepatitis A, IPV, pneumococcal (PCV), and varicella

24. When MMR vaccine is not given the same day as varicella vaccine, what should be the minimum interval between administrations?
    a. 7 days
    b. 14 days
    c. 21 days
    d. 28 days

25. The client is 4 months old and was seen in the emergency department of the local hospital 3 days ago and was diagnosed with a cold and an ear infection. She is taking amoxicillin, an antibiotic, as prescribed for the ear infection and has generally improved. Her immunization record shows that she received hepatitis B vaccine on day 2 of life. At age 2 months, she received hepatitis B, DTaP, Hib, pneumococcal (PCV), rotavirus, and IPV vaccines. If the nurse elected to immunize the client today, what vaccines should be administered?
    a. pneumococcal and influenza
    b. hepatitis B, DTaP, Hib, rotavirus, and IPV
    c. DTaP, Hib, and influenza
    d. DTaP, Hib, pneumococcal (PCV), rotavirus, and IPV

26. A 4-month-old client's parent reports that after her first dose of DTaP, the client experienced some redness and tenderness at the injection site in her left thigh. With this in mind, what should the nurse administer?
    a. DTaP again, because these are common side effects, not contraindications
    b. DT in the right thigh
    c. DTaP subcutaneously instead of intramuscularly to prevent muscle soreness
    d. Half the usual dose of DTaP to reduce the likelihood of a reaction

27. After the nurse administers immunizations to a 4-month-old client, the nurse speaks to the client's parent about future immunizations. When should the nurse recommend the client return?
    a. in 2 weeks after she has recovered from her cold and ear infection
    b. at 9 months of age
    c. at 6 months of age
    d. at 12 months of age

28. Before they leave the clinic today, what information should the nurse provide to the parent of a 4-month-old client who just received her immunizations?

    a. Vaccine Information Statements (VIS) for all vaccines administered

    b. an immunization record

    c. a report of adverse reaction form

    d. an appointment card for the next immunization clinic visit

29. What is a good source of health and immunization information for nurses assisting clients before international travel?

    a. the U.S. embassy in the destination country

    b. the Centers for Disease Control and Prevention

    c. the client's travel agent

    d. no source is necessary because there are no special immunization needs for travelers

30. In the case of an anaphylactic reaction to a vaccine, which drug should the nurse have readily available?

    a. epinephrine

    b. acetaminophen

    c. pseudoephedrine

    d. diphenhydramine

31. What information is required by federal law to be provided to any client who will receive any vaccine?

    a. an immunization record

    b. no more than four immunizations on any given day

    c. Vaccine Information Statements

    d. no more than two immunizations at any given visit

32. Which three viruses are combined in the MMR vaccine? (Select all that apply.)

    a. rubella

    b. roseola

    c. measles

    d. mumps

Case Study

Select the best answer.

R.Q., a 70-year-old man, presents to the clinic in late October after having stepped on a nail. He has suffered a puncture wound to the sole of his right foot. He wonders whether he needs a "lockjaw" shot. He says he has not had any shots since he was in the army for a 4-year stint "straight out of high school." He is taking atenolol for hypertension but otherwise does not "go to the doctor much." He has no known medication allergies.

1. What is another name for "lockjaw"?
   a. Bell's palsy
   b. measles
   c. tetanus
   d. rabies

2. What clinical manifestations should the nurse expect to see in someone who has tetanus? (Select all that apply.)
   a. headache
   b. irritability
   c. muscle spasms
   d. blurred vision

3. What vaccine would routinely be administered in this circumstance?
   a. Td
   b. MMR
   c. rabies vaccine
   d. PPV

4. What is the route of administration for the above vaccine?
   a. subcutaneous
   b. intravenous
   c. intramuscular
   d. intradermal

5. Given R.Q.'s age and the time of year, what other vaccine(s) might he also be eligible for?
   a. PPV and zoster
   b. DPT
   c. MMR
   d. rabies

37 Anticancer Drugs

Study Questions

Crossword puzzle: Use the definitions to determine the correct terms.

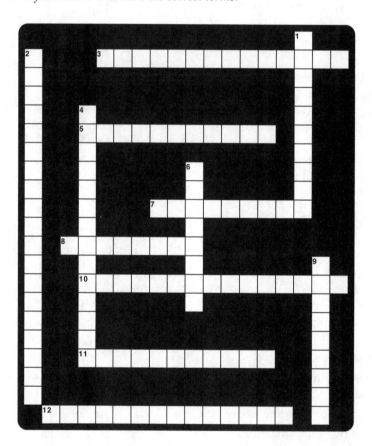

Across

3. Given with high-dose cyclophosphamide to inactivate urotoxic metabolites in the bladder and minimize organ damage
5. Type of drug that kills cancer cells during all phases of the cell cycle
7. Type of chemotherapy where there is a short interval between successive doses of agents (2 words)
8. Type of drug that works on in a specific cell cycle
10. Treatment to be done with chemotherapy (2 words)
11. Type of chemotherapy where two or more agents are used
12. The percent of actively dividing cells (2 words)

Down

1. Type of chemotherapy used to relieve symptoms associated with advanced disease
2. Tumor resistance to chemotherapeutic drugs (2 words)

4. Another term for anticancer drugs
6. Drug that can cause tissue necrosis if it infiltrates into the tissues
9. Cellular death

Match the chemotherapy drugs/terms in Column I with the most appropriate description in Column II.

Column I

____ 13. Angiogenesis inhibitors
____ 14. Aromatase inhibitors
____ 15. Cyclophosphamide (Cytoxan)
____ 16. Doxorubicin (Adriamycin)
____ 17. Dose-dense chemotherapy
____ 18. Fluorouracil (5-FU; Adrucil)
____ 19. Hormonal agents
____ 20. Methotrexate (Trexall)
____ 21. Ways to reduce exposure to chemotherapy
____ 22. Vincristine (Oncovin)

Column II

a. Associated with hemorrhagic cystitis
b. Leucovorin rescue
c. Stomatitis is early sign of toxicity
d. Associated with cardiotoxicity
e. Associated with neurotoxicity
f. Powder-free gloves, mask, impermeable gown
g. Not true chemotherapy agents
h. Prevents growth of new blood vessels
i. Intervals between doses of chemotherapy shortened
j. Block conversion of androgens to estrogen

NCLEX Review Questions

Select the best response.

23. The nurse is working with a client receiving combination chemotherapy. The client asks why she has to take more than one agent. What is the nurse's best response?
    a. "It has better response rates than single-agent chemotherapy."
    b. "It is always more effective than surgery or radiation."
    c. "It is never given with other treatment modalities (e.g., surgery)."
    d. "Survival time is decreased as compared to single-agent chemotherapy."

24. The nurse is teaching a community group about factors that influence the development of cancer in humans. Which is the best information to be included in the teaching?
    a. Aflatoxin is associated with cancer of the lung.
    b. Benzene is associated with cancer of the tongue.
    c. Epstein-Barr virus is associated with cancer of the stomach.
    d. Human papillomavirus is associated with cancer of the cervix.

25. A client is to receive chemotherapy for the treatment of cancer. What should the nurse know concerning the side effects of chemotherapy?
    a. Side effects are minimal because chemotherapy drugs are highly selective.
    b. Side effects are minimal because chemotherapy does not affect normal cells.
    c. Side effects of chemotherapy are caused by toxicities to normal cells.
    d. Side effects of chemotherapy are usually permanent.

26. A male client has advanced cancer that has spread to other areas of his body. He is scheduled to receive palliative chemotherapy. He state that he does not understand why he should have palliative chemotherapy if it won't kill the cancer cells. What is the best response?

    a. "It is given to limit the growth of cancer."

    b. "It will shrink the tumors throughout your body."

    c. "It is done to improve your quality of life."

    d. "It is given to slow the growth of the cancer."

27. A client is scheduled to receive chemotherapy that will cause a low white blood cell count. Which priority nursing actions should the nurse plan?

    a. Assess for a change in temperature.

    b. Assess for an increase in diarrhea.

    c. Assess for evidence of petechiae.

    d. Assess for taste changes.

28. A client has low platelet counts secondary to the administration of chemotherapy. Which nursing actions would be the most appropriate?

    a. Assess for diarrhea and provide small, frequent meals.

    b. Assess intake and output and help the client conserve energy.

    c. Assess for localized infections and monitor breath sounds.

    d. Assess for occult bleeding and apply pressure to injection sites.

29. The nurse is caring for a client who is experiencing diarrhea secondary to chemotherapy. Which important information should be included in client teaching about chemotherapy-related diarrhea?

    a. Eat only very hot or very cold foods.

    b. Increase intake of fresh fruits and vegetables.

    c. Increase intake of high-fiber foods.

    d. Limit caffeine intake.

30. An oncology client is to receive cyclophosphamide (Cytoxan) as part of his chemotherapy protocol. The nurse note on the medical record that the client is taking digoxin (Lanoxin) each morning to treat atrial fibrillation. What should the nurse be aware of when giving these two medications?

    a. Cyclophosphamide decreases digoxin levels.

    b. Cyclophosphamide has no effect on digoxin levels.

    c. Digoxin increases cyclophosphamide levels.

    d. These medications should never be given together.

31. A client in the outpatient oncology clinic is receiving fluorouracil (5-FU; Adrucil) as part of treatment for colon cancer. The physician prescribes metronidazole (Flagyl) to treat trichomoniasis. What should concern the nurse about this order?

    a. 5-FU may decrease the effectiveness of metronidazole.

    b. 5-FU may increase the toxicity of metronidazole.

    c. Metronidazole may decrease the effectiveness of 5-FU.

    d. Metronidazole may increase 5-FU toxicity.

32. A client is to receive doxorubicin (Adriamycin) as part of her chemotherapy protocol. Which assessment finding is the most important for the nurse to assess before administration of Adriamycin?

    a. cardiac status

    b. liver function

    c. lung sounds

    d. mental status

33. A client is receiving cyclophosphamide (Cytoxan), doxorubicin (Adriamycin), and methotrexate (Trexall) (CAM) for the treatment of prostate cancer. During morning rounds, the client complains of feeling short of breath. Physical assessment reveals crackles in both lungs. What is the most likely cause of this clinical manifestation?
    a. Adriamycin
    b. cyclophosphamide
    c. methotrexate
    d. client anxiety

34. A client is to receive fluorouracil (5-FU; Adrucil) as part of a treatment protocol for colon cancer. When teaching the client about this drug, what should the nurse say concerning when the nadir usually occurs in the blood counts?
    a. 1 to 4 days after administration
    b. 5 to 9 days after administration
    c. 10 to 14 days after administration
    d. 15 to 19 days after administration

35. A client has reached the nadir of his blood counts secondary to chemotherapy. Which nursing diagnoses is the most appropriate?
    a. Risk for cardiac failure
    b. Risk for dehydration
    c. Risk for infection
    d. Risk for malnutrition

36. Which nursing outcome would be most appropriate as part of the planning for a client scheduled to receive cyclophosphamide (Cytoxan)?
    a. Client will be free of symptoms of stomatitis.
    b. Client will maintain cardiac output.
    c. Client will limit exposure to sunlight.
    d. Client will maintain blood counts in the desired range.

37. A client is to receive cyclophosphamide (Cytoxan) as part of her cancer treatment. Which nursing intervention should the nurse expect to complete?
    a. Assess for signs of hematuria, urinary frequency, or dysuria.
    b. Decrease fluids to reduce the risk of urate deposition or calculus formation.
    c. Hydrate the client with IV fluids only after administration of cyclophosphamide.
    d. Medicate with an antiemetic only after the client complains of nausea.

38. The nurse is teaching a 29-year-old client about cyclophosphamide (Cytoxan), which will be given as part of her treatment protocol for cancer. Which priority information should be included in the teaching?
    a. Hair loss has never been reported with the use of cyclophosphamide.
    b. Menstrual irregularities and sterility are not expected with this drug.
    c. No special isolation procedures are needed when receiving this chemotherapy.
    d. Pregnancy should be prevented during treatment with cyclophosphamide.

39. The nurse is administering IV fluorouracil (5-FU; Adrucil) to a client in the outpatient oncology clinic. Which nursing intervention would be most appropriate?
    a. 5-FU is a vesicant, so assess for tissue necrosis at the IV site.
    b. Apply heat to the IV site if extravasation occurs.
    c. Assess for hyperpigmentation along the vein in which the drug is given.
    d. Encourage mouth rinses once every 8 hours during chemotherapy.

40. A client receiving cyclophosphamide (Cytoxan), epirubicin (Ellence), and fluorouracil (5-FU; Adrucil) (CEF) has experienced severe nausea, vomiting, and diarrhea over the past week. He has lost 5.5 pounds. Which nursing diagnosis would be most appropriate?

   a. Knowledge deficit related to chemotherapeutic regimen

   b. Pain secondary to diarrhea

   c. Risk for altered nutrition

   d. Risk for infection secondary to low WBC counts

41. The nurse is teaching a client about doxorubicin (Adriamycin), which she will receive as part of her treatment for breast cancer. Which statement made by the client indicate that she needs additional teaching?

   a. "Adriamycin is a severe vesicant."

   b. "My blood counts will be checked."

   c. "My cardiac status will be closely monitored."

   d. "This drug may make my urine turn blue."

42. The nurse is administering doxorubicin (Adriamycin) to a client in the outpatient oncology clinic. What is priority information to include in the client teaching?

   a. Blood counts will most likely remain normal.

   b. Complete alopecia rarely occurs with this drug.

   c. Report any shortness of breath, palpitations, or edema to your doctor.

   d. Tissue necrosis usually occurs 2 to 3 days after administration.

43. The nurse is administering doxorubicin (Adriamycin) to a client diagnosed with cancer. What should the nurse keep in mind with regard to tissue necrosis associated with this drug?

   a. Tissue necrosis may occur 3 to 4 weeks after administration.

   b. Tissue necrosis occurs immediately after administration.

   c. Tissue necrosis occurs 2 to 4 days after administration.

   d. Tissue necrosis rarely occurs with this drug.

44. One week ago in the outpatient oncology clinic, a client received his first cycle of chemotherapy consisting of cyclophosphamide (Cytoxan), doxorubicin (Adriamycin), and fluorouracil (5-FU; Adrucil) (CAF). He returns to the clinic today for follow-up. Which nursing intervention would be most appropriate at this time?

   a. Culture the IV site and send a specimen to the laboratory for analysis.

   b. Monitor blood counts and laboratory values.

   c. Offer analgesics for pain and evaluate effectiveness.

   d. Teach the client about good skin care.

45. The nurse is preparing IV vinblastine (Velban), bleomycin (Blenoxane), and cisplatin (Platinol) (VBP) for administration to a client on the nursing unit. Which precaution should the nurse take when hanging chemotherapy?

   a. Wear a clean cotton gown.

   b. Wear shoe covers.

   c. Wear a hair net.

   d. Wear powder-free gloves.

46. A client is being discharged after receiving IV chemotherapy. Which statement made by the client indicates a need for additional teaching?

   a. "Chemotherapy is excreted in my bodily fluids."

   b. "I will not need to know how to check my temperature."

   c. "My spouse should wear gloves when emptying my urinal."

   d. "The chemotherapy will remain in my body for 2 to 3 days."

47. The nurse is preparing to administer chemo-therapy, which can cause severe nausea and vomiting, to a client in the outpatient clinic. Which nursing action would be most appropriate?

    a. Give an antiemetic before administering the chemotherapy.

    b. Withhold any antiemetic drugs until the client complains of nausea.

    c. Give an antiemetic only after the client has vomited.

    d. Offer the client a glass of ginger ale to prevent nausea.

48. A client is admitted to the hospital 1 week after receiving teniposide (VP-16) in the outpatient oncology clinic. On physical assessment, the nurse notes the presence of petechiae, ecchymoses, and bleeding gums. Which nursing diagnosis would be most appropriate?

    a. Risk for fatigue

    b. Risk for infection

    c. Risk for bleeding

    d. Risk for falls

49. A client with breast cancer is scheduled to receive anastrozole (Arimidex), an aromatase inhibitor. Which priority information should be included in the client teaching?

    a. Aromatase inhibitors block the peripheral conversion of androgens to estrogens.

    b. Aromatase inhibitors are used to treat tumors that are not hormonally sensitive.

    c. Aromatase inhibitors are used only in premenopausal women with breast cancer.

    d. Aromatase inhibitors are used only in postmenopausal women with breast cancer.

50. A client is scheduled to receive vincristine (Oncovin) as part of treatment for his cancer. The medication record for the client indicates that he is receiving phenytoin (Dilantin) to control a seizure disorder. What should the nurse monitor in this client?

    a. headaches

    b. increased blood pressure

    c. renal failure

    d. seizures

51. A client is scheduled to receive vincristine as part of her treatment for non-Hodgkin's lymphoma. She reports that she takes bromelain (pineapple extract) at home to prevent constipation. What should the nurse monitor in this client?

    a. urine output

    b. blood glucose levels

    c. CBC

    d. BUN and creatinine levels

52. A client in the outpatient oncology clinic has developed mucositis secondary to cancer therapy. Which statement made by the client would indicate that she needs additional teaching about mucositis?

    a. "I will rinse my mouth out frequently with normal saline."

    b. "I will try using ice pops or ice chips to help relieve mouth pain."

    c. "I will use a mouthwash that has an alcohol base."

    d. "I will use a soft toothbrush."

53. A client presents with neutropenia secondary to cancer therapy. Which nursing diagnosis would be the most appropriate?

    a. Risk for cardiac failure

    b. Risk for dehydration

    c. Risk for infection

    d. Risk for malnutrition

Case Study

Select the best answer.

The nurse is caring for C.Z., who is receiving high doses of cyclophosphamide (Cytoxan).

1.   C.Z. says that she does not believe her cancer therapy is effective and that she would like to start taking garlic and echinacea because she has heard they help to enhance the immune system. What is the nurse's best response?

   a.   "If you believe they will help you during this treatment, then you should take them."

   b.   "We will need to check with your physician before you take those herbal products."

   c.   "Those herbal products can negatively affect the chemotherapeutic agent you are taking and should be avoided."

   d.   "Those herbal products will supplement your chemotherapeutic agent, and you should take them in moderate doses."

2.   When caring for C.Z., what assessment should always be included?

   a.   vital signs with temperature

   b.   pupil reactivity

   c.   Babinski reflex

   d.   skin turgor

3.   Which laboratory values should be monitored in C.Z. on a weekly basis?

   a.   LDH levels

   b.   CBC with differential

   c.   electrolytes

   d.   arterial blood gases

4.   C.Z. is concerned about the side effect of hemorrhagic cystitis. What should she do to decrease the risk of this alteration?

   a.   Decrease fluid intake to 1000 mL/day.

   b.   Increase fluid intake to 2-3 L/day.

   c.   Request that the physician prescribe a diuretic.

   d.   Drink two glasses of cranberry juice daily.

5.   The nurse is preparing a teaching plan for C.Z. Which priority information should be included? (Select all that apply.)

   a.   "Do not take herbal preparations or OTC drugs before consulting your health care provider."

   b.   "Take the medication early in the day to prevent its accumulation in the bladder at night."

   c.   "Avoid pregnancy for 3 to 4 months after completing the medication."

   d.   "Use some form of contraception while taking this medication."

   e.   "Report any elevation in temperature or blood in the urine to your physician immediately."

38 Targeted Therapies to Treat Cancer

Study Questions

Complete the following word search. Clues are given in Questions 1–7. Circle your responses.

```
U S R O T C A F N O I T P I R C S N A R T B
H O Z Q M W P G H G Y G P K L G Q V V J F K
Y S G W X V E A S T R R V N I B P C Y C Q J
S N E U F S G E T O A O Y O B R X D L V M K
P I V S W P M K R H R R W K O J X N M J F Z
B L T Y T Y E X D S W J G T C F Y Y U W A N
R C B U Z Y J J Z E A A E E H Z V A D E V Z
I Y X N L A A K L K G A Y W T F F Y Q D D X
C C E W V V E J Q J S O F S R E A G P J T F
Z N O I T A L Y R O H P S O H P D C U H F Z
U R F J Z S E N M N A N B T Q Q E K T V U J
T B S P A T D E G R A D A T I O N X Z O P R
P C E L L U L A R R E C E P T O R S Y X R U
H M N O I T C U D S N A R T L A N G I S K Y
```

1. The _____ _____ receptors on the cell membrane can activate tyrosine kinases, which then turn on signal transduction pathways promoting cell division.

2. _____ _____ is a method of communication that allows events, conditions, and substances outside of the cell to influence it.

3. Tyrosine kinases are a family of enzymes that activate other substances by adding a phosphate molecule, a process known as _____.

4. _____ _____ for cell division are substances that enter the nucleus and signal the cell that mitosis is needed.

5. _____ are part of a family of proteins that, when active, stimulate the cell to move through the cell cycle.

6. A _____ is a large complex of proteins in cell fluid (cytoplasm) and cell nucleus that regulates protein expression and the _____ of damaged or old proteins within the cell.

7. _____ therapy for cancer that takes advantage of biological features, such as _____, _____, _____, or other molecular proteins of cancer cells that either are not present or are present in much smaller quantities in normal cells.

NCLEX Review Questions

Select the best response.

8. What occurs in cancer tumor cells when the EGFR-TK signal is inappropriately turned on?
    a. proliferation
    b. invasion
    c. angiogenesis
    d. metastasis

9. During the first dose of trastuzumab (Herceptin), the client complains of shortness of breath and pruritus. What is the best action by the nurse?
    a. Decrease the infusion rate by 50% and notify the physician.
    b. Stop the infusion and manage the reaction.
    c. Review the pretreatment MUGA scan.
    d. Disconnect the IV and attach a 0.22-micron filter.

10. What is the rationale for administering bevacizumab in a client with metastatic colon cancer?
    a. enhance the client's immune response
    b. modulate an inflammatory response
    c. increase apoptosis
    d. inhibit formation of blood supply

11. Iressa most frequently causes which toxicities?
    a. acneiform rash
    b. diarrhea
    c. myelosuppression
    d. nausea and vomiting

12. An oncology client is to begin treatment for NSCLC with administration of gefitinib. The nurse notes on his medical record that the client is also taking warfarin daily for atrial fibrillation. What should concern the nurse about the client taking gefitinib and warfarin?
    a. Gefitinib increases the effects of warfarin.
    b. It may reach toxic levels when given concurrently with warfarin.
    c. It is never given to a client taking anticoagulants.
    d. Gefitinib may require a dose increase when taken with warfarin.

13. A client in the outpatient oncology clinic is receiving sunitinib as part of his treatment for GIST. The physician prescribes metronidazole to treat trichomoniasis. What should concern the nurse about taking these medications concurrently?
    a. Sunitinib may decrease the effectiveness of metronidazole.
    b. Sunitinib may lead to toxic levels of metronidazole.
    c. Metronidazole may decrease the effectiveness of sunitinib.
    d. Metronidazole may potentiate sunitinib toxicity.

14. A client is beginning therapy with the EGFR erlotinib (Tarceva) for NSCLC. Which is the most important status for the nurse to assess before beginning therapy with this targeted agent?
    a. cardiac status
    b. liver function
    c. lung sounds
    d. mental status

15. A client is admitted to the hospital 1 week after receiving teniposide (VP-16) in the outpatient oncology clinic. On physical assessment, the nurse notes the presence of petechiae, ecchymosis, and bleeding gums. Which nursing diagnoses would be most appropriate?
    a. Risk for fatigue
    b. Risk for infection
    c. Risk for bleeding
    d. Risk for falls

16. Which nursing outcomes would be most appropriate as part of the planning for a client about to begin therapy with the oral MKI sorafenib? (Select all that apply.)

    a. Client will be free of symptoms of stomatitis.

    b. Client will be free of cardiac dysfunction.

    c. Client will maintain skin integrity.

    d. Client will maintain adequate fluid balance.

17. Which nursing outcomes would be most appropriate as part of the planning for a client scheduled to begin treatment with imatinib (Gleevec)? (Select all that apply.)

    a. Client will maintain adequate nutrition and hydration status.

    b. Client will maintain cardiac output.

    c. Client will maintain blood counts in the desired range.

    d. Client will maintain renal function.

Case Study

Select the best answer.

C.L. is being treated with bevacizumab for metastatic breast cancer. She presents to the clinic for her third treatment.

1. The nurse is getting ready to hang the IV infusion. When checking the medication, the nurse notices that the medication is mixed in D_5W. What should concern the nurse about this combination?

    a. Nothing; it is the appropriate combination.

    b. This medication should be combined only with $D_{50}W$.

    c. This medication should be combined only with lactated Ringer's.

    d. This medication should be combined only with .9% normal saline.

2. Before hanging C.L.'s IV, the nurse draws blood for laboratory tests. Which tests should the nurse expect to be ordered? (Select all that apply.)

    a. CBC with differential

    b. BUN and creatinine

    c. electrolytes

    d. liver enzymes

3. The nurse offers C.L. crackers and ginger ale before starting the IV infusion. C.L. asks why she is being offered soda and crackers. What is the best answer?

    a. "The soda and crackers will help to keep your energy up while receiving the treatment."

    b. "The soda and crackers are available in case you get hungry during the IV infusion."

    c. "The soda and crackers should help decrease the nausea you might have during the IV."

    d. "The soda and crackers will decrease the diarrhea associated with this treatment."

4. As the nurse is hanging the medication, C.L. asks how this drug will work against her cancer. What is the best answer?

    a. "This drug blocks the further metastasis of the cancer throughout the body."

    b. "This drug blocks microvascular growth and inhibits metastatic disease progression."

    c. "This drug stimulates vascular growth so the body's immune system can attack the cancer wherever it is."

    d. "This medication blocks cellular division and growth of the cancer."

5. Before C.L. is discharged, what priority teaching should she receive? (Select all that apply.)

    a. She should contact her health care provider if she has a fever, chills, persistent sore throat, weight gain, chest pain, or shortness of breath.

    b. She should contact her health care provider if she has black tarry stools or vomit that looks like coffee grounds.

    c. She should avoid direct sunlight and tanning beds and wear sunscreen when outside.

    d. She should avoid taking NSAIDs for any reason.

    e. She should avoid drinking any hot fluids to help prevent burns.

39 Biologic Response Modifiers

Study Questions

Crossword puzzle: Use the definitions to determine the correct terms.

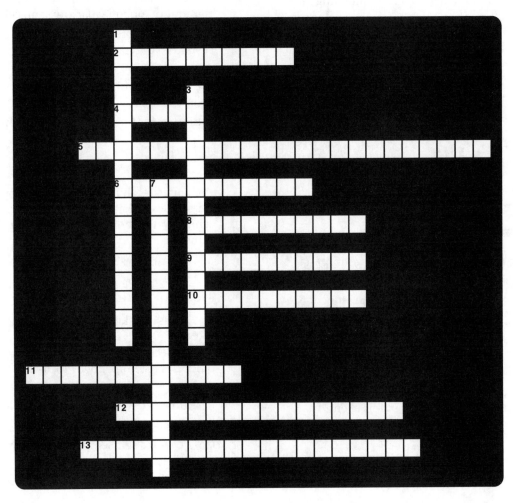

Across
2. Stimulates megakaryocyte and thrombocyte production
4. Lowest value of formed blood cells
5. White blood cell count × % of neutrophils + % of bands (3 words)
6. A family of proteins released by WBCs when exposed to pathogens
8. Process of adding a polyethylene glycol [PEG] molecule to another molecule
9. A naturally occurring substance that interferes with the ability of viruses to reproduce

10. Destructive to tumor cells
11. Increases the number of macrophages in the body
12. Suppression of bone marrow activity
13. Process that uses mice to mass-produce monoclonal antibodies (2 words)

Down

1. Type of factor that stimulates or regulates the growth, maturation, and differentiation of bone marrow stem cells (2 words)
3. Stimulates red blood cell production in response to hypoxia
7. Condition where there are not enough platelets

Match the description in Column II with the appropriate term in Column I.

Column I

____ 14. Colony-stimulating factors (CSFs)
____ 15. Erythropoietin
____ 16. Granulocyte colony–stimulating factor (G-CSF)
____ 17. Granulocyte-macrophage colony–stimulating factor (GM-CSF)
____ 18. Neumega (oprelvekin)

Column II

a. Glycoprotein that regulates the production of neutrophils within the bone marrow
b. Proteins that stimulate growth and maturation of bone marrow stem cells
c. Glycoprotein produced by kidneys in response to hypoxia
d. Supports survival, clonal expression, and differentiation of hematopoietic progenitor cells
e. Indicated for prevention of severe thrombocytopenia

NCLEX Review Questions

Select the best response.

19. What are the primary functions of BRMs? (Select all that apply.)
    a. enhance host immunologic function
    b. destroy tumor activities
    c. improve liver functioning
    d. promote differentiation of stem cells

20. The client is receiving G-CSF therapy. What is a priority assessment in this client?
    a. bone pain
    b. urinary retention
    c. flu-like syndrome
    d. rash

21. A client is receiving GM-CSF therapy. The nurse knows that attention is focused on which system both during and after these infusions?
    a. cardiac system
    b. respiratory system
    c. central nervous system
    d. musculoskeletal system

22. What special preparation and administration of EPO is recommended? (Select all that apply.)
    a. Inject less than 3 mL volume/injection.
    b. Do not re-enter the vial.
    c. Discard unused portion; no preservatives.
    d. Warm vial to room temperature.

23. What is the dose-limiting side effect of IFN alfa Roferon?
    a. malaise
    b. chills
    c. fever
    d. fatigue

24. A 64-year-old client has hairy cell leukemia that is being treated with the IFN alfa Roferon. The client reports all of the following gastrointestinal side effects. Which side effect is considered the dose-limiting toxicity for the gastrointestinal system?
    a. taste alteration
    b. anorexia
    c. xerostomia
    d. diarrhea

25. A 64-year-old client has hairy cell leukemia that is being treated with the IFN alfa Roferon. The client reports neurologic side effects. What is most appropriate response to the client's questions?
    a. "These side effects rarely occur."
    b. "These side effects are reversible after the drug is stopped."
    c. "These side effects are not reversible."
    d. "The worst effect is mild confusion."

26. When is the best time to administer a BRM?
    a. at bedtime
    b. 2 hours after meals
    c. with meals
    d. 1 hour before meals

27. Which laboratory values should be monitored specific to concerns related to assessing renal and hepatic function? (Select all that apply.)
    a. BUN
    b. creatinine
    c. transaminase
    d. bilirubin

28. What dermatologic effects should the nurse assess for in a client taking alfa IFNs? (Select all that apply.)
    a. vesicle formation
    b. alopecia
    c. irritation at injection site
    d. pruritus

29. What is priority health teaching information for a 64-year-old client who has hairy cell leukemia that is being treated with the IFN alfa Roferon and her significant others? (Select all that apply.)
    a. that most BRM side effects disappear within 72–96 hours after discontinuation of therapy
    b. that the client may return for another demonstration of drug administration techniques
    c. that the client should report any unusual weight gain
    d. information on the effect of BRM-related fatigue on ADLs, including sexual activity

30. For what conditions should GM-CSF be administered to clients? (Select all that apply.)
    a. ANC <500/mm^3
    b. autologous BMT recipient
    c. allogenic BMT recipient
    d. 2 weeks after high-dose chemotherapy administration

Case Study

Select the best answer.

J.G. is a 67-year-old client diagnosed with metastatic renal cell carcinoma. His medical oncologist has prescribed interleukin-2 (IL-2). J.G. weighs 150 pounds, and he will receive 600,000 International Units/kg (0.037 mg/kg) intravenously every 8 hours for 5 days (total of 14 doses of IL-2). He will have a 9-day rest after the initial 14 doses and then receive another 14 doses. Pretreatment laboratory work includes CBC, serum electrolytes, and renal and liver function tests. Client education will focus on review of treatment schedule, side effect profile, and postinfusion management.

1.   In addition to his cancer, J.G. has congestive heart failure (CHF). How would this underlying condition affect nursing care?

   a.   There would be no change in nursing care as the cardiac system is not affected by this client's medication.

   b.   The nurse will have to monitor I & O and respiratory status.

   c.   The nurse will monitor vital signs and CBC results.

   d.   The nurse should monitor peripheral pulses and pedal edema.

2.   J.G. calls his oncology nurse 3 days after receiving the last dose of IL-2. He is complaining of dizziness, pruritus, and urinary retention. What should the nurse advise him?

   a.   To use Benadryl tablets and take oatmeal baths for the itching and to run water in the sink when trying to urinate.

   b.   To return to the office to be evaluated by his health care provider.

   c.   To use Benadryl cream on the areas of itching and to run water in the sink when trying to urinate.

   d.   To report this to his health care provider when he returns for his next treatment.

3.   Eight days after receiving IL-2, J.G. experiences confusion and lethargy. What should the nurse expect for this client?

   a.   The client will be required to increase his oral intake and start taking a multivitamin.

   b.   The client will be hospitalized for IV fluids and further evaluation.

   c.   The health care provider will most likely delay the next scheduled treatment.

   d.   The client will be encouraged to take epoietin-alfa [Procrit] to increase his Hct level.

40 Drugs for Upper Respiratory Disorders

Study Questions

Match the term in Column I to the description in Column II.

Column I

_____ 1.   Antihistamines
_____ 2.   Antitussives
_____ 3.   Decongestants
_____ 4.   Expectorants

Column II

a.   Act on the cough-control center in the medulla

b.   Loosen bronchial secretions so they can be removed by coughing

c.   H₁ blockers or H₁ antagonists

d.   Stimulate the alpha-adrenergic receptors, producing vascular constriction in the nasal capillaries

Complete the following word search. Clues are given in questions 5-16. Circle your responses.

```
A N T I T U S S I V E S R B C I D F B C S Q
C R X J F H H J N E F Q S S O R K V H O D F
U R I N A R Y H M A V M I I M S S Q M M I E
T M S W X B E Z U R R K T J M Q V F I M U X
E F Q I K P H B I O P X I K O U T L N O L Q
R P H H N F E J O U A H G X N P L M I N F L
H J Z B K U N M P U E S N Y C H P Y M C R B
I Q C E F X S M C W N F Y P O M U L A O O R
N C O N S T R I C T E D R K L V K P L L R W
I Y W Z V P E S T I J Q A D D E V W M D E D
T A R E N O T R B I U T L A X Z W B T Q T U
I M F R O O M H J E S E D A T I O N S T A X
S Y J R T W O T O F O U R U C J R G H A W O
O W S I T I L L I S N O T E T U C A H G T N
```

5.   Upper respiratory infections (URIs) include the following five conditions: _____, _____, _____, _____, and _____.

6.   The most common cause of URIs is _____.

7.   On average, adults have _____ to _____ colds per year.

8.   When the H₁ receptor is stimulated, smooth muscle lining the nasal cavity is _____.

9.   Second-generation antihistamines differ from first-generation antihistamines because they do not cause _____.

10. Clients taking antihistamines need to be monitored for signs and symptoms of _____ dysfunction.

11. After constant use of a nasal spray, _____ congestion is likely to occur.

12. Do NOT use nasal sprays for children younger than _____ years of age.

13. The drug group that acts on the cough control center in the medulla is _____.

14. A nondrug expectorant available to everyone is _____.

15. In emergency situations such as anaphylaxis, antihistamines (are/are not) helpful. (Circle correct answer.)

16. Drug therapy for acute laryngitis has (minimal/optimal) impact on the condition. (Circle correct answer.)

NCLEX Review Questions

Select the best response.

17. Antihistamines are another group of drugs used for the relief of cold symptoms. What properties of this medication result in decreased secretions?
    a. cholinergic
    b. anticholinergic
    c. analgesic
    d. antitussive

18. Compared to first-generation antihistamines, second-generation antihistamines have a lower incidence of which side effect?
    a. vomiting
    b. tinnitus
    c. drowsiness
    d. headache

19. The FDA has ordered removal of all cold remedies containing which drug?
    a. propranolol
    b. dextromethorphan
    c. guaifenesin
    d. phenylpropanolamine

20. What is the recommended dosage of diphenhydramine (Benadryl)?
    a. 25-50 mg q4-6h
    b. 25-50 mg daily
    c. 50-100 mg q4-6h
    d. 100 mg daily

21. What is one of the effects of Benadryl?
    a. antihypertensive
    b. anticoagulant
    c. antitussive
    d. anticonvulsant

22. Benadryl blocks which histamine receptor?
    a. H_1
    b. H_2
    c. B_1
    d. B_2

23. A client taking Benadryl breastfeeds her infant daughter. What advice should the nurse give her?
    a. Large amounts of the drug pass into milk; breastfeeding is not recommended.
    b. The drug does not affect breastfeeding.
    c. Small amounts of the drug pass into breast milk; breastfeeding is not recommended.
    d. Breastfeeding is recommended.

24. The health teaching plan for a client taking Benadryl should include the side effects of the drug. What might the nurse assess in a client experiencing a side effect? (Select all that apply.)
    a. drowsiness
    b. disturbed coordination
    c. urinary retention
    d. tinnitus

25. What is the advantage of systemic decongestants over nasal sprays and drops?
    a. They are less costly.
    b. They provide longer relief.
    c. They have fewer side effects.
    d. They are preferred by older persons.

26. Which expectorant is frequently an ingredient in cold remedies?
    a. guaifenesin
    b. ephedrine
    c. hydrocodone
    d. promethazine

27. What nursing interventions should be implemented for the common cold? (Select all that apply.)
    a. Monitor vital signs.
    b. Observe color of bronchial secretions; antibiotics may be needed.
    c. Monitor reaction; codeine preparations for cough suppression can lead to physical dependence.
    d. Encourage adequate fluid intake.

28. What groups of drugs are used to treat cold symptoms? (Select all that apply.)
    a. decongestants
    b. antitussives
    c. expectorants
    d. indoles
    e. antihistamines

29. Decongestants are contraindicated for clients with which of the following? (Select all that apply.)
    a. hyperthyroidism
    b. cardiac disease
    c. obesity
    d. diabetes mellitus
    e. hypertension

30. Which priority information should be included in teaching a client who is taking medications for a common cold? (Select all that apply.)
    a. Use 4 puffs of nasal spray for a full 10 days.
    b. Read labels for OTC drugs for any interactions with current medications.
    c. Antibiotics are also needed to fight a common cold virus.
    d. Do not drive during initial use of a cold remedy containing an antihistamine.
    e. Take cold remedies with a decongestant for a better night's sleep.

Case Study

Select the best answer.

S.Y. is 80 years old and states, "My head is all filled up. I need something to open it up." A decongestant, Afrin, is ordered. S.Y. reports having numerous other medications in the bathroom cabinet.

1. What is the recommended dose and schedule for administration of Afrin?
    a. 1-2 gtts in each nostril daily
    b. 1-2 gtts in each nostril twice a day
    c. 2-3 gtts in each nostril daily
    d. 2-3 gtts in each nostril twice a day

2. What is the recommended length of time for use of Afrin?
    a. 2-3 days
    b. 3-5 days
    c. 5-8 days
    d. 8-10 days

3. What possible side effects might be assessed in S.Y.?
    a. rebound congestion
    b. headaches
    c. nausea
    d. constipation

4. What priority measures should the nurse advise S.Y. to implement to avoid rebound congestion? (Select all that apply.)
    a. Use the medication only for the recommended period of time.
    b. Limit use as much as possible.
    c. Use only as directed.
    d. Use as often as you need it.

5. What dietary restrictions should S.Y. observe?

    a. Don't drink alcohol when taking this medication.

    b. Don't drink orange juice when taking this medication.

    c. Don't drink grapefruit juice when taking this medication.

    d. Don't drink caffeinated beverages when taking this medication.

    decaff

6. What is the best advice the nurse can give S.Y. about the use of over-the-counter cold preparations? (Select all that apply.)

    a. "Check with your health care provider before using."

    b. "Make sure to read the drugs labels carefully."

    c. "Use the products only as directed."

    d. "Use the preparations as often as needed."

41 Drugs for Lower Respiratory Disorders

Study Questions

Match the drug in Column I with its category in Column II.

Column I

D 1. Acetylcysteine

F 2. Zafirlukast

B 3. Albuterol

C 4. Dexamethasone

A,b 5. Epinephrine

b 6. Arformoterol tartrate

Column II

a. Alpha adrenergic

b. Beta adrenergic

c. Glucocorticoids

d. Mucolytic

e. Steroids

f. Leukotrienes

Complete the following.

7. The substance responsible for maintaining bronchodilation is _____.

8. In acute bronchospasm caused by anaphylaxis, the drug administered subcutaneously to promote bronchodilation and elevate the blood pressure is _____.

9. The first line of defense in an acute asthmatic attack are the drugs categorized as _____.

10. Isuprel, one of the first drugs to treat bronchospasm, is a (selective/nonselective) beta$_2$ agonist. (Circle correct answer.)

11. Sympathomimetics cause dilation of the bronchioles by increasing _____.

12. Theophylline (increases/decreases) the risk of digitalis toxicity. (Circle correct answer.)

13. When theophylline and beta$_2$-adrenergic agonists are given together, a _____ effect can occur.

14. The half-life of theophylline is (shorter/longer) for smokers than for nonsmokers. (Circle correct answer.)

15. Aminophylline, theophylline, and caffeine are _____ derivatives used to treat _____.

16. The drug commonly prescribed to treat unresponsive asthma is _____.

17. Cromolyn (Intal) is used as _____ treatment for bronchial asthma. It acts by inhibiting the release of _____.

18. A serious side effect of cromolyn is _____.

19. The newer drugs for asthma are more selective for _____ receptors.

20. The leukotriene receptor antagonist considered safe for use in children 6 years and older is _____.

21. The preferred time of day for the administration of Singulair is _____.

22. The usual dose of Singulair for an adult is _____ and for a child is _____ administered without food.

23. A group of drugs used to liquefy and loosen thick mucous secretions is _____.

24. With infection resulting from retained mucous secretions, a(n) _____ may be prescribed.

NCLEX Review Questions

Select the best response.

25. A 54-year-old client is receiving treatment for chronic obstructive pulmonary disease (COPD). The client's medication is delivered via a metered-dose inhaler. Related health teaching would include which priority information?
    a. Test the inhaler first to see if the spray works.
    b. Shake the inhaler well just before use.
    c. Refrigerate the inhaler.
    d. Hold the inhaler upside down.

26. What facts about an inhaler drug dose should the nurse be aware of? (Select all that apply.)
    a. lower than an oral dose
    b. higher than an oral dose
    c. fewer side effects than an oral dose
    d. onset of action more rapid than that of an oral dose

27. How many minutes should a client wait after using a bronchodilator and before using a glucocorticoid preparation?
    a. 1
    b. 3
    c. 5
    d. 10

28. A client experiencing an acute asthmatic attack was given an IV loading dose of aminophylline. The client is now receiving oral Theo-Dur. How often is the medication generally administered?
    a. q2h
    b. q3-4h
    c. q6-12h
    d. daily

29. What is the usual adult dose of Theo-Dur?
    a. 100-200 mg q8-12h
    b. 200-300 mg q8-12h
    c. 300-400 mg q8-12h
    d. 400-500 mg q8-12h

30. Which serum theophylline level should concern the nurse?
    a. 5 mcg/mL
    b. 10 mcg/mL
    c. 20 mcg/mL
    d. 30 mcg/mL

31. Which assessment finding in a client taking Theo-Dur is associated with the medication? (Select all that apply.)
    a. tachycardia
    b. insomnia and restlessness
    c. cardiac dysrhythmias
    d. urinary retention

32. Dietary influences for a client taking Theo-Dur include which of the following? (Select all that apply.)
    a. increased metabolism with low-carbohydrate diet
    b. decreased elimination with high-carbohydrate diet
    c. increased elimination with high-carbohydrate diet
    d. increased metabolism with high-protein diet

33. Which person(s) should not use Theo-Dur? (Select all that apply.)
    a. 45-year-old with hypertension
    b. 63-year-old with severe cardiac dysrhythmias
    c. 29-year-old with peptic ulcer disease
    d. 18-year-old with uncontrolled seizure disorder

34. What specific nursing interventions should be implemented for a client taking Theo-Dur? (Select all that apply.)
    a. Provide hydration.
    b. Monitor vital signs.
    c. Observe for confusion.
    d. Weigh daily.

35. What should be included in the health teaching plan for a client taking Theo-Dur? (Select all that apply.)
    a. Stop smoking.
    b. Remove mouth piece and cough.
    c. Do not use OTC products.
    d. Avoid caffeine products.

36. What are the side effects of long-term use of glucocorticoids? (Select all that apply.)
    a. hypoglycemia
    b. impaired immune response
    c. fluid retention
    d. hyperglycemia

37. Which anticholinergic drug has few systemic effects and is administered by aerosol?
    a. Amcort
    b. Aristocort
    c. Atrovent
    d. Theo-Dur

38. Drug selection and dosage for older adults with an asthmatic condition need to be considered. The use of large, continuous doses of a beta$_2$-adrenergic agonist may cause which side effect in the older adult?
    a. urinary retention
    b. bronchoconstriction
    c. constipation
    d. tachycardia

39. Which herb should be avoided by clients taking theophylline products?
    a. feverfew
    b. ephedra
    c. ginkgo
    d. garlic

40. When the client who has COPD has questions about using the inhaler, which priority information should the nurse include in a review of inhaler administration? (Select all that apply.)
    a. Keep lips secure around mouthpiece and inhale while pushing top of canister once.
    b. Hold breath for a few seconds, remove mouthpiece, and exhale slowly.
    c. Wait 5 minutes and repeat the procedure if a second inhalation is required.
    d. Cleanse all washable parts of inhaler equipment daily.
    e. Teach client to monitor heart rate.

41. When providing health teaching for the client who has COPD, the nurse discusses the side effects that may occur with the use of bronchodilators. What possible clinical manifestations should the client be aware of? (Select all that apply.)
    a. bradycardia
    b. nervousness
    c. tremors
    d. insomnia
    e. palpitations

42. Which medication when prescribed with Theo-Dur should concern the nurse? (Select all that apply.)
    a. beta-blockers
    b. digitalis
    c. stool softeners
    d. lithium
    e. phenytoin

Case Study

Select the best answer.

S.E., age 15 years, has severe asthma. She is being treated with theophylline and an inhaled glucocorticoid.

1. S.E. would like to know why she can't use her inhaled glucocorticoids to treat her severe asthmatic attacks. What is the nurse's best answer?
    a. "You can feel free to use your steroid inhaler for asthma attacks."
    b. "You can't take this medication for asthma attacks as it takes 30 minutes to work."
    c. "You can't take this medication for asthma attacks as it takes a certain blood level for this medication to work."
    d. "You can't take steroids for asthma attacks as it can take up to 4 hours to be effective."

2. The nurse is teaching S.E. how to take her theophylline. When should this medication be taken?
    a. 30 minutes before a meal
    b. 1 hour after a meal
    c. with meals
    d. at bedtime

3. The nurse is teaching S.E. about her oral inhalers. What possible side effects should S.E. be aware she might experience? (Select all that apply.)
    a. hoarseness
    b. dry mouth
    c. white spots in the oral cavity
    d. coughing
    e. headaches

4. S.E. is concerned about the side effects of the oral inhaler. What actions can she take to prevent or diminish the incidence of side effects? (Select all that apply.)
    a. Use a spacer on the inhaler.
    b. Increase her fluid intake.
    c. Rinse out her mouth after using the inhaler.
    d. Use the inhaler only as needed.

5. S.E. will be taking steroids for a long period of time. Which side effects should she be informed she might experience? (Select all that apply.)
    a. increased blood glucose levels
    b. fluid retention
    c. thickening of the skin on her hands and feet
    d. impaired immune response
    e. increased urine output

42 Cardiac Glycosides, Antianginals, and Antidysrhythmics

Study Questions

Crossword puzzle: Use the definition to determine the pharmacologic/physiologic term.

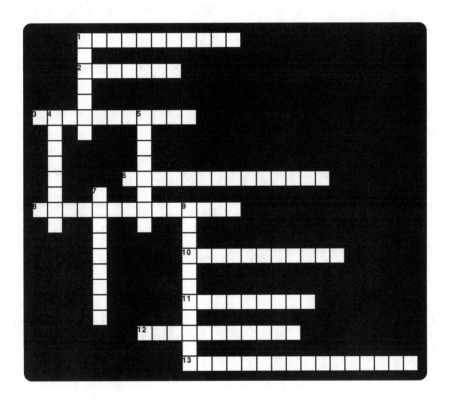

Across

1. Increased carbon dioxide in the blood
2. Amount of blood in the ventricle at the end of diastole
3. Drug category used to treat angina pectoris
6. Myocardium at rest
8. Myocardial contraction
10. Low serum potassium level
11. Peripheral vascular resistance
12. Pulse rate below 60 beats/min
13. Drug group used to treat disturbed heart rhythm

Down

1. Lack of oxygen to body tissues
4. Drug group used to control angina pain by relaxing coronary vessels
5. Lack of blood supply to the (heart) muscle
7. Cardiac _____ causes cardiac muscles to contract more efficiently
9. Pulse rate above 100 beats/min

Complete the following.

14. Heart failure occurs when the myocardium (strengthens/weakens) and (shrinks/enlarges), which causes the heart to lose its ability to pump blood through the heart and circulatory system. (Circle correct answers.)

15. With heart failure there is a(n) (increase/decrease) in preload and afterload. (Circle correct answer.)

16. Another name for heart failure is _____ failure.

17. Cardiac glycosides are also called _____ _____.

18. The action of antianginal drugs is to increase blood flow and to (increase/decrease) oxygen supply or to (increase/decrease) oxygen demand by the myocardium. (Circle correct answers.)

19. Name three of the four effects of digitalis preparations on the heart muscle (myocardium): _____, _____, and _____.

20. Beta blockers and calcium channel blockers (decrease/increase) the workload of the heart. (Circle correct answer.)

21. Nitroglycerin (NTG) is not swallowed because _____, thereby decreasing it effectiveness.

22. NTG sublingually acts within _____ minutes. Administration may be repeated _____ times.

23. The most common side effect of NTG is _____.

24. The drug group that may be used as an antianginal, antidysrhythmic, and antihypertensive is _____.

25. A calcium channel blocker that is effective in the long-term treatment of angina and has the side effect of bradycardia is _____.

26. Beta blockers and calcium channel blockers should not be discontinued without health care provider approval. Withdrawal symptoms may include _____ and _____.

27. Classic angina occurs when the client is _____.

28. Unstable angina (preinfarction) has the following pattern of occurrence: _____ _____.

29. Variant angina (Prinzmetal's angina) occurs when the client _____.

30. Prinzmetal's angina is due to _____ of the vessels.

31. The major systemic effect of nitrates is _____.

32. Cardiac dysrhythmias can result from (hypoxia/hyperoxia) and (hypocapnia/hypercapnia). (Circle correct answers.)

33. Examples of antidysrhythmics include _____, _____, and _____.

34. Clients taking antidysrhythmics should avoid _____ and _____.

The nurse should obtain a history of herbs the client is taking. This is especially true for clients taking digoxin. Match the herbs in Column I with their effects on digoxin in Column II.

Column I

____ 35. St. John's wort
____ 36. Ephedra
____ 37. Metamucil
____ 38. Aloe
____ 39. Goldenseal
____ 40. Ginseng

Column II

a. Increased risk of digitalis toxicity
b. Decreased digoxin absorption
c. Decreased effects of digoxin
d. Falsely elevated digoxin levels

NCLEX Review Questions

Select the best response.

41. What are digitalis preparations effective for treating?
    a. bowel obstruction
    b. congestive heart failure (CHF)
    c. thrombophlebitis
    d. urinary tract infection

42. Phosphodiesterase inhibitors are used to treat CHF by inhibiting the enzyme phosphodiesterase. What do these agents promote?
    a. positive inotropic response
    b. negative inotropic response
    c. vasoconstriction
    d. increased serum sodium and potassium levels

43. What is an example of a phosphodiesterase inhibitor?
    a. digoxin
    b. isosorbide dinitrate (Isordil)
    c. amlodipine (Norvasc)
    d. inamrinone lactate (Inocor)

44. What is the best way to describe a dysrhythmia?
    a. absence of heart rhythm
    b. disturbed heart rhythm
    c. heart rhythm greater than 200 beats/min
    d. functional heart rate

45. Quinidine was the first antidysrhythmic used to treat cardiac dysrhythmias; however, it has many side effects. Procainamide (Pronestyl, Procanbid), another antidysrhythmic, causes less cardiac depression than quinidine. What is the classification of each of these medications?
    a. beta blockers
    b. calcium channel blockers
    c. fast sodium channel blocker IB
    d. fast sodium channel blocker IA

46. What are the actions of quinidine and procainamide?
    a. slow conduction and shorten repolarization
    b. slow conduction and prolong repolarization
    c. increase conduction and prolong repolarization
    d. increase conduction and shorten repolarization

47. What type of drug is propranolol (Inderal)?
    a. nonselective beta blocker
    b. cardioselective beta blocker
    c. calcium channel blocker
    d. fast sodium blocker

48. Which antidysrhythmic drug should be used during life-threatening situations to convert ventricular fibrillation to normal sinus rhythm when lidocaine and procainamide are ineffective?
    a. phenytoin (Dilantin)
    b. tocainide
    c. atropine
    d. bretylium

49. What are actions of antidysrhythmics? (Select all that apply.)
    a. block adrenergic stimulation of the heart
    b. increase myocardial contractility
    c. decrease myocardial contractility
    d. increase recovery time of the myocardium

50. What is lidocaine (Xylocaine) primarily used to treat?
    a. bradycardia
    b. ventricular dysrhythmias
    c. atrial dysrhythmias
    d. heart block

51. What is a common problem experienced by individuals who are taking verapamil?
    a. tachycardia
    b. bradycardia
    c. headache
    d. nausea

52. What is the most potent calcium blocker?
    a. nicardipine (Cardene)
    b. diltiazem (Cardizem)
    c. verapamil (Calan)
    d. nifedipine (Procardia)

53. Clients taking calcium blockers need to have which laboratory values monitored?
    a. BUN
    b. creatinine
    c. liver enzymes
    d. urinary output

54. Abnormal atrial natriuretic peptide (ANP) and brain natriuretic peptide (BNP) levels indicate which disease process?
    a. emphysema
    b. peptic ulcer
    c. colon cancer
    d. heart failure

55. An 80-year-old client is taking digoxin daily along with several other medications. The client's BNP is 420 pg/mL. What should concern the nurse about this level?
    a. Nothing; it is within normal/reference range.
    b. It is slightly elevated.
    c. It is markedly elevated.
    d. It is below the normal/reference range for his age.

56. Which condition should the nurse watch for if a digitalis preparation is prescribed?
    a. CHF
    b. atrial flutter
    c. emphysema
    d. atrial fibrillation

57. What is the usual maintenance dose of digoxin?
    a. 0.125-0.25 mg/day
    b. 0.5-1 mg/day
    c. 0.04-0.06 mg/day
    d. 0.4-0.6 mg/day

58. Within which range would the nurse want to maintain a client's serum digoxin level?
    a. 0.15-0.5 ng/mL
    b. 0.5-2 ng/mL
    c. 2-3.5 ng/mL
    d. 3.5-4 ng/mL

59. Which clinical manifestations should the nurse assess in a client taking digoxin if there is concern about digitalis toxicity? (Select all that apply.)
    a. anorexia
    b. diarrhea
    c. bradycardia
    d. visual disturbances

60. Which is the antidote for digitalis toxicity?
    a. protamine
    b. vitamin K
    c. digoxin immune Fab
    d. gamma globulin

61. The nurse is reviewing the client's MAR. Which medications on the MAR should concern the nurse given that the client is taking digitalis? (Select all that apply.)
    a. furosemide (Lasix)
    b. cortisone
    c. nitroglycerin
    d. potassium-wasting diuretics

62. What specific nursing intervention should be implemented specific to taking the pulse of a client taking digoxin?
    a. Measure at the radial site for 30 seconds.
    b. Measure at the radial site for 60 seconds.
    c. Listen at the apical site for 30 seconds.
    d. Listen at the apical site for 60 seconds.

63. Which foods may a client taking digoxin include in the diet? (Select all that apply.)
    a. fruits
    b. potatoes
    c. fruit juice
    d. sausage

64. What priority information should be included in the teaching plan for a client taking digoxin? (Select all that apply.)
   a. Take blood pressure daily.
   b. Read drug labels carefully.
   c. Eat foods high in potassium.
   d. Report pulse rate <60 beats/min.

65. Which drugs may be used to treat heart failure? (Select all that apply.)
   a. vasodilators
   b. angiotensin-converting enzyme (ACE) inhibitors
   c. beta blockers
   d. diuretics

66. A client is receiving NTG sublingually for anginal pain. The nurse monitors the client's vital signs. Which assessment finding is associated with antianginal drugs? (Select all that apply.)
   a. hypotension
   b. hypertension
   c. increased heart rate
   d. decreased heart rate

67. What is the most commonly seen side effect a client may experience when taking NTG?
   a. faintness
   b. dizziness
   c. headache
   d. weakness

68. What priority health teaching should be given to a client taking NTG? (Select all that apply.)
   a. A biting sensation indicates that the NTG tablet is fresh.
   b. The NTG should be stored away from light.
   c. The contents of an opened bottle of NTG remain effective for approximately 6 months.
   d. If pain persists after five tablets, notify the health care provider immediately.

69. A Nitro transdermal patch is prescribed for a client taking NTG sublingually for anginal pain. How often is the patch applied?
   a. q6h
   b. q12h
   c. q24h
   d. q48h

70. A client is prescribed atenolol (Tenormin) 50 mg daily. What type of drug is this?
   a. nonselective beta blocker
   b. cardioselective beta blocker
   c. calcium channel blocker
   d. adrenergic stimulant

71. How should the nurse evaluate the effects of atenolol on angina?
   a. By asking the client if the presence of angina pain has subsided.
   b. By checking for the presence of bronchoconstriction because of atenolol.
   c. By determining if the client's urinary output has decreased.
   d. By monitoring the client's blood pressure for hypertension.

72. The client is taking acebutolol (Sectral) 200 mg b.i.d. for irregular heart rate. The client asks the nurse how often she should take the drug. What is the nurse's best response?
   a. "Once a day."
   b. "Twice a day."
   c. "Three times a day."
   d. "Every other day."

73. Which type of drug is acebutolol (Sectral)?
   a. nonselective beta blocker
   b. cardioselective beta blocker
   c. calcium channel blocker
   d. fast sodium channel blocker

74. The nurse is instructing a client on how to take Sectral. What instruction should be included on stopping this medication?

    a. "Notify the doctor within a week after stopping the drug."

    b. "If you run out, ask a friend to lend you a tablet until the drug can be refilled."

    c. "Do not abruptly stop taking Sectral or you risk an adverse reaction."

    d. "Have the drug refilled no later than a month after taking the last dose."

75. Which possible side effects of Sectral should the nurse mention to a client? (Select all that apply.)

    a. dizziness

    b. nausea

    c. possible impotence

    d. hypertension

76. After a month, the nurse evaluates a client's response to Sectral. Which specific things should be included in the nurse's assessment? (Select all that apply.)

    a. vital signs

    b. presence of side effects

    c. compliance (whether the client is taking the drug as ordered)

    d. urinary output

77. Which nursing interventions related to digoxin administration should be included in client teaching? (Select all that apply.)

    a. Check the apical pulse rate before administering digoxin.

    b. Check the sodium level before administering digoxin.

    c. Instruct the client to report side effects of digoxin, such as pulse rate greater than 100 beats/min.

    d. Advise the client who is taking a potassium-wasting diuretic such as thiazide to eat foods rich in potassium.

    e. Advise the client to avoid taking the herb St. John's wort because it can decrease the absorption of digoxin.

78. The nurse is administering a nitrate drug for angina pectoris. Which nursing interventions should be implemented? (Select all that apply.)

    a. Instruct the client to swallow the sublingual nitrate during chest pain.

    b. Inform the client that headaches may occur when first taking a nitrate product.

    c. Instruct the client not to ingest alcohol while taking a nitrate drug.

    d. Tell the client that sublingual nitroglycerin 0.4 mg may be taken every half hour during chest pain.

    e. Tell the client that if the chest pain is not alleviated with a nitroglycerin tablet after repeating the dose three times, the health care provider should be immediately notified.

79. Which condition(s) can lead to cardiac dysrhythmias? (Select all that apply.)

    a. hypoxia

    b. hypocapnia

    c. electrolyte imbalance

    d. excess catecholamines

    e. vertigo

Case Study

Select the best answer.

J.B., 61 years old, has had several attacks of angina pectoris. J.B. has nitroglycerin gr 1/150 sublingual tablets to relieve acute attacks, and metoprolol (Lopressor) 25 mg b.i.d. has been prescribed. Vital signs: BP 154/88 mm Hg, P 82 beats/min, R 26 breaths/min.

1. What are priority nursing interventions for J.B. regarding the use of NTG tablets? (Select all that apply.)

    a. Take the NTG at the onset of angina pain.

    b. If pain is not relieved in 5 minutes, repeat dose every 5 minutes for a total of 3 doses.

    c. If still experiencing pain after 15 minutes, immediately contact your health are provider.

    d. Swallow the tablet if the first tablet does not totally relieve the pain.

    e. Chew the tablet to speed pain relief.

2. Which vital signs should be measured in J.B.? (Select all that apply.)

    a. blood pressure

    b. heart rate

    c. respiratory rate

    d. temperature

3. Which should J.B. take if he has asthma? (Select all that apply.)

    a. metoprolol

    b. propranolol

    c. amlodipine

    d. nifedipine

4. What nonpharmacologic measures should the nurse include in the health teaching for J.B.? (Select all that apply.)

    a. Use relaxation techniques.

    b. Get adequate rest.

    c. Do not smoke.

    d. Decrease use of salt.

    e. Exercise when you feel up to it.

43 Diuretics

Study Questions

Crossword puzzle: Use the definitions to determine the correct terms.

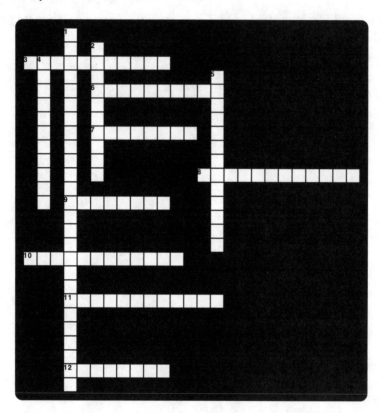

Across

3. Excretion of increased amount of sodium via the urine
6. Concentration of body fluids
7. Most frequently prescribed osmotic diuretic
8. Main side effect of potassium-sparing diuretics
9. Increased production of urine
10. One disease for which a health care provider will prescribe diuretics
11. Term for above-normal levels of potassium
12. Term for decreased production of urine

Down

1. Decreases intraocular pressure in clients with glaucoma (3 words)
2. Potassium-wasting diuretic
4. Hormone that affects the body's sodium levels
5. Term for above-normal levels of blood glucose

List the possible abnormal serum chemistry test results associated with thiazides.

Laboratory Test	Abnormal Results
13. Potassium	
14. Magnesium	
15. Calcium	
16. Chloride	
17. Bicarbonate	
18. Uric acid	
19. Blood sugar	
20. Blood lipids	

NCLEX Review Questions

Select the best response.

21. Which of the following groups of diuretics are frequently prescribed to treat hypertension and congestive heart failure? (Select all that apply.)
    a. osmotic
    b. potassium-sparing
    c. loop
    d. thiazides

22. When compared with thiazides, how are loop (high-ceiling) diuretics different?
    a. They are more effective as antihypertensives.
    b. They are more potent as diuretics.
    c. They promote potassium absorption.
    d. They cause calcium reabsorption.

23. Herb-diuretic interaction should be assessed by the nurse. Which herb may increase blood pressure when it is taken with a thiazide diuretic?
    a. St. John's wort
    b. licorice
    c. ginkgo
    d. ginger

24. What is the pharmacologic action of Aldactone?
    a. increase potassium and sodium excretion
    b. promote potassium retention and sodium excretion
    c. promote potassium, sodium, and calcium retention
    d. promote potassium excretion and sodium retention

25. What is the classification of spironolactone (Aldactone)?
    a. potassium-wasting diuretic
    b. potassium-sparing diuretic
    c. osmotic diuretic
    d. thiazide diuretic

26. The client had an acute myocardial infarction 6 months ago. He was prescribed spironolactone (Aldactone) 25 mg daily to aid in treating an irregular heart rate. What should the nurse suspect is the reason the client was prescribed Aldactone?
    a. It retains more sodium for heart contraction.
    b. It excretes potassium to lessen circulatory (serum) potassium level.
    c. It retains circulatory (serum) potassium for the heart muscle.
    d. It retains calcium for heart contraction.

27. A client who is taking Aldactone after an acute myocardial infarction requests assistance with his diet. Which foods should the nurse recommend? (Select all that apply.)
    a. lean meat
    b. bananas
    c. apples
    d. squash

28. When evaluating the effects of Aldactone, what should the nurse be sure to monitor?
    a. serum potassium level
    b. complete blood count (CBC)
    c. serum lipoproteins
    d. blood glucose level

29. The client had an acute myocardial infarction 6 months ago. He was prescribed spironolactone (Aldactone) 25 mg daily to aid in treating an irregular heart rate. The client's serum potassium level should be monitored periodically. If the serum potassium level is 5.5 mEq/L, what is a priority intervention to be implemented?
    a. The Aldactone dose should be reduced or stopped and the client instructed to decrease intake of foods rich in potassium.
    b. The Aldactone dose should be continued and the client encouraged to eat fruits, vegetables, and meats.
    c. The Aldactone dose should be increased and the client instructed to decrease foods rich in potassium.
    d. Instruct the client to continue the prescribed Aldactone dose and report any signs or symptoms of hypokalemia.

30. What individual is the best candidate to take acetazolamide (Diamox)?
    a. 50-year-old with open-angle glaucoma
    b. 75-year-old with narrow-angle glaucoma
    c. 60-year-old with acute glaucoma
    d. 58-year-old with acute heart failure

31. What type of acid-base imbalance could occur if a client is taking high doses of Diamox or uses the drug constantly?
    a. respiratory acidosis
    b. respiratory alkalosis
    c. metabolic alkalosis
    d. metabolic acidosis

32. Why would a client be prescribed Diamox to take when mountain climbing?
    a. for maintaining potassium levels
    b. for preventing high-altitude sickness
    c. for preventing dehydration
    d. for increasing endurance when climbing mountains

33. How often is HydroDIURIL generally scheduled to be taken?
    a. q2h
    b. q4h
    c. q6h
    d. daily

34. What is the usual dose of HydroDIURIL?
    a. 25-100 mg/day
    b. 100-150 mg/day
    c. 150-200 mg/day
    d. 200-250 mg/day

35. What is the optimal time to administer diuretics?
    a. at bedtime
    b. with meals
    c. on an empty stomach
    d. in the morning

36. While an 80-year-old client is taking HydroDIURIL, which laboratory values should be monitored? (Select all that apply.)
    a. serum calcium
    b. uric acid
    c. blood sugar
    d. alkaline phosphatase
    e. BUN

37. The nurse assesses the client taking Hy-droDIURIL for side effects. What might the nurse expect to see if the client is experiencing side effects? (Select all that apply.)
    a. electrolyte imbalances
    b. dizziness
    c. diarrhea
    d. headache

38. Which drug-lab values interactions are caused by thiazides? (Select all that apply.)
    a. enhance action of lithium
    b. enhance hypertensive state when used with alcohol
    c. potentiate other antihypertensives
    d. cause hypokalemia

39. What foods should the nurse recommend that the client taking HydroDIURIL include in his diet? (Select all that apply.)
    a. oranges
    b. dates
    c. apples
    d. bananas

40. What is priority health teaching information that should be included in a health teaching plan for the client taking HydroDIURIL? (Select all that apply.)
    a. maintaining nutrition
    b. advising the client to arise slowly to a standing position
    c. monitoring pulse and respiratory rates
    d. weighing daily

41. In which client are thiazide diuretics contraindicated for use?
    a. 40-year-old with emphysema
    b. 68-year-old with arteriosclerotic cardiovascular disease
    c. 45-year-old with renal failure
    d. 72-year-old with liver failure

42. The nurse should encourage clients taking a loop (high-ceiling) diuretic to include which foods in their diet? (Select all that apply.)
    a. fresh and dry fruits
    b. ice cream
    c. potato skins
    d. peanut butter
    e. bread

43. Which nursing intervention(s) should be implemented for clients who are hypertensive and receiving a thiazide diuretic? (Select all that apply.)
    a. Assess extremities for pitting edema.
    b. Monitor lung sounds.
    c. Monitor laboratory results.
    d. Encourage fluids.
    e. Monitor vital signs.

Case Study

Select the best answer.

A.D., age 56 years, is hypertensive. She has maturity-onset diabetes mellitus. Vital signs: blood pressure 162/90 mm Hg, pulse 90 beats/min, respiratory rate 24 breaths/min. A.D. was prescribed hydrochlorothiazide (HydroDIURIL) 50 mg daily.

1. A.D. is prescribed an oral antidiabetic (hypoglycemic) drug. What should concern the nurse about this drug being added to A.D.'s drug regimen?
    a. The client's blood glucose level will decrease so her antidiabetic medication will have to be increased.
    b. The client's blood glucose level will increase so her antidiabetic medication will have to be increased.
    c. The client's diuresis will increase so her diuretic will have to be increased
    d. The client's diuresis will decrease so her diuretic will have to be decreased.

2. What type of diuretic is hydrochlorothiazide (HydroDIURIL)?
    a. thiazide
    b. loop
    c. osmotic
    d. potassium-sparing

3. What are the similarities and differences in the actions of thiazide diuretics and loop diuretics?

    a. Thiazides act on the loop of Henle and the loop diuretics act on the collecting tubule.

    b. Thiazides act on the distal tubule and the loop diuretics act on the loop of Henle.

    c. Thiazides work on the collecting tubule and the loop diuretics act on the loop of Henle.

    d. Thiazides work on the distal tubule and the loop diuretics work on the collecting ducts.

4. What is the impact of thiazide diuretics and loop diuretics on blood electrolytes?

    a. Thiazides increase potassium while loop diuretics increase sodium.

    b. Thiazides increase sodium while loop diuretics lower the serum calcium levels.

    c. Thiazides increase serum calcium levels while loop diuretics lower calcium levels.

    d. Thiazides increase magnesium levels while loop diuretics lower magnesium levels.

5 . What priority instruction should be provided to A.D. before discharge? (Select all that apply.)

    a. She will need to check her blood glucose levels more frequently.

    b. She will need to eat foods rich in potassium.

    c. She will have to increase her sodium intake.

    d. She should change positions slowly to prevent a blood pressure drop.

    e. She should use sunscreen whenever she is outside.

Digoxin 0.25 mg daily was added to A.D.'s drug regimen. Her serum potassium level is 3.7 mEq/L.

6. What should concern the nurse about this value?

    a. Nothing; it is within the normal values.

    b. It could lead to digitalis toxicity.

    c. It is too low for digitalis to work properly.

    d. It will lead to increased diuresis.

7. The nurse is assessing A.D. and notes that she has a heart rate of 60 beats/min, is not eating, and has blurred vision. What should the nurse suspect is occurring in this client?

    a. decreasing potassium levels

    b. decreasing fluid volume

    c. digitalis toxicity

    d. potassium toxicity

44 Antihypertensives

Study Questions

Crossword puzzle: Use the definitions to determine the correct terms.

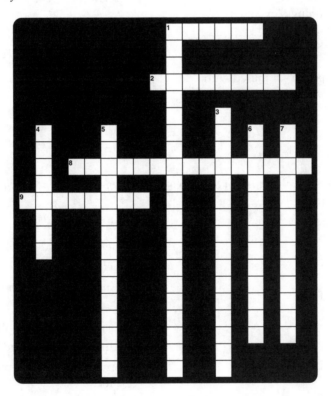

Across
1. Site of ANP and BNP release
2. Most common antihypertension agent for stage I disease
8. Nonpharmacologic method to decrease blood pressure (2 words)
9. Frequent side effect of ACE inhibitors

Down
1. A type of antihypertensive drug for clients who can't take ACE inhibitors (3 words)
3. Cultural group that does not respond well to beta blockers (2 words)
4. An example of a cardioselective alpha blocker
5. Can be combined with an ACE inhibitor (2 words)
6. An arteriolar vasodilator used in a hypertensive crisis
7. Vital sign that should be taken prior to starting an antihypertensive (2 words)

Complete the following.

10. When hypertension cannot be controlled by nonpharmacologic means, antihypertensive drugs may be prescribed. Three of the sympatholytic groups are _____, _____, and _____.

11. Three additional categories of antihypertensives in addition to the sympatholytics are _____, _____, and _____.

12. The Joint National Committee on Prevention, Detection, Evaluation, and Treatment of High Blood Pressure (JNC-7) uses three classifications for defining elevated systolic blood pressure (SBP): _____, _____, and _____.

13. Thiazide diuretics may be combined with other antihypertensive agents such as _____ and _____.

14. Many antihypertensive drugs can cause fluid retention. To decrease body fluid, the drug group often administered with antihypertensive drugs is _____.

15. A client with a blood pressure of 182/105 mm Hg has what stage of hypertension according to JNC-7? _____

16. Beta-adrenergic blockers reduce cardiac output by diminishing the sympathetic nervous system response. With continued use of beta blockers, vascular resistance is (increased/diminished) and blood pressure is (lowered/increased). (Circle correct answers.)

17. Atenolol and metoprolol are examples of (cardioselective/noncardioselective) antihypertensive drugs. (Circle correct answer.)

18. The alpha blockers are useful in treating hypertensive clients with lipid abnormalities. The effects they have on lipoproteins include _____ and _____.

Match the generic drug name in Column I with the category of antihypertensive in Column II.

Column I

_____ 19. Captopril

_____ 20. Verapamil

_____ 21. Prazosin

_____ 22. Methyldopa

_____ 23. Hydralazine

_____ 24. Candesartan

Column II

a. Beta blocker

b. Selective alpha blocker

c. Angiotensin antagonist (ACE inhibitor)

d. Calcium blocker

e. Centrally acting sympatholytic

f. Direct-acting vasodilator

g. Angiotensin II receptor antagonist (A-II blocker)

NCLEX Review Questions

Select the best response.

25. The JNC-7 has developed guidelines for determining hypertension. What are the blood pressure readings for someone who is in the category of prehypertension?
    a. less than 120 mm Hg/less than 80 mm Hg
    b. 120-139 mm Hg/80-89 mm Hg
    c. 140-159 mm Hg/90-99 mm Hg
    d. greater than 160 mm Hg/greater than 100 mm Hg

26. A cardioselective beta-adrenergic blocker is also known by which other term?
    a. alpha blocker agent
    b. beta blocker agent
    c. alpha-beta blocker agent
    d. beta-angiotensin agent

27. What client would be most suited for treatment with a nonselective alpha-adrenergic blocker?
    a. 50-year-old with mild to moderate renal failure
    b. 55-year-old with a severe hypertension caused by adrenal medulla tumor
    c. 45-year-old with hyperlipidemia
    d. 46-year-old with type II diabetes

28. Where in the body do direct-acting vasodilators act to decrease blood pressure?
    a. smooth muscles of the blood vessels
    b. skeletal muscles
    c. renal tubules
    d. cardiac valves

29. With use of direct-acting vasodilators, sodium and water are retained, and peripheral edema occurs. Which category of drugs should be given to avoid fluid retention?
    a. anticoagulants
    b. antidysrhythmics
    c. cardiac glycosides
    d. diuretics

30. Which are actions of angiotensin II receptor blockers (ARBs)? (Select all that apply.)
    a. blocks angiotensin II
    b. increases sodium retention
    c. causes vasodilation
    d. decreases peripheral resistance

31. An ARB can be combined with the thiazide diuretic HydroDIURIL. What is the purpose of combining these two drugs?
    a. decrease rapid blood pressure drop
    b. promote potassium retention
    c. enhance the antihypertensive effect by promoting sodium and water loss
    d. increase sodium and water retention for controlling blood pressure

32. ARBs may be prescribed for hypertensive clients instead of an ACE inhibitor. What is the most limiting factor in the use of ACE inhibitors?
    a. coughing
    b. sneezing
    c. dizziness
    d. shortness of breath

33. Which client's orders should the nurse question if the client was prescribed an ACE inhibitor?
    a. 49-year-old Hispanic man
    b. 60-year-old Asian woman
    c. 45-year-old white woman
    d. 48-year-old African-American woman

34. ACE inhibitors can be effective for treating hypertension in African Americans if the ACE inhibitor is given with which other drug?
    a. beta blocker
    b. calcium blocker
    c. angiotensin II blocker
    d. diuretic

35. Herb-drug interactions may occur if the client is taking certain herbal supplements. An herb history should be obtained. What may occur in an individual who also uses ma huang or ephedra with an antihypertensive drug?
    a. an increase in the hypertensive state
    b. a decrease or counteraction of the effects of the antihypertensive drug
    c. an increase in the hypotensive effects of the antihypertensive drug
    d. no effect on the action of the antihypertensive drug

36. Captopril is from which group of antihypertensives?
    a. beta blocker
    b. calcium blocker
    c. direct-acting vasodilator
    d. angiotensin antagonist (ACE inhibitor)

37. What is the action of captopril?
    a. dilation the arteries
    b. inhibit angiotensin II (a vasoconstrictor)
    c. increase in sodium and water excretion
    d. inhibit the alpha receptors

38. What is the protein-binding power of captopril?
    a. highly protein-bound
    b. moderately to highly protein-bound
    c. moderately protein-bound
    d. low protein-bound

39. A 59-year-old client has essential hypertension. He is taking captopril 25 mg t.i.d. If the client takes captopril with a highly protein-bound drug, what might occur?
    a. There will be no drug displacement, because captopril is not highly protein-bound.
    b. There will be moderate drug displacement of captopril, which is moderately to highly protein-bound.
    c. Captopril and the highly protein-bound drug will compete for protein sites.
    d. The concentration of captopril will be increased.

40. A client takes captopril with nitrates, diuretics, or adrenergic blockers. What might the nurse assess in this client?
    a. hypertensive reaction
    b. hypotensive reaction
    c. no effect
    d. hypoglycemic reaction

41. Which group of individuals should not be prescribed captopril?
    a. children
    b. Caucasians
    c. older adults
    d. African Americans

42. If a client takes captopril with a potassium-sparing diuretic, what might occur?
    a. hypokalemia
    b. hyperkalemia
    c. hypocalcemia
    d. hypercalcemia

43. A client states that he wishes to stop taking captopril for his hypertension. How might the nurse respond?
    a. "Yes, you could stop taking captopril now because your blood pressure has been normal."
    b. "Yes, you can stop taking the drug for a month and see how it affects your blood pressure."
    c. "No, you should not stop taking the drug until you speak with your health care provider because the drug is controlling your blood pressure."
    d. "Yes, you may stop taking captopril if you exercise regularly and avoid salt."

44. A client's antihypertensive drug was changed from captopril to nifedipine (Procardia) 10 mg t.i.d. What type of antihypertensive drug is nifedipine?
    a. beta blocker
    b. calcium blocker
    c. angiotensin antagonist
    d. centrally acting sympatholytic

45. What is the protein-binding power of nifedipine?
    a. highly protein-bound
    b. moderately to highly protein-bound
    c. moderately protein-bound
    d. low protein-bound

46. The nurse is assessing the client with essential hypertension following the shift report. What might the nurse assess if the client is experiencing side effects from his medications? (Select all that apply.)
    a. dizziness
    b. lightheadedness
    c. headache
    d. increased blood pressure

47. Amlodipine (Norvasc) is what type of drug?
    a. diuretic
    b. ACE inhibitor
    c. angiotensin II blocker
    d. calcium channel blocker

48. What action does Norvasc have in the body?
    a. vasoconstriction
    b. vasodilation
    c. increased peripheral vascular resistance
    d. peripheral clotting

49. What is the protein-binding power of Norvasc?
    a. highly protein-bound
    b. moderately protein-bound
    c. low protein-bound
    d. has a very short half-life

50. The client taking Norvasc complains of swelling in his ankles. What is the nurse's best response to his concern?
    a. "Swelling is common when taking Norvasc. You should cut the tablet in half to reduce your dosage."
    b. "You should not be taking that drug because of your age. I will see what other antihypertensive drug you can take."
    c. "Swelling may occur with Norvasc. I will contact your health care provider to determine if the drug should be changed or if another drug should be added."
    d. "You should stop taking the drug for several days and check that the swelling has decreased."

51. What classification of drug is Zebeta?
    a. diuretic
    b. beta blocker
    c. calcium blocker
    d. ACE inhibitor

52. What classification of drug is Procardia?
    a. diuretic
    b. beta blocker
    c. calcium blocker
    d. ACE inhibitor

53. What classification of drug is Pindolol?
    a. diuretic
    b. beta blocker
    c. calcium blocker
    d. ACE inhibitor

54. What are the advantage(s) of using beta-adrenergic blockers as an antihypertensive? (Select all that apply.)
    a. increase serum electrolyte levels
    b. minimize hypoglycemic effect
    c. maintain renal blood flow
    d. help prevent bronchoconstriction
    e. can be abruptly discontinued without causing rebound symptoms
    f. prevent hypolipidemia

55. ARBs have gained popularity for treating hypertension. Which are example(s) of ARB agents? (Select all that apply.)
    a. irbesartan (Avapro)
    b. losartan potassium (Cozaar)
    c. valsartan (Diovan)
    d. lisinopril (Prinivil)
    e. metoprolol (Lopressor)

56. A new antihypertensive agent/group, the direct renin inhibitors, has been approved by the FDA for treatment of hypertension. Which statement(s) best describe(s) this drug? (Select all that apply.)
    a. It is effective for treating severe hypertension.
    b. It can be combined with another antihypertensive drug such as an ARB.
    c. It can cause hypokalemia when taken as a monotherapy drug.
    d. Aliskiren (Tekturna) is an example of a direct renin inhibitor.
    e. Telmisartan (Micardis) is an example of a direct renin inhibitor.
    f. Diazoxide (Hyperstat) is an example of a direct renin inhibitor.

Case Study

Select the best answer.

S.H., 82 years old, has essential hypertension. He is taking atenolol (Tenormin) 25 mg daily and hydrochlorothiazide 25 mg daily. His vital signs are BP 138/88 mm Hg, P 74 beats/min, R 22 breaths/min. He lives by himself and is visited by a caregiver for 4 hours each morning and 4 hours each evening. The caregiver assists S.H. with his medication and food.

1. What type of antihypertensive agent is atenolol (Tenormin)?
    a. alpha-adrenergic blocker
    b. beta-blocker
    c. calcium blocker
    d. ACE inhibitor

2. S.H. asks the nurse, "How does the atenolol decrease my blood pressure?" What is the best answer the nurse can give?
    a. "It blocks the heart from stimulation by the cranial nerves."
    b. "It decreases the responsiveness of the renin-angiotensin-aldosterone system."
    c. "It blocks the beta$_1$-adrenergic receptors in the heart."
    d. "It increases urinary output."

3. Why would this drug be ordered for S.H.?
    a. It helps to lower blood pressure by blocking the renin system.
    b. It helps to lower blood pressure by increasing the heart rate.
    c. It helps to lower the blood pressure by decreasing fluid volume.
    d. It helps to lower blood pressure by also blocking the alpha-adrenergic receptors.

4. What type of electrolyte imbalance may occur with the use of hydrochlorothiazide?
    a. hypercalcemia
    b. hypocalcemia
    c. hyperkalemia
    d. hypokalemia

5. What important client teaching points should the nurse discuss with S.H.'s caregiver? (Select all that apply.)
    a. That it is important for S.H. to adhere to the drug regimen.
    b. That S.H. should be sure to eat potassium-rich foods daily.
    c. That the caregiver should check S.H.'s blood pressure every day.
    d. That S.H. should get adequate amounts of rest and exercise for someone his age.

6. When administering medications, the nurse should be careful not to confuse atenolol and amlodipine. What change might occur if amlopidine is given instead of atenolol?
    a. hyperglycemia
    b. excessive potassium and fluid loss
    c. hypernatremia and fluid retention
    d. increased heart rate and fluid volume loss

7. The nurse is assessing S.H. If he were experiencing side effects of atenolol, what might the nurse assess? (Select all that apply.)

   a. dizziness
   b. diarrhea
   c. fatigue
   d. slow heart rate
   e. cold extremities

8. For S.H., which laboratory tests should be monitored regularly? (Select all that apply.)

   a. serum electrolytes
   b. BUN and creatinine levels
   c. liver enzymes
   d. cardiac enzymes

9. S.H.'s caregiver is very interested in herbal supplements and wants to know what will happen if S.H. takes licorice, goldenseal, parsley, and hawthorne. What should the nurse know about these supplements? (Select all that apply.)

   a. Hawthorne may decrease the effects of beta-blockers.
   b. Licorice antagonizes the effects of antihypertensive drugs.
   c. Goldenseal may increase the effects of antihypertensives.
   d. Parsley may increase the cause of hypotension when taken with an antihypertensive drug.

10. What priority teaching information should the nurse provide to S.H.'s caregiver upon discharge from the hospital? (Select all that apply.)

   a. "Do not use any OTC preparations or herbs without consulting his health care provider."
   b. "S.H. needs a Medic-Alert bracelet just in case he needs to go to the hospital without you."
   c. "Be sure to increase S.H.'s fluid volume intake."
   d. "Be sure S.H. remains on a low-fat, low-salt diet."

45 Anticoagulants, Antiplatelets, and Thrombolytics

Study Questions

Complete the following word search. Clues are given below. Circle your responses.

```
J B S J A G G R E G A T I O N U O
V M L K I N W P O F L W Y W W I L
A S I S Y L O N I R B I F Q H E D
D V T N G M X L U S P C G X Z T U
Q F S R R W A R L K C Q U U H S S
B T L K O H B P V D G H Z I H I E
Q S R A P K V W D Q C G E F S Q A
W T P N Q F E J W G L V D M I O U
T A N T I C O A G U L A N T I D U
Q F Y X K C K P Y M K H H H B A W
J F U C I T Y L O B M O R H T G Y
```

a. Clumping together of platelets to form a clot
b. Inhibits blood clot formation
c. Breakdown of fibrin for preventing clot formation
d. Lack of blood supply to tissues
e. Category of drugs used to destroy blood clot formation
f. Antiplatelets are prescribed to prevent myocardial infarction and _____

Locate and circle the abbreviations for:

g. International Normalized Ratio
h. Low-molecular-weight heparin
i. Deep vein thrombosis
j. Prothrombin time

Complete the following.

1. A thrombus can form in a(n) _____ and in a(n) _____.

2. Anticoagulants are used to inhibit _____.

3. Anticoagulants and thrombolytics (have/ do not have) the same action. (Circle correct answer.)

4. The most frequent use of heparin is to prevent _____.

5. Heparin can be given (orally/subcutaneously/intravenously). (Circle correct answers.)

6. The new low molecular weight heparins (LMWHs) are derivatives of _____. The advantage of the use of LMWHs is to _____.

7. The International Normalized Ratio (INR) is a laboratory test to monitor the therapeutic effect of (warfarin/heparin). (Circle correct answer.)

8. Heparin can (decrease/increase) the platelet count, causing thrombocytopenia. (Circle correct answer.)

9. A thrombus disintegrates when a thrombolytic drug is administered within _____ hours following an acute myocardial infarction.

10. The action of the thrombolytic drugs streptokinase and urokinase is the conversion of _____ to _____.

11. The major complication with the use of thrombolytic drugs is _____.

12. A synthetic anticoagulant that indirectly inhibits thrombin production but is closely related in structure to heparin and LMWH is _____.

Match the drug in Column I with its drug group in Column II.

Column I

____ 13. Warfarin
____ 14. Aspirin
____ 15. Enovaparin (Lovenox)
____ 16. Dalteparin sodium (Fragmin)
____ 17. Protamine sulfate
____ 18. Clopidogrel (Plavix)
____ 19. Streptokinase
____ 20. Bivalirudin (Angiomax)
____ 21. Alteplase (tissue plasminogen activator [tPA])

Column II

a. Anticoagulant: LMWH
b. Direct thrombin inhibitor (parenteral)
c. Coumarin
d. Antiplatelet
e. Anticoagulant antagonist
f. Thrombolytic

NCLEX Review Questions

Select the best response.

22. What is the action of anticoagulants?
    a. dissolve blood clots
    b. administered with thrombolytics to dissolve blood clots
    c. prevent new clot formation
    d. promote clot formation

23. The nurse has several clients receiving warfarin therapy. Which INR should concern the nurse?
    a. 1.4
    b. 1.8
    c. 2.0
    d. 3.0

24. What is one of the primary reasons LMWHs are prescribed?
    a. prevention of cerebrovascular accident, or stroke
    b. enhancement of the action of warfarin
    c. prevention of deep vein thrombosis after knee or hip replacement surgery
    d. prevention of GI bleeding caused by a peptic ulcer

25. Which drug is not an LMWH?
    a. ardeparin (Normiflo)
    b. danaparoid (Organan)
    c. tinzaparin sodium (Innohep)
    d. clopidogrel (Plavix)

26. What is an example of an antiplatelet agent for angioplasty and acute coronary syndrome?
    a. abciximab
    b. protamine sulfate
    c. warfarin
    d. aminocaproic acid

27. Which statement best describes clopidogrel (Plavix)?
    a. It is more effective when prescribed singly as an antiplatelet drug.
    b. It is more effective when prescribed with aspirin after MI and stroke.
    c. It is an inexpensive antiplatelet drug for stroke.
    d. It is an antiplatelet drug that can be used instead of an anticoagulant drug.

28. The effects of heparin are monitored by which of the following laboratory test(s)?
    a. CBC and WBC
    b. PTT and aPTT
    c. PT and INR
    d. BUN

29. Enoxaparin sodium is an anticoagulant used to prevent and treat deep vein thrombosis and pulmonary embolism. To which category does this drug belong?
    a. standard heparin
    b. LMWH
    c. oral anticoagulant
    d. thrombolytic

30. In the event of hemorrhage, which medication is most likely to be administered intravenously?
    a. urea
    b. cimetidine
    c. phenytoin
    d. protamine sulfate

31. What is the protein-binding power of warfarin?
    a. highly protein-bound
    b. moderately to highly protein-bound
    c. moderately protein-bound
    d. low protein-bound

32. The client is given heparin for early treatment of deep vein thrombophlebitis. Later, warfarin (Coumadin) is prescribed. If the client is taking a highly protein-bound drug with warfarin, what might occur?
    a. no drug displacement of warfarin or the highly protein-bound drug
    b. moderate drug displacement of warfarin, which is moderately protein-bound
    c. drug displacement of warfarin, which is also highly protein-bound
    d. drug displacement of the highly protein-bound drug but not displacement of warfarin

33. Which medication is administered to decrease bleeding and increase clotting for bleeding resulting from excess free Coumadin?
    a. vitamin E
    b. vitamin K
    c. glucagon
    d. calcium gluconate

34. Which medication, if given with heparin, should concern the nurse? (Select all that apply.)
    a. aspirin
    b. oral hypoglycemics
    c. phenytoin
    d. over-the-counter antacid

35. What priority information should be included in the health teaching plan for a client taking Coumadin for early treatment of deep vein thrombophlebitis? (Select all that apply.)
    a. importance of compliance with ongoing laboratory test regimen
    b. importance of reporting bleeding to the health care provider
    c. importance of taking aspirin instead of other analgesics for headache
    d. the importance of using an electric razor versus a conventional razor to shave

36. A 51-year-old client in the emergency department is receiving streptokinase. What might the nurse assess in a client who is experiencing an allergic reaction to this drug? (Select all that apply.)
    a. nausea
    b. hives
    c. dyspnea
    d. bronchospasm

37. Which drug should the nurse have readily available as an antidote if a client experiences an allergic reaction to streptokinase?
    a. aminocaproic acid (Amicar)
    b. Apsac
    c. alteplase (tPA)
    d. calcium gluconate

38. Which nursing actions are best to include when caring for a client taking streptokinase? (Select all that apply.)
    a. Record vital signs and report changes.
    b. Observe for signs and symptoms of bleeding.
    c. Monitor liver enzymes.
    d. Assess for reperfusion dysrhythmias.

39. In which disorders are anticoagulants recommended for use? (Select all that apply.)
    a. coronary thrombosis
    b. renal failure
    c. pulmonary embolism
    d. cerebrovascular accidents (CVAs)
    e. esophageal varices

40. Which priority nursing interventions should be implemented for clients taking warfarin? (Select all that apply.)
    a. Use a firm toothbrush when cleaning teeth and gums.
    b. Suggest the client carries a medical ID card or wears ID jewelry indicating that he/she is taking warfarin.
    c. Inform the client that smoking does not influence warfarin dose.
    d. Instruct the client that the health care provider should be notified before taking OTC drugs.
    e. Inform the client that many herbal products interact with warfarin.
    f. Advise the client to report bleeding, such as petechiae, ecchymoses, purpura, tarry stools, bleeding gums, or expectoration of blood.

41. Which priority nursing interventions should be included for all clients receiving anticoagulants? (Select all that apply.)
    a. Regularly monitor vital signs.
    b. Monitor drug specific lab values. PTT
    c. Monitor client for bleeding—check gums, puncture sites, increases in bruising.
    d. Keep antagonists readily available.
    e. Protect the client from injury.

Case Study

Select the best answer.

B.C., age 63 years, had a myocardial infarction. While hospitalized, he received heparin 5000 units subcutaneously q6h for 5 days. Heparin is available as 5000 units/mL and 10,000 units/mL. On the fifth day, warfarin 5 mg daily was started. His INR is 2.7.

1. The nurse is administering B.C.'s heparin, and B.C. asks why he can't take the medication as a pill. What is the best response?
   a. "You can take it as a pill. We will prescribe it for you when you are discharged."
   b. "You can take it as a pill later. Right now we must increase your blood level of the medication."
   c. "This medication is poorly absorbed in the gut, so it has to be given by injection to have any impact."
   d. "This medication is not available in an oral form. It is supplied only as an injection."

2. What laboratory testing is used to monitor heparin doses?
   a. PTT and aPTT
   b. INR
   c. Hgb and Hct
   d. CBC

3. Which laboratory finding should concern the nurse caring for B.C.?
   a. aPTT 100 seconds
   b. aPTT 75 seconds
   c. PTT 75 seconds
   d. PTT 90 seconds

4. How many tablet(s) of warfarin (Coumadin) should the nurse administer to B.C. per day if each tablet contains 2.5 mg of warfarin?
   a. ½ tablet
   b. 1 tablet
   c. 1½ tablets
   d. 2 tablets

5. What should the nurse assess for if suspecting that B.C. is experiencing side effects associated with use of warfarin? (Select all that apply.)
   a. bleeding—gums, skin, gastric
   b. anorexia
   c. diarrhea
   d. headache
   e. fever

6. What client teaching is essential for B.C. when he is taking warfarin? (Select all that apply.)
   a. "Use a soft toothbrush, and don't brush your teeth too vigorously."
   b. "Assess your skin for increased bruising and bleeding."
   c. "Keep appointments with your health care provider to check INR."
   d. "Keep your medication follow-up appointments."
   e. "Place padding on your home's floor to protect you in case you fall."

46 Antihyperlipidemics and Peripheral Vasodilators

Study Questions

Crossword puzzle: Use the definitions to determine the correct terms.

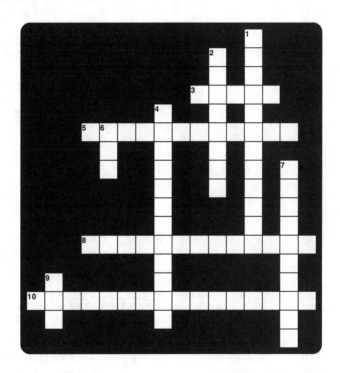

Across

3. Time frame before antilipidemic medications lower cholesterol levels
5. One of the bad types of cholesterol
8. Vitamin that is effective in lowering low-density lipoproteins (LDLs) (2 words)
10. Area of the most common discomfort associated with antilipidemics

Down

1. Herb taken for intermittent claudication (2 words)
2. A nonpharmacologic intervention that decreases LDLs and increases high-density lipoproteins (HDLs)
4. A high level of this has been related to cardiovascular disease and stroke
6. Abbreviation for the "friendly" lipoproteins
7. A decreased libido may be experienced with this drug
9. This should be decreased in dietary intake with high cholesterol

Match the drug in Column I with its drug group in Column II.

Column I	Column II
___ 11. Colestipol hydrochloride	a. Statins
___ 12. Gemfibrozil (Lopid)	b. Bile-acid sequestrant
___ 13. Atorvastatin (Lipitor)	c. Fibrates
___ 14. Simvastatin (Zocor)	d. Cholesterol absorption inhibitors
___ 15. Cholestyramine resin (Questran)	
___ 16. Ezetimibe (Zetia)	

NCLEX Review Questions

Select the best response.

17. Elevated apolipoproteins can be an indicator of LDL and coronary heart disease (CHD). Which Apo is an indicator of low-density lipoprotein that could lead to CHD?
    a. Apo A-1
    b. Apo A-2
    c. Apo B
    d. Apo C

18. What would the nurse observe if she were assessing a client for a severe side effect of a statin drug?
    a. rhabdomyolysis
    b. headache
    c. diarrhea
    d. convulsions

19. Homocysteine is a protein in the blood that has been linked to cardiovascular disease and stroke. What other negative action may it also promote?
    a. blood clotting
    b. urine retention
    c. increased blood flow
    d. lowering of lipid levels

20. Which herb has been taken for intermittent claudication, although it has not been approved by the FDA?
    a. St. John's wort
    b. ginkgo biloba
    c. ginger
    d. ginseng

21. What is the standard preferred level of overall cholesterol?
    a. less than 100 mg/dl
    b. less than 150 mg/dl
    c. less than 200 mg/dl
    d. less than 250 mg/dl

22. What is the standard preferred level of LDL?
    a. less than 50 mg/dl
    b. less than 80 mg/dl
    c. less than 130 mg/dl
    d. less than 150 mg/dl

23. What is the standard preferred level of HDL?
    a. greater than 24 mg/dl
    b. greater than 45 mg/dl
    c. greater than 60 mg/dl
    d. greater than 100 mg/dl

24. Why might a client's serum lipids not drop after 2 months of a low-fat and low-cholesterol diet?
    a. The client most likely did not adhere to the diet.
    b. Diet modification usually decreases cholesterol levels by only 10% to 30%.
    c. The client lost less than 10 pounds on the diet.
    d. The client's exercise program should have been increased.

25. A client is prescribed simvastatin (Zocor). She asks if she can eat whatever she wants now that she's taking Zocor. What is the nurse's best response?
    a. "Yes, you may eat whatever you want as long as you take Zocor."
    b. "Diet is not an important factor if you take Zocor and exercise."
    c. "You should maintain a low-fat and low-cholesterol diet and exercise."
    d. "With Zocor, diet is not important, but you should lose weight through exercise."

26. Vasodilan is prescribed for peripheral vascular disease. It is also prescribed for treatment of which conditions? (Select all that apply.)
    a. transient ischemic attack
    b. Raynaud's disease
    c. Buerger's disease
    d. Paget's disease

27. What is the usual dose of Vasodilan?
    a. 10-20 mg t.i.d.
    b. 20-30 mg t.i.d.
    c. 30-40 mg t.i.d.
    d. 40-50 mg t.i.d.

28. What priority information should the nurse include in the health teaching plan for a client taking Vasodilan for peripheral vascular disease? (Select all that apply.)
    a. Take medications with meals.
    b. Avoid use of alcohol and smoking.
    c. Do not take aspirin.
    d. Monitor for side effects including flushing, headache, and dizziness.
    e. Take your blood pressure weekly.

29. Which antilipidemics other than the statins are prescribed for reducing cholesterol and LDL levels? (Select all that apply.)
    a. bile-acid sequestrants
    b. alpha-adrenergic antagonists
    c. direct thrombin inhibitors
    d. nicotinic acid
    e. antiplatelets
    f. cholesterol absorption inhibitors

30. What type of medication is rosuvastatin (Crestor)? (Select all that apply.)
    a. HMG-CoA reductase inhibitor
    b. cholesterol absorption inhibitor
    c. statin drug
    d. combination of two antilipidemics
    e. bile-acid sequestrant

31. The client is receiving Crestor 5 mg PO daily. Crestor 10 mg tablets are available. How many tablets should the nurse administer?
    a. ½ tablet
    b. 1 tablet
    c. 1½ tablets
    d. 2 tablets

Case Study

Select the best answer.

R.T.'s cholesterol level is 267 mg/dl. Her LDL level is 146 mg/dl, and her HDL level is 44 mg/dl. She is 36 years old. R.T. was initially prescribed atorvastatin (Lipitor) 10 mg daily, and later the dosage was increased to 20 mg daily.

1. R.T. wants to know why she as been prescribed a medication to lower her cholesterol. She says that her levels are "not that bad." What is the nurse's best response?
    a. "You're right; your cholesterol level isn't that bad. Let me check with the physician."
    b. "Your cholesterol level is just a little too high, and it needs to be lowered."
    c. "Your cholesterol level should be less than 200 mg/dl, and yours is higher than that."
    d. "Your cholesterol is very high and the physician wants to decrease it to less than 100 mg/dl."

2. Why is R.T. receiving atorvastatin?
    a. increase her HDL level
    b. decrease her cholesterol level
    c. decrease her HDL level
    d. increase her LDL level

3. R.T. wants to know what to do if she decides she wants to get pregnant. What is the nurse's best response?

    a. "You should get your cholesterol level lower before you decide to get pregnant."

    b. "You should have no problems getting pregnant while taking this medication."

    c. "You should not get pregnant while taking this medication."

    d. "If you decide to get pregnant, we will need to decrease the amount of medication you're currently taking."

4. What is the protein-binding power of atorvastatin?

    a. highly protein-bound

    b. moderately to highly protein-bound

    c. moderately protein-bound

    d. low protein-bound

5. If R.T. was taking a highly protein-bound drug with atorvastatin, what might occur?

    a. no drug displacement of atorvastatin or the highly protein-bound drug

    b. moderate drug displacement of atorvastatin

    c. drug displacement of atorvastatin and the other drug

    d. drug displacement of the highly protein-bound drug but not of atorvastatin

6. R.T. wants to know when she should take atorvastatin. How should the nurse respond?

    a. Weekly

    b. Every third day

    c. Every other day

    d. Daily at any time chosen by the patient

7. What laboratory test(s) should be monitored while R.T. is taking atorvastatin? (Select all that apply.)

    a. serum lever enzymes

    b. Hgb and Hct

    c. WBC

    d. cholesterol levels

8. What client teaching is essential for R.T.'s drug therapy? (Select all that apply.)

    a. R.T. should be encouraged to lose weight with a calorie-restriction diet.

    b. R.T. should eat foods that are low in cholesterol and saturated fat.

    c. R.T. should have her liver enzymes checked periodically.

    d. R.T. should maintain her follow-up appointments with health care provider.

    e. R.T. should increase her level of exercise if possible.

47 Drugs for Gastrointestinal Tract Disorders

Study Questions

Match the words in Column I with the description they are most associated with in Column II.

Column I

_____ 1. Adsorbents
_____ 2. Cannabinoids
_____ 3. Chemoreceptor trigger zone (CTZ)
_____ 4. Emetics
_____ 5. Opiates
_____ 6. Osmotics
_____ 7. Purgatives

Column II

a. Harsh cathartics that cause a watery stool with abdominal cramping
b. Induces vomiting (used after poisoning)
c. Hyperosmolar laxatives
d. Relieves chemotherapy-induced nausea/vomiting
e. Lies near the medulla
f. Adsorbs bacteria or toxins that cause diarrhea
g. Decreases intestinal motility, thereby decreasing peristalsis

Select the best response.

8. Which area(s) in the brain cause(s) vomiting when stimulated? (Select all that apply.)
   a. chemoreceptor trigger zone
   b. vomiting center
   c. nausea center
   d. vertigo center

9. What are the groupings of prescriptive antiemetics? (Select all that apply.)
   a. antihistamines
   b. anticholinergics
   c. opioids
   d. cannabinoids
   e. phenothiazines

10. How do most of the antiemetics work?
    a. They stimulate the dopamine receptors in the brain associated with vomiting.
    b. They simulate the histamine receptors which are associated with nausea.
    c. They block the acetylcholine receptors associated with vomiting.
    d. They block the norepinephrine receptors associated with nausea.

11. Which group of drugs should not be used until the cause of vomiting is identified?
    a. antihistamines
    b. anticholinergics
    c. phenothiazines
    d. absorbents

12. Which are nonpharmacologic methods to decrease nausea and vomiting? (Select all that apply.)
    a. Provide the client with weak tea to drink.
    b. Have the client sip flattened carbonated beverages.
    c. Provide the client with gelatin to eat.
    d. Have the client breathe out of the mouth rather than through the nose.

13. How long before traveling should the client take an over-the-counter (OTC) antihistamine such as Dramamine or a prescribed scopolamine transdermal patch?
    a. 15 minutes
    b. 30 minutes
    c. 45 minutes
    d. 60 minutes

14. The nurse has a pregnant client who asks what to do about morning sickness. What options should the nurse teach the client? (Select all that apply.)
    a. "Take an OTC antiemetic."
    b. "Sip flattened carbonated beverages."
    c. "Take an opioid."
    d. "Sip weak tea."

15. Which drugs are most commonly used to treat motion sickness?
    a. anticholinergics
    b. antihistamines
    c. cannabinoids
    d. osmotics

16. What is the major ingredient of the cannabinoids?
    a. morphine
    b. alcohol
    c. marijuana
    d. amphetamines

17. For which disease is diphenidol (Vontrol) recommended for symptoms of nausea, vomiting, and vertigo?
    a. Bell's palsy
    b. Parkinson's disease
    c. Meniere's disease
    d. renal disease

18. In addition to antiemetic effects, what does benzquinamide do?
    a. increase blood pressure
    b. decrease cardiac output
    c. increase heart rate
    d. decrease temperature

19. What should the nurse expect to occur after the administration of charcoal?
    a. vomiting
    b. gagging
    c. absorption of the poison
    d. abdominal pain

20. Which drugs are classified as antidiarrheals? (Select all that apply.)
    a. opiates
    b. proton pump inhibitors
    c. adsorbents
    d. anticholinergics

21. The client is receiving an opium preparation. Which common side effect might the nurse see in this client?
    a. diarrhea
    b. vomiting
    c. constipation
    d. abdominal cramping

22. What should concern the nurse caring for client who has been taking opiates and opiate-related drugs for an extensive period of time? (Select all that apply.)
    a. abuse
    b. major side effects
    c. tolerance
    d. misuse

23. What type of stool should the nurse expect in a client taking a laxative?
    a. hard and dry
    b. watery
    c. soft
    d. soft and watery

24. Which are types of laxatives/cathartics? (Select all that apply.)
    a. osmotic
    b. contact
    c. bulk-forming
    d. emollients
    e. stool softeners

25. How do contact laxatives/cathartics increase peristalsis?
    a. By increasing water in the gut
    b. By stimulating more smooth muscle contraction
    c. By irritating the gut
    d. By slowing the movement of food through the gut

26. What is the action of emollients in the intestine?
    a. irritation of the mucosa
    b. increasing peristalsis
    c. decreasing movement of food through the gut
    d. water accumulation

27. The prescription of saline cathartics should be questioned in which client?
    a. 38-year-old with diabetes
    b. 52-year-old with heart failure
    c. 48-year-old with PVD
    d. 50-year-old with COPD

28. Should the nurse be concerned about a client becoming dependent on bulk-forming laxatives?
    a. Yes; these types of laxatives significantly decrease peristalsis.
    b. No; there is no risk for dependence.
    c. Yes; the gut will no longer absorb the needed fluid for normal bowel movements.
    d. No; the gut will recover over time from changes due to this laxative.

29. The client is taking a mineral oil laxative. What should concern the nurse if the client takes this for a long period of time?
    a. decreased absorption of fat-soluble vitamins A, D, E, and K
    b. decreased absorption of fat-soluble vitamins A, C, E
    c. increased absorption of fats
    d. increased absorption of vitamin D

30. What priority instruction should be given to a client experiencing constipation? (Select all that apply.)
    a. "Increase water intake and eat foods rich in fiber."
    b. "Avoid cathartic-like drugs, which may cause electrolyte imbalance."
    c. "Increase the amount of exercise you do regularly."
    d. "Know that laxatives may cause urine discoloration."
    e. "Take a laxative every day until regularity returns."

NCLEX Review Questions

Select the best response.

31. What is an expected action of opiates?
    a. absorb toxic materials
    b. decrease intestinal motility
    c. gently stimulate peristalsis
    d. stimulate the chemoreceptor trigger zone

32. Which client should not use a laxative/cathartic?
    a. 60-year-old with heart disease
    b. 55-year-old with Parkinson's disease
    c. 48-year-old with cirrhosis
    d. 65-year-old with a bowel obstruction

33. A 50-year-old client is receiving prochlor-perazine (Compazine) for nausea and vomiting. Which dosage and route of Compazine should concern the nurse? (Select all that apply.)
    a.   5-10 mg q3-4h IM prn
    b.   10 mg SR PO q12h
    c.   5-25 mg supp every 4 hours PRN
    d.   25 mg q3h PRN

34. What might the nurse assess in a client experiencing side effects of Compazine? (Select all that apply.)
    a.   hypotension
    b.   excessive saliva
    c.   agitation
    d.   urinary retention

35. What priority nursing interventions should be implemented for a client receiving Compazine for nausea and vomiting? (Select all that apply.)
    a.   obtaining history of vomiting
    b.   monitoring vital signs and bowel sounds
    c.   encouraging fluids
    d.   maintaining oral hygiene

36. Which priority information should be included in the health teaching plan for a client receiving Compazine for nausea and vomiting? (Select all that apply.)
    a.   "You may wish to try nonpharmacologic methods to help the side effects."
    b.   "You should try to stay busy to keep your mind off the nausea."
    c.   "You should avoid driving or operating hazardous machinery while taking Compazine."
    d.   "You should avoid alcohol while you are taking Compazine."

37. A client is taking dronabinol (Marinol) for nausea and vomiting caused by cancer chemotherapy. How should this drug be administered?
    a.   1-3 hours before and for 24 hours after chemotherapy
    b.   12 hours before and for 24 hours after chemotherapy
    c.   q3-4h PRN
    d.   q6h PRN

38. What is the usual adult dose of dronabinol?
    a.   1-2 mg
    b.   3-4 mg
    c.   5-7 mg
    d.   8-10 mg

39. Which client should not be prescribed antidiarrheals?
    a.   65-year-old with congestive heart failure
    b.   56-year-old with COPD
    c.   46-year-old with diabetes
    d.   66-year-old with liver disease

40. The client is experiencing severe diarrhea. What should the nurse monitor? (Select all that apply.)
    a.   electrolytes
    b.   vital signs
    c.   bowel sounds
    d.   WBC count

41. Which drug is a somatostatin analogue frequently prescribed for metastatic cancer-related severe diarrhea?
    a.   loperamide
    b.   octreotide (Sandostatin)
    c.   docusate potassium (Dialose)
    d.   psyllium

42. How much water should the nurse teach a client to mix with a bulk-forming laxative?
    a.   4 oz
    b.   8 oz
    c.   12 oz
    d.   16 oz

43. Use of opiate-related drugs for severe diarrhea may cause which side effects? (Select all that apply.)
    a.   drowsiness
    b.   constipation
    c.   paralytic ileus
    d.   urinary frequency
    e.   abdominal cramping

44. Which food products should a client with diarrhea avoid? (Select all that apply.)
    a. fried foods
    b. clear liquids
    c. bottled water
    d. raw vegetables
    e. milk products

45. Which foods should the nurse should encourage a client with constipation to eat? (Select all that apply.)
    a. hard cheese
    b. oat bran
    c. whole grains
    d. fresh fruit
    e. water

Case Study

Select the best answer.

L.B., age 85 years, comes to the clinic complaining, "I can't move my bowels." L.B. lives independently in a studio apartment in housing for older persons. Two months ago, she fell and fractured her hip. She is currently taking digoxin, an antacid, and a narcotic PRN for pain.

1. The nurse knows that constipation is a major problem in older persons. What are possible contributing factors to L.B.'s problem? (Select all that apply.)
    a. insufficient water intake
    b. poor dietary habits
    c. fecal impaction
    d. ignoring the urge to defecate
    e. regular exercise
    f. current medications

It is determined that L.B. does not have a fecal impaction, and bisacodyl 10 mg PO is ordered.

2. Is this dose within the therapeutic range? If no, why not? If so, what time of day should it be taken?
    a. Yes, in the morning.
    b. Yes, at the noon meal.
    c. No, it is too low.
    d. No, it is too high.

3. What is the mode of action of bisacodyl?
    a. It stimulates water absorption by the gut.
    b. It stimulates peristalsis through irritation of the gut.
    c. It stimulates the gut to increase the bulk of the stool.
    d. It stimulates peristalsis through effect on the gut's smooth muscles.

4. What is the mode of action of bulk-forming laxatives?
    a. They increase water drawn into the intestine.
    b. They stimulate peristalsis through irritation of the gut.
    c. They stimulate the gut to increase the bulk of the stool.
    d. They stimulate peristalsis through effect on the gut's smooth muscles.

5. Which clients should not use bisacodyl? (Select all that apply.)
    a. 30-year-old with intestinal/biliary obstruction
    b. 45-year-old with appendicitis
    c. 50-year-old with diabetes
    d. 60-year-old with CAD

6. The nurse is teaching L.B. about food and drug interactions. Which priority information should be part of L.B.'s health teaching? (Select all that apply.)

    a. "Limit the use of antacids because they decrease the effect of your medications."

    b. "Don't take the medications with milk or other dairy beverages."

    c. "Take your medications with orange or grapefruit juice."

    d. "Take your medications along with histamine blockers."

7. What specific instructions should the nurse give L.B. related to taking bisacodyl? (Select all that apply.)

    a. "Take the tablet with 8 ounces of water."

    b. "Do not take this drug within 1 hour of taking another drug."

    c. "Chew the tablet to help increase its absorption."

    d. "Take this drug early in the day to avoid disruption of sleep."

48 Antiulcer Drugs

Study Questions

Match the descriptor in Column I with the drug/factor in Column II. Use each term only once.

Column I

_____ 1. Risk factor for the development of peptic ulcer disease (PUD)

_____ 2. Neutralizes gastric acid

_____ 3. Inhibition of gastric acid secretion

_____ 4. Associated with recurrence of PUD

_____ 5. Used as mucoprotective in conjunction with NSAIDs

_____ 6. Binds free protein in base of ulcer

_____ 7. Eradication rates require addition of this antimicrobial

_____ 8. Causes antidiarrheal effect of some antacids

_____ 9. OTC agent used in combination to eradicate *H. pylori*

_____ 10. H$_2$ antagonist with multiple drug interactions

Column II

a. Pepto-Bismol

b. Magnesium hydroxide

c. *Helicobacter pylori*

d. Sucralfate

e. Cimetidine

f. Omeprazole

g. Misoprostol

h. Smoking

i. Antacids

j. Metronidazole

Match the drug in Column I with the category to which it belongs in Column II.

Column I

_____ 11. Rabeprazole

_____ 12. Ranitidine

_____ 13. Glycopyrrolate

_____ 14. Nizatidine

_____ 15. Esomeprazole magnesium

_____ 16. Sucralfate

_____ 17. Magaldrate

_____ 18. Famotidine

Column II

a. Anticholinergics

b. Antacid

c. Proton pump inhibitor

d. Histamine 2 blocker

e. Pepsin inhibitors

NCLEX Review Questions

Select the best response.

19. When is the most ideal time to administer an antacid?
    a. with meals and 1 hour after
    b. 1 hour before meals
    c. 1 and 3 hours after meals
    d. with meals

20. For best results, antacids should be taken with how many ounces of water?
    a. 2-4
    b. 4-6
    c. 6-8
    d. at least 8

21. Which drugs are often used in the treatment of gastric and duodenal ulcers?
    a. histamine blockers
    b. antacids
    c. pepsin inhibitors
    d. tranquilizers

22. Which group of drugs is used to prevent acid reflux in the esophagus? (Select all that apply.)
    a. antacids
    b. pepsin inhibitors
    c. prostaglandin analogues
    d. histamine blockers

23. Propantheline bromide (Pro-Banthine) belongs to which drug group?
    a. tranquilizers
    b. anticholinergics
    c. suppressors of gastric acid
    d. antacids

24. For best results, when should the nurse recommend Pro-Banthine to be administered?
    a. with meals
    b. before meals
    c. 2 hours after meals
    d. with two glasses of fluid

25. A client is being treated for peptic ulcers. She is taking Pro-Banthine. She is also receiving an antacid. When is the best time to administer the antacid?
    a. with belladonna
    b. 2 hours before meals
    c. 2 hours after meals
    d. with meals

26. Cimetidine may cause an increase in which laboratory tests?
    a. platelets
    b. BUN
    c. WBCs
    d. blood sugar

27. The enhancement of which drug effect is due to cimetidine?
    a. inhibiting hepatic metabolism
    b. inhibiting renal excretion
    c. prolonging the half-life
    d. displacing protein-binding sites

28. What is a synthetic prostaglandin analogue used for the prevention and treatment of peptic ulcers?
    a. Pepcid
    b. Zantac
    c. Indocin
    d. Cytotec

29. Which drug inhibits gastric acid secretions to a greater extent than histamine antagonists?
    a. Prilosec
    b. Pepcid
    c. Pro-Banthine
    d. Quarzan

30. Which drugs are proton pump inhibitors? (Select all that apply.)
    a. esomeprazole (Nexium)
    b. pantoprazole (Protonix)
    c. rabeprazole (AcipHex)
    d. none of the above

31. The client is taking Pro-Banthine. What side effects might the nurse assess? (Select all that apply.)
    a. bradycardia
    b. dry mouth
    c. constipation
    d. urinary retention
    e. decreased gastric secretions

32. Which assessment findings in a client taking cimetidine (Tagamet) should concern the nurse? (Select all that apply.)
    a. headache
    b. back pain
    c. nausea
    d. loss of libido
    e. gynecomastia

33. Which drugs or categories of drugs should concern the nurse if they are prescribed with cimetidine? (Select all that apply.)
    a. laxatives
    b. oral anticoagulants
    c. propranolol (Inderal)
    d. phenytoin (Dilantin)
    e. fluconazole (Diflucan)

Case Study

Select the best answer.

S.S., 63 years old, has a high-stress job as a county judge. She complains of abdominal distress after eating. She is currently taking aluminum hydroxide (Amphojel) 600 mg q4h (while awake).

1. Is this an appropriate dose for S.S. given her problems with stress and abdominal pain after eating?
    a. No; the administration times are wrong.
    b. No; the dose is too low.
    c. The amount is appropriate but the administration times are wrong.
    d. Yes, a high dosage is required for this client.

2. How should S.S. be taught to take this medication?
    a. every 4 hours with milk
    b. 1 hour ac and at bedtime
    c. 1 hour pc and at bedtime
    d. with meals and at bedtime

3. S.S. asks if there is a specific fluid she should use when taking this medication. What is the nurse's best response?
    a. "You should thoroughly chew the medication and then follow it with any fluid that you like."
    b. "You should swallow the pill whole with water or milk."
    c. "You should thoroughly chew the medication and then follow with water."
    d. "You should swallow the pill whole with any fluid you like."

4. S.S. is skeptical that this medication will relieve her gastric upset. She asks the nurse how this medication works. What is the nurse's best answer?
    a. "It works by neutralizing gastric acid."
    b. "It works by inhibiting histamine and the histamine receptors."
    c. "It works with gastric acid to form a protective barrier."
    d. "It blocks gastric acid production."

5. What other medications or category of medications, if prescribed for S.S., should be of concern to the nurse? (Select all that apply.)
    a. benzodiazepines
    b. isoniazid
    c. digitalis
    d. nizatidine
    e. phenytoin

6. What is a common side effect of aluminum hydroxide?
    a. diarrhea
    b. headache
    c. constipation
    d. abdominal pain

7. Which individual should not take aluminum hydroxise?
    a. 78-year-old with hypokalemia
    b. 56-year-old with hypernatremia
    c. 70-year-old with hypophosphatemia
    d. 45-year-old with hyperkalemia

8. The nurse is teaching S.S. about her medication and the amount of stress in her life. What priority dietary recommendations should the nurse give S.S.? (Select all that apply.)
    a. Avoid caffeine-containing beverages.
    b. Use salt sparingly.
    c. Avoid alcoholic beverages.
    d, Avoid orange and apple juice.

9. What priority health teaching should the nurse provide to S.S.? (Select all that apply.)
    a. "Don't use the prescribed drug every time you have gastric upset. Use it only as prescribed."
    b. "Drink at least 2 to 4 ounces of water after taking your antacid."
    c. "I will teach you how to use relaxation techniques to deal with stress."
    d. "You should have a glass of wine on the really stressful days."

49 Drugs for Eye and Ear Disorders

Study Questions

Complete the following word search. Clues are given in questions 1-15. Circle your responses.

```
C X C P I A I R U N A L K L W G Z C G M G P A A U N D Z Q Z F R
L N F E A I S X L A G O G D K K Y X P K V N P V S O P R Z D R I
S R O T I B I H N I E S A R D Y H N A C I N O B R A C L T E M Z
U E A S M S T V R P Z P D S D E U E I X X W A N E T L Q Q H L W
A Y D L F O I J C W D U S Z V H B Z T D N Y E M M J V L B Y N Y
K R E N M X N T E A R S B Q U P T E P C P R T G L G O L K D S P
L R S I E C T C I N C R E A S E T O B Z D V P B T O Q K D R N O
T S F L S I R M S V A M O C U A L G V L E T C J S U I J G A Q M
S B K U A I A J H C I Y O B B L J Z I J O Z H M I L W F X T Y T
N T J W E J O T W Z I T D Y K T M H F D O O O C C V Y P C I H K
I U X A R Z C W T R D T C O B H C F D S S T D V Z W H Y U O S U
Q W V A C C U T O I S V E N B B U N C E I S E S T C X A M N B H
N J Z V N Z L M I N B C V R U N N R S C C J B J U C L E P C P P
R D V Y I D A M A S W W E W U J G W S H C R H M K G C N F F Y I
L N P O E P R Y V B V N C A R I N I I B U N E L A Y A S Y R V Y
X L T Q S S B R R J A Q P I P K D O E I F O H A P X K R I D R O
E E B T E M F X G K L S E V S Y W E C R E Y W U S X Z T G Y D Q
Z C L R T W I P Z Q E A Y J X P D R J R O W F B I E R S P J O S
O B U L Q L B Z V N B D T U Y X D A Q Z Y F V X P L W G I Y V W
L Q X E W H C E A C Y C L O P L E G I C S K T O N U W I X W T F
```

1. Topical anesthetics are used during an eye exam and before removal of a _____ from the eye.

2. Lubricants are used to moisten contact lenses and/or to replace _____.

3. Miotics are used to lower _____ pressure.

4. Carbonic anhydrase inhibitors were developed as _____. They are effective in treating _____.

5. Osmotic drugs are used to (decrease/increase) the amount of aqueous humor. (Circle correct answer.)

6. Mannitol is contraindicated for clients with the condition of _____ or _____.

7. Diabetic clients taking Glyrol require monitoring of _____.

8. The drug group used to paralyze the muscles of accommodation is _____.

9. BufOpto atropine is frequently used for refraction in _____.

10. Instruct clients with glaucoma to avoid atropine-like drugs because they (decrease/increase) intraocular pressure. (Circle correct answer.)

11. Antiinfectives are used to treat infections of the eye, including inflammation of the membrane covering the eyeball and lining the eyelid known as _____.

12. Drugs that interfere with production of carbonic acid, leading to decreased aqueous humor formation and decreased intraocular pressure, belong to the group _____.

13. Beta-adrenergic blockers used to treat open-angle glaucoma may (increase/decrease) the effect of systemic beta blockers. (Circle correct answer.)

14. The group of eye medications contraindicated in persons allergic to sulfonamides is _____.

15. The volume of vitreous humor is reduced by the _____ group of drugs.

Match the term in Column I with its definition in Column II.

Column I

____ 16. Conjunctivitis
____ 17. Optic
____ 18. Cerumen
____ 19. Lacrimal duct
____ 20. Miosis
____ 21. Otic

Column II

a. Passage that carries tears into the nose
b. Contraction of the pupil
c. Ear
d. Eye
e. Inflammation of the membrane covering the eyeball
f. Earwax

NCLEX Review Questions

Select the best response.

22. The client has a medication ordered to dilate his eyes. Such a medication belongs to which group of drugs?
    a. mydriatics
    b. osmotics
    c. carbonic anhydrase inhibitors
    d. ceruminolytics

23. The client is taking a carbonic anhydrase inhibitor. The nurse will assess for which side effect associated with this group of drugs?
    a. nausea
    b. increased blood pressure
    c. renal calculi
    d. urinary retention

24. Which drug is most effective in treating glaucoma in African-American clients?
    a. latanoprost (Xalatan)
    b. bimatoprost (Lumigan)
    c. travoprost (Travatan)
    d. unoprostone (Rescula)

25. The client is taking a prostaglandin analogue, and the nurse assesses for the most common adverse reaction. To find this, what should the nurse assess in this client?
    a. light intolerance
    b. ocular hyperemia
    c. conjunctivitis
    d. blurred vision

26. The client had her ears irrigated. To determine the results of this irrigation, visualization of which structure is required?
    a. semicircular canals
    b. tympanic membrane
    c. external acoustic meatus
    d. auricle

27. Preparations that are helpful for loosening wax from the ear canal belong to which group?
    a. carbonic anhydrase inhibitors
    b. osmotics
    c. prostaglandin analogues
    d. ceruminolytics

28. The client is receiving Isopto-Eserine eye drops for treatment of glaucoma. The nurse should assess the client for which possible side effects? (Select all that apply.)
    a. headache
    b. nausea
    c. brow pain
    d. decreased vision

29. What priority nursing interventions should be included in the care for the client receiving Isopto-Eserine eye drops for treatment of glaucoma? (Select all that apply.)
    a. monitoring for postural hypotension
    b. assessing for increased bronchial secretions
    c. increasing fluid intake
    d. maintaining oral hygiene

30. What health teaching should be provided for the client receiving Isopto-Eserine eye drops for treatment of glaucoma? (Select all that apply.)
    a. The client should ensure that the first dose is administered by the health care provider.
    b. The client should be sure to follow up with tonometry readings.
    c. The client should increase daily caloric intake.
    d. The client should understand the importance of regular medical supervision.

31. Which solutions are commonly used to irrigate the ear? (Select all that apply.)
    a. Burow's solution
    b. hydrogen peroxide 3%
    c. hypotonic HCl solution 10%
    d. acetic acid

32. A 7-year-old client is receiving Bactrim (trimethoprim/sulfamethoxazole) for an inner-ear infection. Which are the best nursing interventions to include while caring for this client? (Select all that apply.)
    a. obtaining culture and sensitivity
    b. assessing for hematuria and oliguria
    c. restricting fluids
    d. monitoring intake and output

33. What should the nurse do when administering ear drops to a young child? (Select all that apply.)
    a. Pull down and back on the auricle.
    b. Pull up and back on the auricle.
    c. Tilt head to unaffected side.
    d. Instill medication at room temperature.

Case Study

Select the best answer.

D.Z. is 82 years old and comes to the office for her regular glaucoma follow-up. She denies any problems but admits to having blurred vision. She reports self-administration of pilocarpine, 2 gtt q4h.

1. D.Z. asks the nurse how pilocarpine works. What is the nurse's best answer?
    a. "It causes the pupil to contract."
    b. "It causes stimulation of the pupillary and ciliary sphincter muscles."
    c. "It increases urine output; thus, it is able to reduce the pressure in the eye."
    d. "It changes the size of the iris."

2. What should concern the nurse about the dose that D.Z. reports taking?
    a. Nothing; it is within the normal range for her age.
    b. It is too low of a dose.
    c. It is too high of a dose.
    d. It is a medication that should not be given to this client.

3. If the dose is too high, what is the best action by the nurse?

   a. Skip the next dose.

   b. Contact the health care provider.

   c. Decrease the dosage.

   d. Skip the next two doses.

4. What should the nurse suspect is the most likely cause of D.Z.'s blurred vision?

   a. side effects of her medication

   b. age

   c. gender

   d. lack of vitamins

5. Which client(s) should be monitored closely for systemic absorption of pilocarpine? (Select all that apply.)

   a. 50-year-old with CAD

   b. 48-year-old with asthma

   c. 67-year-old with diabetes

   d. 50-year-old with an infection

6. As part of the assessment, the nurse asks D.Z. if she experiences other side effects of pilocarpine. Which side effects should D.Z. be asked about? (Select all that apply.)

   a. eye pain

   b. nausea/vomiting/diarrhea

   c. increased salivation and sweating

   d. tremors

   e. increased serum glucose

7. What priority information should be included in client teaching for D.Z.? (Select all that apply.)

   a. "Avoid driving while your vision is impaired."

   b. "Be sure to keep your follow-up appointments with your health care provider."

   c. "Do not suddenly stop taking the medication."

   d. "Be sure to monitor your urine output daily."

50 Drugs for Dermatologic Disorders

Study Questions

Match the term in Column I with the correct description in Column II.

Column I

_____ 1. Macule

_____ 2. Vesicle

_____ 3. Plaque

_____ 4. Papule

Column II

a. Round, palpable lesion <1 cm in diameter

b. Hard, rough, raised lesion; flat on top

c. Flat lesion with varying color

d. Raised lesion filled with fluid and <1 cm in diameter

Label the structures of the skin.

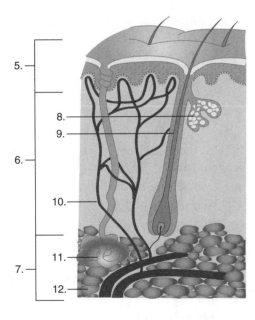

5. _____

6. _____

7. _____

8. _____

9. _____

10. _____

11. _____

12. _____

Match the condition in Column I to the drug that treats it in Column II.

Column I

____ 13.   Psoriasis

____ 14.   Burns

____ 15.   Acne

Column II

a.   Tetracycline

b.   Isotretinoin

c.   Azelaic acid

d.   Estrostep

e.   Alefacept

f.   Silver sulfadiazine

NCLEX Review Questions

Select the best response.

16.   The client has severe acne. Which types of drugs are most frequently used to treat this condition?

    a.   antibiotics and glucocorticoids

    b.   antibiotics and coal tar products

    c.   podophyllum and anthralin

    d.   Sulfamylon and keratolytics

17.   Psoriasis affects what percentage of the population in the United States?

    a.   1%-2%

    b.   3%-4%

    c.   5%-6%

    d.   10%

18.   Psoriatic scales are loosened with which medications?

    a.   podophyllum

    b.   antibiotics

    c.   keratolytics

    d.   benzoyl peroxide

19.   Which drugs are most commonly used to treat moderate to severe psoriasis?

    a.   antibiotics

    b.   biologic agents

    c.   keratolytics

    d.   silver nitrate

20.   How is azelaic acid administered?

    a.   orally

    b.   topically

    c.   subcutaneously

    d.   intramuscularly

21.   Which is the most common cause of contact dermatitis?

    a.   irritation

    b.   burns

    c.   inhalation

    d.   smoke

22.   A moderately severe sunburn is an example of what degree burn?

    a.   first

    b.   second

    c.   third

    d.   full thickness

23.   What is the usual dose of tetracycline for acne vulgaris?

    a.   250-500 mg b.i.d.

    b.   500-1000 mg b.i.d.

    c.   500 mg daily

    d.   1 g daily

24.   What is a major side effect of tetracycline?

    a.   urinary retention

    b.   photosensitivity

    c.   hypersensitivity

    d.   hepatotoxicity

25. The nurse is planning health teaching about tetracycline for an 18-year-old client. Which drug interactions should be included in the client's teaching? (Select all that apply.)

    a. Tetracycline increases the effects of oral anticoagulants.

    b. Tetracycline decreases the effects of oral contraceptives.

    c. Tetracycline increases the effects of oral contraceptives.

    d. Antacids decrease absorption of tetracycline.

26. What priority information should be provided to the client taking tetracycline for acne vulgaris? (Select all that apply.)

    a. Do not use harsh skin cleansers.

    b. Report adverse effects.

    c. Eat a diet high in fiber.

    d. Alert the health care provider if pregnant or possibly pregnant.

27. To control severe psoriasis, which anticancer drug may be prescribed?

    a. benzoyl

    b. tretinoin

    c. etretinate

    d. methotrexate

28. Which FDA-approved drug is for the treatment of baldness?

    a. tretinoin

    b. methoxsalen

    c. etretinate

    d. minoxidil

29. Which medications may be used to treat contact dermatitis? (Select all that apply.)

    a. Burow's solution

    b. calamine

    c. Percocet

    d. Benadryl

30. Which antipruritics are used in the treatment of contact dermatitis? (Select all that apply.)

    a. Peri-Colace

    b. fluconazole

    c. Decadron

    d. Aristocort

31. Which drugs are known to cause alopecia? (Select all that apply.)

    a. antineoplastic agents

    b. sulfonamides

    c. selected NSAIDs

    d. oral contraceptives

Case Study

Select the best answer.

C.S., 2 years old, has a third-degree burn over her right chest and shoulder and second-degree burns on her hands caused when she hit the handle of a pot filled with boiling water. Mafenide acetate is ordered to be applied to chest, shoulder, and hands in a 1/16-inch layer, b.i.d.

1. What are the depths and characteristics of third-degree burns?

    a. blistering, with little to no pain

    b. pearly white skin, charred, no pain

    c. erythema (redness), painful

    d. mottled, blistering, intense pain

2. Should the nurse be concerned about the dosage prescribed for C.S.? If so, why?

    a. No, as it is appropriate for this child's age and type of burn.

    b. Yes, as it is too low a dose for this type of burn.

    c. Yes, as it is too high a dose for this type of burn.

    d. Yes, it is a toxic level given this child's age.

3. What is the mode of action of mafenide acetate?

    a. It interferes with bacterial protein synthesis.

    b. It inhibits bacterial cell wall synthesis.

    c. It causes lysis of the cellular contents.

    d. It interferes with cell wall permeability.

4. What other drug is used for the prevention and treatment of sepsis in second- and third-degree burns?

    a. There is no other drug that has this action

    b. nitrofurazone

    c. adalimumab

    d. silver sulfadiazine

5. Which nursing assessments should be a priority when caring for C.S.? (Select all that apply.)

    a. assessment for infection

    b. assessment of vital signs

    c. assessment of fluid status

    d. assessment and treatment for pain

    e. assessment of blood glucose level

6. Which are priority interventions for C.S.? (Select all that apply.)

    a. Use aseptic technique.

    b. Monitor for acid-base changes.

    c. Assess for drug side effects.

    d. Administer pain medications before burn medications.

7. What possible side effects of mafenide acetate should the nurse discuss with C.S.'s family? (Select all that apply.)

    a. rash

    b. urticaria

    c. swelling

    d. headache

    e. increased blood glucose

8. What priority health teaching is important to include for C.S.'s family? (Select all that apply.)

    a. Require a return demonstration for aseptic technique.

    b. Require a return demonstration for application of medications and dressings.

    c. Stress the importance of hand exercises.

    d. Require a return demonstration of arterial blood gas measurement.

51 Endocrine Drugs: Pituitary, Thyroid, Parathyroid, and Adrenal Disorders

Study Questions

Match the information in Column I with the correct term in Column II.

Column I

_____ 1. Growth hormone hypersecretion after puberty

_____ 2. Anterior pituitary gland

_____ 3. Initials for adrenocorticotropic hormone

_____ 4. Initials for antidiuretic hormone

_____ 5. Severe hypothyroidism in children

_____ 6. Ductless glands that produce hormones

_____ 7. Growth hormone hypersecretion during childhood

_____ 8. Cortisol hormone secreted from the adrenal cortex

_____ 9. Pituitary gland

_____ 10. Aldosterone hormone secreted from the adrenal cortex

_____ 11. Severe hypothyroidism in adults

_____ 12. Posterior pituitary gland

_____ 13. Toxic hyperthyroidism because of hyperfunction of the thyroid gland

_____ 14. T$_4$ hormone secreted by the thyroid gland

_____ 15. T$_3$ hormone secreted by the thyroid gland

Column II

a. ADH

b. Gigantism

c. Mineralocorticoid

d. Neurohypophysis

e. Triiodothyronine

f. Acromegaly

g. Myxedema

h. Endocrine

i. Adenohypophysis

j. ACTH

k. Thyrotoxicosis

l. Thyroxine

m. Glucocorticoid

n. Cretinism

o. Hypophysis

Match the description from Column II with the applicable term in Column I.

Column I

____ 16.   Hyperglycemia

____ 17.   Buffalo hump

____ 18.   Hypoglycemia

____ 19.   Seizures

____ 20.   Fatigue

____ 21.   Impaired clotting

____ 22.   Cataract formation

____ 23.   Hypotension

____ 24.   Hypervolemia

____ 25.   Peptic ulcer

Column II

a.   Adrenal hyposecretion

b.   Adrenal hypersecretion

Match the nursing intervention in Column I with the correct rationale related to glucocorticoid drug administration in Column II.

Column I

____ 26.   Monitor vital signs.

____ 27.   Monitor weight after taking a cortisone preparation for more than 10 days.

____ 28.   Monitor laboratory values, especially blood glucose and electrolytes.

____ 29.   Instruct the client to take the cortisone with food.

____ 30.   Advise the client to eat foods rich in potassium.

____ 31.   Instruct the client not to abruptly discontinue cortisone preparation.

____ 32.   Report changes in muscle strength and signs of osteoporosis.

____ 33.   Teach client to report signs and symptoms of drug overdose.

Column II

a.   Cortisone increases sodium retention and increases blood pressure.

b.   Adrenal crisis may occur if cortisone is abruptly stopped.

c.   Glucocorticoid drugs promote loss of potassium.

d.   Weight gain occurs with cortisone use as a result of water retention.

e.   Glucocorticoid drugs promote sodium retention, potassium loss, and increased blood glucose.

f.   Cortisone promotes loss of muscle tone and loss of calcium from bone.

g.   Glucocorticoid drugs may cause moon face, puffy eyelids, edema in the feet, dizziness, and menstrual irregularity at high doses.

h.   Glucocorticoid drugs can irritate the gastric mucosa and may cause peptic ulcer.

NCLEX Review Questions

Select the best response.

34. A 49-year-old client is being treated for hypothyroidism. The client is taking levothyroxine (Synthroid) 100 mcg/day. What should concern the nurse about the client's dose of Synthroid?

    a. Nothing; it is within the normal maintenance dose.

    b. Nothing; someone the client's age should start at a low dose.

    c. It is too low for the client's age.

    d. It is too high a dose for the client's age.

35. How soon after starting levothyroxine (Synthroid) should the client report feeling its effects?

    a. 3-4 days

    b. 4-7 days

    c. 1-3 weeks

    d. 3-5 weeks

36. The nurse assesses the client for symptoms of hyperthyroidism. Which are symptoms of hyperthyroidism? (Select all that apply.)

    a. tachycardia

    b. tinnitus

    c. chest pain

    d. excessive sweating

37. The nurse is speaking to the client with hypothyroidism about avoiding foods that can inhibit thyroid secretion. Which statement(s) indicate(s) that the client understands the teaching? (Select all that apply.)

    a. "I hate to give up strawberries, but I want to feel better."

    b. "I don't like cabbage anyway, so I won't miss eating it."

    c. "Radishes burn my tongue, so no great loss if I should avoid them."

    d. "I don't eat string beans as they give me gas, so I won't miss them."

38. What time of day should the nurse teach the client to take Synthroid?

    a. before breakfast

    b. with breakfast

    c. after breakfast

    d. with lunch

39. What is priority information to include in the health teaching plan for the client with hypothyroidism? (Select all that apply.)

    a. Take medication at the same time each day.

    b. Wear a Medic-Alert information device.

    c. Increase food and fluid intake.

    d. Avoid over-the-counter (OTC) drugs.

40. A 56-year-old client is taking prednisone for an exacerbation of arthritic knee pain. What is the usual dose of prednisone?

    a. 0.5-6 mg/day

    b. 5-60 mg/day

    c. 60-100 mg/day

    d. 100-125 mg/day

41. While a 56-year-old client is taking prednisone, which laboratory values should be closely monitored?

    a. magnesium

    b. potassium

    c. hemoglobin

    d. hematocrit

42. When is the best time to take prednisone?

    a. before meals

    b. with meals

    c. 1 hour after meals

    d. at bedtime

43. Which drug(s) should be used with caution when taking prednisone? (Select all that apply.)

    a. NSAIDs, including aspirin

    b. potassium-wasting diuretics

    c. acetaminophen

    d. oral anticoagulants

44. What are priority nursing interventions to implement in the care of a 56-year-old client taking prednisone? (Select all that apply.)
    a. Monitor vital signs.
    b. Monitor for signs and symptoms of hypokalemia.
    c. Obtain a complete medication history.
    d. Follow the physical therapy regimen.

45. Which statement by a 56-year-old client taking prednisone indicates that she needs more education about her medications?
    a. "I will take glucocorticoids only as ordered."
    b. "I should wear a Medic-Alert device or carry a card."
    c. "I will make sure I force fluids daily."
    d. "I will not abruptly stop taking my medication."

46. When an herbal laxative such as cascara or senna and herbal diuretics such as celery seed or juniper are taken with a corticosteroid, what imbalance may occur?
    a. hypervolemia
    b. hyperkalemia
    c. hypokalemia
    d. hypernatremia

47. What changes can occur when ginseng is taken with a corticosteroid?
    a. CNS depression
    b. CNS stimulation and insomnia
    c. serum potassium excess
    d. counteraction of the effects of the corticosteroid

48. Which drug would the nurse anticipate using for a procedure to diagnose adrenal gland dysfunction?
    a. metyrapone (Metopirone)
    b. mitotane (Lysodren)
    c. ketoconazole (Nizoral)
    d. prednisolone (Delta-Cortef)

49. The nurse advises a client to avoid potassium loss by eating which foods? (Select all that apply.)
    a. nuts
    b. meats
    c. vegetables
    d. dried fruits
    e. milk products

50. Which drugs are known to interact with Synthroid? (Select all that apply.)
    a. digitalis
    b. diuretics
    c. anticoagulants
    d. acetaminophen
    e. oral antidiabetics

51. The nurse assesses a client for the side effects of prednisone. What assessment findings may be present? (Select all that apply.)
    a. edema
    b. anorexia
    c. hypertension
    d. mood changes
    e. increased blood sugar

Case Study

Select the best answer.

M.N., age 52 years, is taking prednisone 10 mg t.i.d. for an acute neurologic problem. She also has a cardiac problem and is taking digoxin 0.25 mg daily and hydrochlorothiazide 25 mg daily. Her serum potassium level is 3.2 mEq/L.

1. What should concern the nurse about M.N.'s prednisone dosage?
    a. Nothing; it is within the normal range.
    b. Nothing; it is OK for her to take a low dose.
    c. It is too high for her health issues.
    d. It is too low for her health issues.

2. What electrolyte imbalance may occur with the use of prednisone and hydrochlorothiazide?

    a. hypernatremia

    b. hypokalemia

    c. hypercalcemia

    d. hypomagnesemia

3. How could M.N.'s electrolyte imbalance be avoided? (Select all that apply.)

    a. Change her medications.

    b. Have her eat potassium-rich foods.

    c. Add a potassium supplement to her drug regimen.

    d. Increase her fluid intake.

4. What effect could hypokalemia have on digoxin?

    a. It may cause digoxin toxicity.

    b. It will decrease the effectiveness of digoxin.

    c. It has no impact on digoxin.

    d. It increases the effectiveness of digoxin.

5. When discontinuing prednisone, why is it recommended that the doses be tapered?

    a. The adrenal cortex will overproduce steroids so it should be discontinued quickly.

    b. The adrenal cortex needs time to begin production and secretion of cortisol.

    c. It will allow the client to get used to not taking medications.

    d. It will significantly change her urine output and will require an immediate reduction of fluid intake.

6. What priority information should the nurse include in the teaching plan for M.N.? (Select all that apply.)

    a. Take the prednisone with food.

    b. Eat foods rich in potassium.

    c. Avoid persons with respiratory infections.

    d. Report side effects to your health care provider.

    e. Discontinue the medication when you feel better.

52 Antidiabetics

Study Questions

Match the term in Column I with its definition in Column II.

Column I

____ 1.   Diabetes mellitus

____ 2.   Insulin

____ 3.   Hypoglycemic reaction

____ 4.   Type 1 diabetes

____ 5.   Type 2 diabetes

____ 6.   Ketoacidosis

____ 7.   Lipodystrophy

____ 8.   Polydipsia

____ 9.   Polyphagia

____ 10. Polyuria

____ 11. Dawn phenomenon

Column II

a.   Increased hunger

b.   Type of diabetes with some beta cell function

c.   Increased urine output

d.   Hyperglycemia on awakening

e.   Diabetic acidosis

f.   Disease resulting from deficient glucose metabolism

g.   Increased thirst

h.   Protein secreted from the beta cells of the pancreas

i.   Tissue atrophy

j.   Type of diabetes with no beta-cell function

k.   Reaction to low blood glucose

Select the best answer.

12. What are the major symptoms that characterize diabetes? (Select all that apply.)
    a. polyuria
    b. polyphagia
    c. polyposia
    d. polydipsia
    e. polyrrhea

13. Which drugs may cause hyperglycemia? (Select all that apply.)
    a. prednisone
    b. epinephrine
    c. levothyroxine
    d. hydrochlorothiazide

14. What is the rationale for rotation of insulin injection sites?
    a. prevents polyuria
    b. prevents rejection of insulin
    c. prevents an allergic reaction
    d. prevents lipodystrophy

15. What is the only type of insulin that may be administered IV?
    a. NPH
    b. Detemir
    c. Lantus
    d. Regular

16. Which clinical manifestations may be seen in a client experiencing a hypoglycemic (insulin) reaction? (Select all that apply.)

    a. headache

    b. nervousness

    c. tremor

    d. excessive perspiration

    e. tachycardia

    f. abdominal pain

17. Which clinical manifestations may be seen in a client experiencing diabetic ketoacidosis (hyperglycemia)? (Select all that apply.)

    a. thirst

    b. polyuria

    c. bradycardia

    d. Kussmaul's sign

    e. dry mucous membranes

    f. fruity breath odor

18. In maturity-onset, or type 2, diabetes, the oral antidiabetic (hypoglycemic) drug group that stimulates beta cells to secrete more insulin is sulfonylureas. For juvenile-onset, or type 1, diabetes, oral hypoglycemics (are/ are not) prescribed. (Circle correct answer.)

19. Which information should be included in health teaching for clients taking insulin? (Select all that apply.)

    a. Recognize signs of hypoglycemic reaction.

    b. Adhere to the prescribed diet.

    c. Take insulin as prescribed.

    d. Monitor blood glucose level.

    e. Be sure to exercise.

    f. Keep appointments with health care provider.

    g. Alter insulin dose based on how you're feeling.

20. Which information should be included in health teaching for clients taking oral antidiabetic (hypoglycemic) drugs? (Select all that apply.)

    a. Monitor blood glucose levels.

    b. Take medications at prescribed time.

    c. Adhere to prescribed diet.

    d. Monitor weight.

    e. Participate in regular exercise.

Match the terms in Column I with their definitions in Column II.

Column I

____ 21. NPH insulin

____ 22. Lipoatrophy

____ 23. Sulfonylureas

____ 24. Glucagon

____ 25. Lispro insulin

Column II

a. oral hypoglycemic drug group

b. hyperglycemic hormone that stimulates glycogenolysis

c. intermediate- acting insulin

d. long-acting insulin

e. tissue atrophy

f. rapid-acting insulin

Match the nursing intervention in Column I with its rationale in Column II.

Column I

_____ 26. Monitor blood glucose levels.

_____ 27. Instruct the client to report signs
and symptoms of "insulin shock"
(hypoglycemic reaction).

_____ 28. Inform the client to have orange juice
or a sugar-containing drink available if
a hypoglycemic reaction occurs.

_____ 29. Instruct the client to check the blood
sugar daily.

_____ 30. Instruct the client to adhere to the
prescribed diet.

_____ 31. Instruct family members on how to
administer glucagon by injection for a
hypoglycemic reaction.

_____ 32. Advise the client to obtain a medical
alert card or tag.

Column II

a. Done to make sure it is within normal levels.

b. Orange juice or a sweetened beverage adds
sugar to the body for insulin utilization.

c. Diet is prescribed to according to amount of
insulin given per day.

d. Signs and symptoms include nervousness,
tremors, cold and clammy skin, and slurred
speech.

e. Client may be unable to swallow orange
juice.

f. Needed in case of a severe hypoglycemic reaction where the client may be unconscious.

g. Prevents incidences of hyper- and hypoglycemia.

NCLEX Review Questions

Select the best response.

33. Site and depth of insulin injection affect absorption. In which site is insulin absorption
is greater?

a. ventrogluteal and abdominal areas

b. deltoid and abdominal areas

c. deltoid and rectus femoris areas

d. dorsogluteal and ventrogluteal areas

34. Lipoatrophy is a complication that occurs
when insulin is injected repeatedly in one
site. What is the physiologic effect that occurs?

a. a depression under the skin surface

b. a raised lump or knot on the skin surface

c. rash at a raised area on the skin surface

d. bruising under the skin

35. Where should the client who takes insulin
daily be taught to store the insulin?

a. in the refrigerator

b. in a cool place

c. wrapped in aluminum

d. in the light

36. How should the nurse or client prepare insulin prior to administration?

a. shaking the bottle well

b. allowing air to escape from the bottle

c. rolling the bottle in the hands

d. adding diluent to the bottle

37. The nurse is preparing to give a client his
daily insulin. What is the best action by the
nurse?

a. Prepare two separate injections.

b. Prepare one injection; draw up regular
insulin first.

c. Prepare one injection; draw up NPH
insulin first.

d. Prepare one injection; draw up both
simultaneously and mix well.

38. Which type of syringe should be used to
administer a client's daily insulin dose of 6
units of U100 Regular and 14 units of U100
NPH?

a. 2 mL syringe

b. 5 mL syringe

c. U40 insulin syringe

d. U100 insulin syringe

39. The client needs to develop a "site rotation pattern" for insulin injections. The American Diabetes Association suggests which action(s)? (Select all that apply.)

    a. Choose an injection site for a week.

    b. Inject insulin each day at the injection site at 1½ inches apart.

    c. Change the injection area of the body every day.

    d. With two daily injection times, use the right side in the morning and the left side in the evening.

40. When should the nurse expect that the client may experience a hypoglycemic reaction to Regular insulin if administration occurs at 0700 hours?

    a. 0800-0900 hours

    b. 0900-1300 hours

    c. 1300-1500 hours

    d. 1500-1700 hours

41. How long after NPH administration would the nurse expect the client's insulin to peak?

    a. 1-2 hours

    b. 2-6 hours

    c. 6-12 hours

    d. 12-15 hours

42. Lantus is a long-acting insulin. Which statements best describe Lantus? (Select all that apply.)

    a. It is given in the evening.

    b. Some clients complain of pain at the injection site.

    c. It is safe because hypoglycemia cannot occur.

    d. It is available in a 3 mL cartridge insulin pen.

43. Insulin resistance can be a problem for some clients taking insulin. What changes may cause insulin resistance? (Select all that apply.)

    a. antibody development in clients taking animal insulin over time

    b. clients taking increased units of Humulin insulin over time

    c. clients who are allergic to dust, mold, cat dander, and other allergens

    d. clients with diabetes who are malnourished

44. What is a method to determine if the client has insulin resistance?

    a. chemistry laboratory tests

    b. urinalysis to check for glucose

    c. skin test with different insulin preparations

    d. history of other allergies

45. The insulin pump, though expensive, has become popular in the management of insulin. What does the nurse know about this method of insulin delivery?

    a. It is more effective for use by the type 2 diabetic client.

    b. It is effective in lessening long-term diabetic complications.

    c. It can be used with modified insulins (NPH) as well as Regular insulin.

    d. It can be used with the needle inserted at the same site for weeks.

46. What is the action of an oral hypoglycemic?

    a. increase the number of insulin cell receptors

    b. increase the number of insulin-producing cells

    c. replace receptor sites

    d. replace insulin

47. The client asks if Dymelor is oral insulin. What is the nurse's best response?

    a. "Yes, it is the same as injected insulin, except it is taken orally."

    b. "Yes, it is similar, but hypoglycemic reactions (insulin shock) do not occur with Dymelor."

    c. "No, it is not the same as insulin, and Dymelor can be taken even when the blood sugar remains greater than 250 mg/dl."

    d. "No, it is not the same as insulin. Dymelor can be used only when there is some beta cell function."

48. Acetohexamide (Dymelor) is a(n) _____ hypoglycemic drug. Its duration of action is _____ than tolbutamide (Orinase).

    a. short-acting; shorter

    b. intermediate-acting; longer

    c. intermediate-acting; shorter

    d. long-acting; longer

49. For what reason should the nurse teach a client who is taking acetohexamide to avoid alcohol?

    a. It causes a poor nutritional state.

    b. It decreased mental alertness.

    c. It causes an inability to drive.

    d. It increases the half-life of acetohexamide.

50. Which effects are representative of second-generation sulfonylureas? (Select all that apply.)

    a. They have less hypoglycemic potency than first-generation sulfonylureas.

    b. Effective doses are less than with first-generation sulfonylureas.

    c. They have less displacement from protein-binding sites by other highly protein-bound drugs.

    d. They increase tissue response and decrease glucose production by the liver.

51. The nonsulfonylureas are used to control serum glucose levels after a meal. What best describes their action?

    a. They raise the serum glucose level following a meal.

    b. They increase the absorption of glucose from the small intestine.

    c. They cause a hypoglycemic reaction.

    d. They decrease hepatic production of glucose from stored glycogen.

52. An example of a nonsulfonylurea is acarbose (Precose), an alpha-glucosidase inhibitor that acts by which mechanism?

    a. By increasing insulin production; thus it can cause a hypoglycemic reaction.

    b. Through inhibiting digestive enzymes in the small intestine, which releases glucose from the complex carbohydrates in the diet (less sugar is available).

    c. By stimulating the beta cells to produce insulin.

    d. Through increasing glucose metabolism.

53. One class of nonsulfonylureas is the thiazolidinedione group. How does this group of oral antidiabetics work?

    a. They promote absorption of glucose from the large intestine.

    b. They increase the uptake of glucose in the liver and small intestine.

    c. They increase insulin sensitivity for improving blood glucose control.

    d. They decrease glucose utilization.

54. The first thiazolidinedione, troglitazone (Rezulin), was removed from the market in 2000. What did this drug cause that led the FDA to remove it from the market?

    a. kidney failure

    b. severe liver dysfunction

    c. blood dyscrasia

    d. peptic ulcer disease

55. Clients taking thiazolidinedione drugs such as pioglitazone (Actos) and rosiglitazone (Avandia) should have which laboratory test(s) monitored?
    a. BUN
    b. hemoglobin and hematocrit
    c. cardiac enzymes
    d. liver enzymes

56. Herb-drug interaction must be assessed by clients taking herbs and antidiabetic agents. How do ginseng and garlic affect insulin or oral antidiabetic drugs?
    a. They decrease the effect of insulin and antidiabetic drugs, causing a hyperglycemic effect.
    b. They can lower the blood glucose level, thus causing a hypoglycemic effect.
    c. They may decrease insulin requirements.
    d. They can be taken with insulin without any effect but can cause a hypoglycemic reaction with oral antidiabetic drugs.

57. What are the recommended guidelines for use of oral antidiabetics? (Select all that apply.)
    a. underweight client
    b. onset at age 40 years or older
    c. normal renal and hepatic function
    d. fasting blood sugar less than 200 mg/dl
    e. diagnosis of diabetes mellitus for <10 years

58. Which drug or category of drugs will interact with a sulfonylurea? (Select all that apply.)
    a. aspirin
    b. antacids
    c. sulfonamides
    d. anticoagulants
    e. anticonvulsants

59. What are contraindications for the use of oral antidiabetic drugs? (Select all that apply.)
    a. pregnancy
    b. breastfeeding
    c. severe infection
    d. type 2 diabetes
    e. renal dysfunction

Case Study

Select the best answer.

N.V., age 39 years, was diagnosed with diabetes mellitus 15 years ago. Symptoms of diabetes occurred 3 weeks after he had hepatitis. N.V. takes 42 units of NPH and 8 units of regular insulin daily.

1. What are the best instructions the nurse can give N.V. concerning insulin injection sites? (Select all that apply.)
    a. Injections should be given at one site for 1 week.
    b. Injections should be given 1½ inches apart within the chosen site.
    c. Injections should be given at one site for 2 weeks.
    d. Injections should be given 1 inch apart within the chosen site.

2. N.V. weighs 72 kg. Is the "average" insulin dosage appropriate for a diabetic client of this weight?
    a. Yes; the "average" dose is appropriate for his age and size.
    b. No; it is too low for his age.
    c. No; it too low for his size.
    d. No; it is too high for his age and size.

3. If N.V. took his insulin at 0800, when is it likely that he might have a hypoglycemic (insulin) reaction?
    a. 0900-1100
    b. 1100-1300
    c. 1300-1500
    d. 1600-1700

4. What are the signs and symptoms of a hypoglycemic reaction of which N.V. should be aware? (Select all that apply.)
    a. nervousness
    b. tremors
    c. cold, clammy skin
    d. slurred speech
    e. seizures
    f. headache

5. What priority client teaching strategies should the nurse include for N.V.? (Select all that apply.)

   a. return demonstration on injection and selection of sites

   b. quizzing the client on dietary limitations

   c. suggesting the use of Medic-Alert

   d. telling the client to be sure to take insulin even during times of stress

6. What priority teaching information should the nurse give N.V. and his significant others about reversing the onset of a hypoglycemic reaction? (Select all that apply.)

   a. the clinical manifestations of hypoglycemic reaction

   b. that N.V. should have orange juice, candy, or soda available at all times

   c. that N.V. must treat hypoglycemia immediately when recognized

   d. that N.V. may decrease insulin administration if he feels fine

53 Female Reproductive Cycle I: Pregnancy and Preterm Labor Drugs

Study Questions

Match the terms in Column I with the definitions in Column II.

Column I

_____ 1. Preeclampsia

_____ 2. Gestational hypertension

_____ 3. HELLP

_____ 4. L/S (lecithin/sphingomyelin) ratio

_____ 5. Eclampsia

_____ 6. Preterm delivery

_____ 7. Progesterone

_____ 8. Surfactant

_____ 9. Teratogens

_____ 10. Tocolytic therapy

Column II

a. New-onset of seizures with preeclampsia

b. Prior to 37 gestational weeks

c. Drug therapy to decrease uterine muscle contractions

d. Maintains the uterine environment to nourish the blastocyst

e. Decreases the incidence of respiratory distress syndrome

f. Hypertension during pregnancy

g. Gestational hypertension with proteinuria

h. Substances that cause developmental abnormalities

i. Predictor of fetal lung maturity and risk for neonatal RDS

j. *Hemolysis, Elevated Liver enzymes, and Low Platelet count*

Select the best answer.

11. Therapeutically prescribed drugs such as antibiotics (are/are not) ordered in lower doses during pregnancy. (Circle correct answer.)

12. What maternal physiologic changes are seen during pregnancy that affect drug dosing? (Select all that apply.)

    a. increased glomerular filtration rate and rapid excretion of drugs

    b. increased liver metabolism of drugs

    c. increased fluid volume

    d. decreased urine output

13. Highly protein-bound drugs (do/do not) readily cross the placenta. (Circle correct answer.)

14. The placenta (does/does not) act as a protective barrier to keep substances from going from the maternal circulation into the fetal circulation. (Circle correct answer.)

15. Drug excretion is (slower/faster) in the fetus than in the mother. (Circle correct answer.)

16. The mechanism by which drugs cross the placenta is similar to the way drugs infiltrate which type of body tissue?
    a. subcutaneous
    b. breast
    c. liver
    d. uterine

17. What are important factors that determine the teratogenicity of any drug ingested during pregnancy? (Select all that apply.)
    a. timing
    b. dosage
    c. duration of exposure
    d. urinary clearance

18. What is the composition of surfactant? (Select all that apply.)
    a. albumin
    b. sphingomyelin
    c. lecithin
    d. thymine

19. What is the purpose of determining the L/S ratio?
    a. It is a predictor of premature labor.
    b. It determines the date of delivery.
    c. It determines the maturity of the fetal lungs.
    d. It determines the ratio of urine output/glomerular filtration rate.

20. What is the purpose of giving betamethasone before delivery?
    a. decrease the incidence of preterm labor (PTL)
    b. promote fetal lung maturity
    c. promote fetal adrenal maturity
    d. promote closure of the patent ductus arteriosus

21. What are the primary treatment goal(s) in gestational hypertension? (Select all that apply.)
    a. prevention of seizures
    b. prevention of HELLP syndrome
    c. delivery of an uncompromised infant
    d. decrease the incidence of PTL

22. What are the most common complaints of pregnancy associated with client requests for medication? (Select all that apply.)
    a. treatment of nausea
    b. nutritional support
    c. decrease urgency and frequency of urination
    d. mild discomforts

23. What test is used to determine that a client with iron deficiency anemia generally has responded to iron supplementation therapy?
    a. increase in Hct and Hgb
    b. increase in liver enzymes
    c. increase in reticulocytosis values
    d. decreased WBC count

24. Vitamin and mineral megadoses during pregnancy (will/will not) improve health. (Circle correct answer.)

25. Cultural variations exist in regard to the use of prenatal vitamins. In which country are some individuals known to view vitamins as a "hot food" to avoid in pregnancy?
    a. Korea
    b. Mexico
    c. France
    d. Saudi Arabia

26. What are nonpharmacologic measures to decrease nausea and vomiting during early pregnancy? (Select all that apply.)
    a. eating crackers, dry toast, cereal, or other complex carbohydrates
    b. drinking ginger tea
    c. avoiding fluids before arising
    d. avoiding fatty or highly seasoned foods
    e. eating a high-protein snack at bedtime

27. What are nonpharmacologic measures preferred for the management of heartburn? (Select all that apply.)

   a. limiting the size of meals

   b. avoiding greasy foods

   c. drinking carbonated beverages frequently

   d. drinking fluids, but not during meals

28. What are priority teaching goals for clients with gestational hypertension? (Select all that apply.)

   a. Instruct client to lie on her right side.

   b. Instruct client to maintain adequate fluid intake.

   c. Instruct client on what to report to her health care provider.

   d. Instruct client to put her feet up when sitting down.

Match the letters of the substance in Column II with the associated adverse effects in Column I. Some substances may have more than one adverse effect.

Column I

____ 29. Increased risk of spontaneous abortion

____ 30. Smaller head circumference without catch-up

____ 31. Hypertonicity, tremulousness in baby

____ 32. Abruptio placentae and premature delivery

____ 33. Degenerative placental lesions

____ 34. Decreased intervillous blood flow

____ 35. Inadequate maternal calorie and protein intake

____ 36. Ataxia, syncope, vertigo

____ 37. Rapidly crosses placenta and causes CNS depression in the fetus

Column II

a. Alcohol

b. Caffeine

c. Cocaine

d. Heroin

e. Methadone

f. Barbiturates

g. Tobacco/nicotine

h. Tranquilizer

NCLEX Review Questions

Select the best response.

38. During pregnancy, the amount of iron necessary is how much compared with that of the prepregnant state?

   a. the same as

   b. twice

   c. triple

   d. one and one-half

39. What might the nurse assess in a client taking iron? (Select all that apply.)

   a. nausea

   b. constipation

   c. epigastric pain

   d. jaundice

40. The client needs increased intake of iron. What foods should the nurse recommend that the client eat? (Select all that apply.)

   a. lettuce

   b. liver

   c. spinach

   d. cereal

41. What is the recommended daily allowance of folic acid for a pregnant woman?
    a. 100-400 mcg
    b. 400-800 mcg
    c. 800-1000 mcg
    d. 1000-1200 mcg

42. To enhance both drugs' effectiveness, when should iron and antacids be administered?
    a. at the same time
    b. 2 hours apart
    c. with the antacid first
    d. with the iron first

43. Which drug is most commonly selected and ingested by clients during pregnancy?
    a. ferrous sulfate
    b. Tigan
    c. Mylanta
    d. acetaminophen

44. Which priority interventions should the nurse implement for the client receiving a beta-sympathomimetic drug?
    a. monitoring maternal and fetal vital signs every 15 minutes when receiving IV dose
    b. monitoring daily weight
    c. being alert to hypoglycemia and hypokalemia in newborn delivered within 5 hours of discontinuing the drug
    d. restricting all fluids

45. The health care provider for the client receiving a beta-sympathomimetic drug should be notified of which findings? (Select all that apply.)
    a. auscultated dysrhythmias
    b. respirations greater than 30 breaths/min
    c. systolic blood pressure greater than 100 mm Hg
    d. fetal baseline heart rate greater than 180 beats/min

46. Health teaching for the client receiving a beta-sympathomimetic drug should include which information? (Select all that apply.)
    a. Palpitations are uncommon.
    b. Notify health care provider of frequent contractions while taking the drug.
    c. Consult health care provider before taking any other medications.
    d. Take medications as directed.

47. Which nursing interventions should a client receiving magnesium sulfate for preeclampsia require? (Select all that apply.)
    a. providing continuous fetal monitoring and documentation every 15 minutes
    b. having airway suction equipment readily available
    c. having antidote calcium gluconate at the bedside
    d. monitoring vital signs every 4 hours

48. While caring for a client receiving magnesium sulfate, about which changes should the nurse notify the health care provider? (Select all that apply.)
    a. absence of patellar reflexes
    b. respirations greater than 15 breaths/min
    c. absent bowel sounds
    d. change in affect

49. Which clinical manifestations would the nurse assess in someone experiencing magnesium toxicity?
    a. rapid decrease in blood pressure and respiratory arrest
    b. rapid increase in blood pressure and increase in respiration rate
    c. sudden fever and somnolence
    d. muscle pain and excessive weight gain

50. The client being treated during labor with magnesium sulfate asks how long she will need this drug. When should the nurse suspect this drug will be discontinued?
    a. at the time of delivery
    b. 1-4 hours after delivery
    c. 24 hours after delivery
    d. 48-72 hours after delivery

51. Antacids may cause drug interactions with which drugs? (Select all that apply.)

    a.　digitalis

    b.　anticonvulsants

    c.　tetracyclines

    d.　iron

52. What may occur with the use of aspirin late in pregnancy?

    a.　increased maternal blood loss at delivery

    b.　low birth weight infant

    c.　increased risk of anemia

    d.　decreased hemostasis in newborn

53. The client is receiving magnesium sulfate IV for gestational hypertension. Which expected side effects from this medication may be assessed? (Select all that apply.)

    a.　flushing

    b.　lethargy

    c.　tachycardia

    d.　slurred speech

    e.　hyperreflexia

Case Study

Select the best answer.

S.B. is a 38-year-old woman who has 5- and 7-year-old children. She is 28 weeks pregnant and has recently separated from her husband of 15 years. S.B. calls the OB triage unit from the local mall where she works. She states that she has been unable to get through to her doctor's office because of busy signals and interruptions by her customers. She says that she is "terrified I might be going into labor." She says that she had a "baby born early" 5 years ago. She says, "This can't be happening again. I have no health benefits with this job. My husband has been out of work due to his company downsizing; he has no benefits either. Plus we are separated. Please tell me what to do now." She adds, "I'm having contractions about every 8 minutes and I feel like there is some kind of pressure inside my lower belly. My children are in school and daycare and will be home three hours from now."

1. What data supplied in S.B.'s brief telephone history support a diagnosis of PTL? (Select all that apply.)

    a.　age

    b.　regular contractions at >10-minute intervals

    c.　28 weeks gestation

    d.　having contractions every 8 minutes

    e.　previous history of PTL

2. What additional data should the nurse collect during evaluation at the triage unit to support the accuracy of the preliminary PTL diagnosis?

    a.　level of cervical dilation and effacement

    b.　outcome of previous preterm delivery

    c.　history of fetal demise or abortions

    d.　age of her absent spouse

3. What risk factors are present that increase the likelihood of the PTL diagnosis for S.B.?

    a.　low socioeconomic status

    b.　smoking

    c.　stress

    d.　possible infection

4. Considering that (1) the nurse is talking with S.B. on the phone while she is at work; (2) preliminary data analysis supports that S.B. is indeed at risk for PTL; and (3) S.B. has not been able to reach her personal health care provider, how should the nurse counsel S.B.? (Select all that apply.)

    a.　Have her drink 1-2 glasses of water per hour and lie down on her left side.

    b.　Have her determine if the fetus is moving or if there is a change in movement.

    c.　Make sure she understands not to put anything in her vagina.

    d.　Ask if someone can meet her children and if she has transportation to the hospital.

5. S.B.'s PTL contractions are not relieved fol-
    lowing the conservative measures suggested.
    Her doctor agrees that S.B. should be direct-
    ed to the OB triage unit for further evalua-
    tion. The decision is made after interview,
    fetal monitoring, and cervical examination
    that S.B. is a suitable candidate for tocolytic
    therapy. Which findings, if they were pres-
    ent, would have contraindicated tocolytic
    therapy for S.B.? (Select all that apply.)

    a. pregnancy of less than 20 weeks gesta-
        tion
    b. bulging or premature rupture of mem-
        branes
    c. confirmed fetal death
    d. evidence of severe fetal compromise
    e. age of the mother

6. The nurse shares with S.B. that the goal in
    tocolytic therapy is to (increase/decrease)
    the level of uterine contractions to stop PTL;
    this allows time for maturation of the lungs
    within the uterine environment. (Circle cor-
    rect answer.)

7. What criteria should determine if subcutane-
    ous tocolytic therapy is successful for this
    client? (Select all that apply.)

    a. Contractions decrease to 6 or fewer per
        hour.
    b. There is no further dilation or efface-
        ment of the cervix.
    c. The membranes are no longer bulging.
    d. There is minimal vaginal bleeding.

8. S.B. is to continue taking oral terbutaline
    after discharge. What is the purpose of con-
    tinuing therapy with this medication?

    a. decrease the incidence of fetal demise
    b. stop or prevent recurrence of PTL
    c. decrease S.B.'s blood pressure
    d. improve S.B.'s respiratory status

9. The high-risk unit nurse has worked with
    S.B. to address identified knowledge deficits,
    emphasizing the importance of medication
    compliance. S.B. states that she knows she
    must take her oral terbutaline on schedule
    but says, "If I go back to work, it is hard
    to get free to go to the bathroom or to the
    breakroom for fluids; it is also difficult to get
    my purse, because we aren't allowed to keep
    purses at the counter where I work." How
    could the nurse help S.B. with her adherence
    to the medication regimen?

    a. Have her put the pill in her pocket
        while at work so she can take it with
        sips of water.
    b. Teach her how to take the pill without
        water.
    c. Have her take the medication with her
        meals.
    d. Let her know she only needs to take the
        medication when she feels abdominal
        discomfort.

10. S.B. realizes that she missed taking a dose
    within the past hour and calls for advice.
    What is the nurse's best response?

    a. Tell her not to worry about it, she can
        just take the next dose at the regular
        time.
    b. Have her take the medication now and
        continue on her regular schedule of
        medications.
    c. Have her double the dose at the next
        scheduled time for administration.
    d. Have her take half of the normal dose
        and continue with her next dose at the
        correct time.

54 Female Reproductive Cycle II: Labor, Delivery, and Preterm Neonatal Drugs

Study Questions

Crossword puzzle: Use the definitions to determine the correct terms.

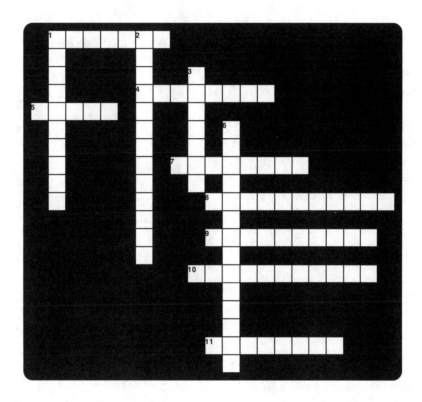

Across

1. Type of pain caused by pressure of the presenting part and stretching of the perineum and vagina
4. Type of anesthesia that achieves pain relief during labor and delivery without loss of consciousness
5. Receptors activated by morphine
7. Softening of the cervix
8. Scoring system to assist in predicting whether labor induction may be successful (2 words)
9. Commonly prescribed synthetic opioid for pain control during labor
10. Tightening and shortening of uterine muscles
11. Cervix and uterus are carried by sympathetic fibers

Down

1. A lipoprotein in the alveoli that works to keep the alveoli open during expiration
2. Rescue administration of surfactant
3. Drug used for labor augmentation
6. Uterine inactivity or hypotonic contractions (2 words)

NCLEX Review Questions

Select the best response.

12. The client is receiving a narcotic-agonist during labor. How long before birth should it be administered to prevent fetal depression?
    a. 30 minutes
    b. 45 minutes
    c. 1-3 hours
    d. 5-6 hours

13. The primary advantage of butorphanol tartrate (Stadol) and nalbuphine (Nubain) is their dose ceiling effect. What does this mean?
    a. Additional doses of the medication do not increase the degree of respiratory depression.
    b. This means that there is no limit as to how much of the drug can be used to obtain the desired effect.
    c. Only one dose is administered to obtain the desired effect.
    d. Both of these medications must be given together to get the dose ceiling effect.

14. The client has received spinal anesthesia for delivery. What should the nurse monitor in this patient?
    a. Hgb and Hct
    b. palpitations
    c. spinal headache
    d. pedal edema

15. What are nursing treatments for postdural headaches? (Select all that apply.)
    a. analgesics
    b. caffeine
    c. decreased fluids
    d. a blood patch

16. When should pain medication be administered to the laboring client using the IV route?
    a. at the beginning of the uterine contraction
    b. in the middle of the uterine contraction
    c. at the end of the uterine contraction
    d. between uterine contractions

17. If the client is abusing narcotics, which drug is commonly used during labor?
    a. Nembutal
    b. Atarax
    c. Stadol
    d. Demerol

18. Which medication is the best to provide reversal of neonatal respiratory depression?
    a. calcium gluconate
    b. calcium carbonate
    c. syrup of ipecac
    d. naloxone (Narcan)

19. Before the administration of general anesthesia, a laboring woman is administered 30 mL of Bicitra. What is the purpose of giving this medication?
    a. prevent nausea and vomiting
    b. decrease gastric acidity
    c. maintain a patent airway
    d. enhance anesthesia induction

20. What should be done before the administration of an epidural?
    a. The woman should receive a bolus of crystalloids, 500-1000 mL IV.
    b. The maternal heart should be monitored for mitral valve disease.
    c. The client should verbally consent to the procedure.
    d. The client should be typed and cross-matched for blood administration.

21. A client is receiving an epidural, and her blood pressure is beginning to drop. What is the first action the nurse should take?
    a. Expect an order to transfuse with 1 unit of packed red cells.
    b. Expect an order to administer 5-15 mg ephedrine IV.
    c. Turn her on her left side.
    d. Administer oxygen 2-4 L by nasal cannula.

22. The woman in labor is questioning the nurse about labor being longer for women who receive an epidural. What is your best response?
    a. "This is not accurate; women who receive epidurals have the same length of labor as those receiving pain relief medications."
    b. "No, women with spinal anesthesia have a longer labor."
    c. "Yes, women do have a longer labor, approximately 15-30 minutes longer; they can feel movement and pressure but not pain."
    d. "Yes, women do have a longer labor, approximately 2-3 hours longer; they have no pain or pressure with epidurals."

23. Scores of which value or greater on the Bishop score are associated with successful labor induction?
    a. 5
    b. 6
    c. 8
    d. 10

24. During which stage of labor do women commonly receive ergot alkaloids?
    a. first
    b. second
    c. third
    d. fourth

25. Before administering methylergonovine (Methergine), which baseline value should be measured?
    a. fetal heart rate
    b. maternal respiratory rate
    c. maternal hourly urinary output
    d. blood pressure

26. With the administration of naloxone (Narcan), what will the woman in labor experience?
    a. increased pain relief
    b. increased pain
    c. increased fetal heart rate decelerations
    d. increased fetal variability

27. The nurse is aware that many factors influence the choice of pain control. What is the most important factor?
    a. intensity of contractions
    b. amount of time likely until delivery
    c. frequency of contractions
    d. client requests

28. What should the nurse know about the use of barbiturates in labor?
    a. They make the delivery time unpredictable.
    b. The narcotic antagonists will not counteract respiratory depression.
    c. Narcotics offer more complete relief.
    d. Active labor is the most appropriate time for their use.

29. Which priority information should be included in client teaching about an analgesic during labor? (Select all that apply.)
    a. expected effects on labor
    b. expected effects on newborn
    c. expected time delivery will occur
    d. restrictions placed on her mobility

30. Which of these statements about the client who receives continuous lumbar epidural block anesthesia in repeated doses is accurate?

    a. Before 8 cm dilation, there is a risk of arresting the first stage of labor.

    b. The method is suitable for vaginal delivery, but not for a cesarean delivery because the density of the block cannot be manipulated.

    c. Following injection, the client needs to be placed flat immediately to ensure dispersion of the local anesthetic toward the diaphragm.

    d. Each time the injection procedure occurs, documentation must be complete.

31. In relation to uterine contractions, how should spinal anesthesia be administered?

    a. before

    b. during

    c. immediately after

    d. 1-2 minutes after

32. Which local anesthetic is metabolized by pseudocholinesterase?

    a. chloroprocaine (Nesacaine)

    b. mepivacaine (Carbocaine)

    c. lidocaine (Xylocaine)

    d. bupivacaine (Marcaine)

33. The nurse assesses a client receiving local anesthetic for side effects. What should the nurse monitor in this client? (Select all that apply.)

    a. palpitations

    b. metallic taste in mouth

    c. nausea

    d. hypertension

34. Which baseline data should the nurse collect on a client having an IV oxytocin induction at 41+ weeks gestation? (Select all that apply.)

    a. pulse rate and blood pressure

    b. deep tendon reflexes

    c. uterine activity

    d. fetal heart rate

35. The nurse observes a client having an IV oxytocin induction at 41+ weeks gestation and her fetus for side effects and adverse reactions to oxytocin. What would the nurse assess?

    a. tetanic uterine contractions

    b. fetal tachycardia

    c. generalized muscular weakness

    d. urinary retention

36. As a precaution, the nurse should have which antidote to oxytocin readily available?

    a. prednisone

    b. Narcan

    c. calcium gluconate

    d. magnesium sulfate

37. The nurse monitors a client having an IV oxytocin induction at 41+ weeks gestation for signs of uterine rupture. What would the nurse assess in a client who has experienced uterine rupture? (Select all that apply.)

    a. hypotension

    b. sudden increased pain

    c. hemorrhage

    d. loss of fetal heart rate

38. Which types of systemic drug groups are used during labor? (Select all that apply.)

    a. NSAIDs

    b. narcotic agonists

    c. ataractics

    d. mixed narcotic agonists-antagonists

39. The client has received a sedative-hypnotic drug and antiemetic/antihistamine for analgesia during labor. This has placed the neonate at risk for which alteration? (Select all that apply.)

    a. decreased fetal heart rate variability

    b. hypotonia

    c. urinary retention

    d. CNS depression

    e. hypothermia

40. The client is complaining of labor pain. This somatic pain is caused by pressure of the presenting part and stretching of the perineum and vagina. This pain is experienced in which stage(s) of labor? (Select all that apply.)
    a. first
    b. latent
    c. active
    d. transition
    e. second
    f. third

41. Which type(s) of anesthesia may be used for cesarean deliveries? (Select all that apply.)
    a. general anesthesia
    b. caudal block
    c. spinal anesthesia
    d. pudenal anesthesia
    e. epidural anesthesia

Case Study

Select the best answer.

K.Z., 28 years old, is the mother of a 2-year-old child. She is 38 weeks pregnant and admitted to the OB unit in active labor. She says, "I'm having contractions about every two minutes. It hurts. Can't you do something?" When questioned further, she rates her pain as 8 on a scale of 1 to 10, describing it as "intense cramping" in "my lower belly." In reviewing her fetal heart rate strip, the nurse notes contractions every 2 to 3 minutes, lasting 50 to 60 seconds and with an intensity of 55 to 65 mm Hg.

1. What objective data supplied support the need for more effective pain management?
    a. uterine contractions every 2-3 minutes with an intensity of 55-65 mm Hg
    b. the intensity of the cramping K.Z. is experiencing in the lower abdomen
    c. the length of the contractions
    d. the number of weeks of pregnancy

2. What additional subjective data support the need for more effective pain management? (Select all that apply.)
    a. rating of pain of 8 on a scale of 1-10
    b. pain described as "intense cramping"
    c. client's statement of "Can't you do something?"
    d. pain lasting more than 2 to 3 minutes

3. K.Z. has asked for an epidural. What factors are contraindications for an epidural? (Select all that apply.)
    a. morbid obesity
    b. severe preeclampsia
    c. coagulation disorders
    d. sepsis
    e. age

4. K.Z. asks the nurse if her labor will be longer with an epidural. What is the nurse's best response?
    a. "No, it will not be longer, as you will no longer be fighting the pain."
    b. "No, it will not be longer, as you will be more relaxed and the cervix can dilate quicker."
    c. "Yes, it will be longer, but only by about 15-30 minutes."
    d. "Yes, it will be several hours longer."

5. Following K.Z.'s admission interview, fetal and uterine monitoring, and cervical examination, she requests pain medication "Now. I can't wait until the epidural, please." Until K.Z. receives the epidural, the health care provider writes an order for nalbuphine (Nubain) IV 10 mg. When will the Nubain be administered in relationship to her uterine contractions?
    a. at the beginning of the contraction
    b. at the peak of the contraction
    c. at the first sign of the contraction easing
    d. immediately after the contraction

6. K.Z. asks where the epidural is injected in her back. What is the nurse's best response?

   a. "It depends on the type of epidural you receive."

   b. "It depends on the level of pain relief you would like."

   c. "In the middle of your back between the dura and pia mater of the spinal cord."

   d. "Near the middle of your back just outside the spinal cord."

7. Before receiving the epidural, K.Z. will receive a bolus of 500-1000 mL of dextrose-free IV fluids. The goal of this bolus of IV fluid is to prevent what from occurring?

   a. increased blood pressure

   b. fetal decelerations

   c. hypotension

   d. pain at the injection site

8. After receiving the epidural, K.Z.'s blood pressure begins to drop. What are immediate nursing actions to address this problem?

   a. Turn her on her left side and put a wedge under her left hip.

   b. Turn her on her right side and put a wedge under her legs.

   c. Increase the rate of her IV administration.

   d. Give her medication for her pain.

9. K.Z.'s blood pressure is continuing to fall. What would the nurse anticipate the health care provider would order?

   a. morphine

   b. to stop the flow of the epidural medication

   c. ephedrine 5-15 mg

   d. rapidly increased fluid intake

10. One hour after delivery, K.Z.'s uterus is boggy and she is saturating a pad within 35 minutes. What medication/dose would the nurse anticipate the health care provider order to be added to K.Z.'s IV fluids?

    a. increased fluids

    b. 10-20 units of Pitocin IV

    c. naxolone

    d. vitamin K

55 Postpartum and Newborn Drugs

Study Questions

Crossword puzzle: Use the definitions to determine the correct terms.

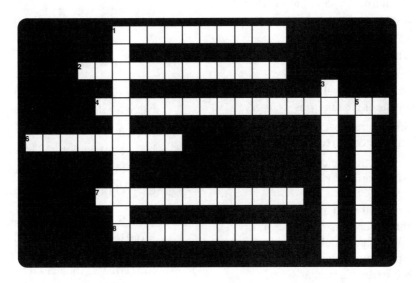

Across

1. The period from delivery until 6 weeks postpartum
2. Provides prophylaxis against eye infections
4. Syndrome where there is transmission of the rubella virus to the fetus via the placenta (2 words)
6. Skin rash caused by an allergic reaction
7. Skin inflammation resulting from contact with an irritating substance or allergen
8. Incision made to enlarge the vaginal opening to facilitate newborn delivery

Down

1. Prevents hemorrhagic disease of the newborn
3. Local anesthetic that can be used for an episiotomy
5. Production and release of milk by mammary glands

NCLEX Review Questions

Select the best response.

9. Which are the most commonly used medications for the relief of perineal pain resulting from episiotomy laceration? (Select all that apply.)
   a. benzocaine
   b. witch hazel compresses
   c. Tucks
   d. mineral oil

10. The nurse is administering a stool softener to a postpartum client. The client asks what the purpose/action of this medication is. What is the nurse's best response?
    a. "To make sure you have a bowel movement before discharge."
    b. "To decrease perineal discomfort and facilitate stool passage postdelivery."
    c. "To decrease the need for eating fiber while in the postpartum period."
    d. "To decrease the incidence of gas, thus decreasing perineal pain."

11. A postpartum client with a repaired fourth-degree laceration has benzocaine topical spray. She asks if she can also use a heat lamp on her perineum for additional comfort. What is the nurse's best answer?
    a. "What a good idea; it will decrease pain while improving healing."
    b. "Yes, you can use a heat lamp to augment the action of benzocaine."
    c. "No, the heat lamp will increase the incidence of bacteria growth."
    d. "No, use of a heat lamp with benzocaine may cause tissue burns."

12. Relief of afterbirth pains may be a concern for the postpartum client. Which factors are associated with an increased risk of afterbirth pains? (Select all that apply.)
    a. primigravida
    b. breastfeeding
    c. multiparity
    d. preeclampsia

13. What interventions can the nurse implement to suppress lactation? (Select all that apply.)
    a. ice packs
    b. tight supportive bra
    c. warm compresses
    d. warm shower water directed to the breasts
    e. lactation

14. When is the best time to administer the standard dose of Rh immune globulin D?
    a. at 28 weeks gestation.
    b. before amniocentesis and at 38 weeks gestation
    c. at 28 weeks gestation and again within 72 hours after delivery
    d. after chorionic villus sampling and at 38 weeks gestation

15. After which procedure should the client receive a microdose of Rh immune globulin D?
    a. amniocentesis
    b. abortion of <13 weeks
    c. abortion of >16 weeks
    d. chorionic villus sampling

16. Which clinical manifestations are commonly reported side effects of the -caine drugs used in local or topical agents ordered for postpartum clients? (Select all that apply.)
    a. stinging
    b. burning
    c. itching
    d. petechiae

17. Which clinical manifestation(s) is/are commonly reported side effects of the hydrocortisone local or topical drugs used in products ordered with occlusive dressings for postpartum clients? (Select all that apply.)
    a. burning
    b. alopecia
    c. folliculitis
    d. swelling

18. Which ophthalmic ointment is administered to the newborn immediately after birth?
    a. erythromycin
    b. bacitracin
    c. gentamicin
    d. penicillin

19. Which priority information should be included in client teaching regarding ophthalmic and parenteral drugs administered to the neonate immediately after birth?
    a. Swelling of eyes usually disappears in the first 24-48 hours.
    b. All parenteral medications can be administered in one injection.
    c. The injection is not painful for the baby.
    d. If the mother has had hepatitis immunizations then the newborn will not receive the hepatitis B immunization.

Case Study

Select the best answer.

M.F., a newly delivered postpartum client, is transported from the labor/delivery suite to the postpartum unit. A nurse fills in and receives the transfer report about M.F. She is Rh-negative and rubella-negative.

1. What information from M.F.'s past and current history must be considered to address the question of whether she will be a candidate for Rh immune globulin D? (Select all that apply.)
    a. M.F.'s age
    b. previous pregnancies and their outcome
    c. the father's Rh status
    d. if M.F. has had Rh immune globulin D in the past
    e. M.F.'s religious beliefs

2. M.F. asks what the Coombs' test is and why her caregivers seem so interested in this test. The nurse explains to M.F. that it screens for the presence of (antigen/antibodies) to the Rh (antigen/antibodies). The outcome is expressed as an (antigen/antibody) titer. The nurse says that Rh immune globulin D candidates are (sensitized/nonsensitized) Rh-negative clients. The goal is, through the use of Rh immune globulin D, to (prevent/establish) her from becoming (sensitized/nonsensitized) by suppressing the active (antigen/antibody) response by coating the (antigen/antibody). (Circle correct answers.)

3. M.F. needs to understand that if the baby she just delivered is Rh (positive/negative), she could, based on factors from her history and/or this pregnancy, labor, and delivery, develop anti-D (antibodies/antigens) as an outcome. Therefore her caregiver's goal is to ascertain that the D (antibody/antigen) is (negative/positive). Likewise, a laboratory report of the baby's blood type and sensitization status (based on detection of red blood cells coated with antibody) is reviewed. If M.F. and the baby both test (positive/negative) for sensitization, general practice is for M.F. to receive Rh immune globulin D within (72/96) hours postpartum to prevent isoimmunization, which could present difficulties for a fetus in a subsequent pregnancy. (Circle correct answers.)

4. M.F.'s history indicated that she is rubella-negative. She is listed in one section of the chart as rubella-immune and in another section of the chart as rubella-susceptible. What would be the most appropriate action by the nurse?
    a. Administer the rubella vaccine to the client.
    b. Obtain a rubella titer to verify her negative status.
    c. Obtain a rubella titer to verify her positive status.
    d. Notify the client's health care provider.

5. M.F. is to receive both Rh immune globulin D and rubella vaccine. What should the nurse explain to M.F. about the interaction of the two drugs?

    a. The client will experience a severe headache for several days after administration.

    b. The client will experience a decreased resistance to the flu virus.

    c. The client will be unable to breastfeed for at least 2 weeks.

    d. The client will have a suppression of rubella antibodies and will need to have a repeat titer in 3 months.

6. Based on her history, what priority information should be given to M.F. as her postdischarge responsibility in regard to the rubella vaccine she has received? (Select all that apply.)

    a. Discuss the importance of using effective contraception for 4 weeks after vaccine administration.

    b. Teach her about her contraceptive of choice and how to appropriately use it.

    c. Tell her she should have a rubella titer drawn 3 months after administration.

    d. Tell her to avoid persons with colds or influenza for the next 3 months.

56 Drugs for Women's Reproductive Health and Menopause

Study Questions

Crossword puzzle: Use the definitions to determine the correct terms.

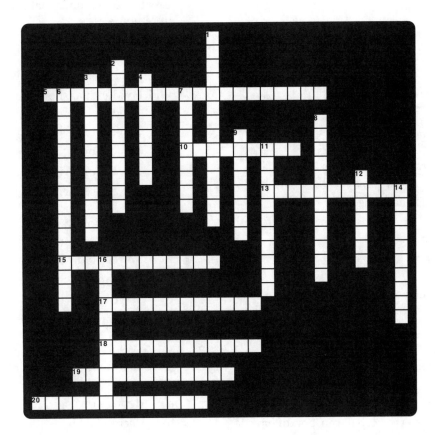

Across

5. Higher dose of estrogen that increases the risk of this of occurring (2 words)
10. Derivative of the steroid testosterone
13. Heavy periods
15. Painful periods
17. Loss of bone mass predisposing client to fractures
18. Surgical removal of the ovaries
19. Medication that stops the pregnancy in the uterus
20. Midcycle pain usually associated with ovulation

Down

1. Infrequent or very light menstruation
2. Painful sexual intercourse
3. Another name for emergency contraception (2 words)
4. Hyperpigmentation of the skin
6. The most commonly used estrogen (2 words)

7. The permanent cessation of menstruation
8. First marketed as RU486
9. The start of spontaneous menstruation
11. Another name for the progestin-only oral contraceptive pill (2 words)

12. Vaginitis from yeast
14. Absence of periods
16. Drug given to cause the uterus to contract and expel the products of conception

Match characteristics associated with the investigational drugs in Column II with the drugs in Column I. Some Column II characteristics may be used more than once.

Column I

____ 21. Misoprostol
____ 22. Methotrexate

Column II

a. Chemotherapeutic agent
b. Ulcer agent
c. Destabilizes uterine lining
d. Creates contractions that shed uterine lining in 24 hours
e. Given 1 week after the first drug

NCLEX Review Questions

Select the best response.

23. Which contraceptive methods are available for poor pill-takers ? (Select all that apply.)
    a. Depo-Provera injection
    b. Ortho-Evra patch
    c. NuvaRing
    d. Implanon

24. Which mode(s) of action is/are correct for emergency contraception? (Select all that apply.)
    a. delays ovulation
    b. interferes with hormones for implantation
    c. causes an abortion
    d. interferes with tubal transport of embryo

25. What are the advantages of oral contraceptives? (Select all that apply.)
    a. relative safety
    b. ease of use
    c. low cost
    d. high degree of effectiveness

26. Which individual should not take oral contraceptives?
    a. 20-year-old who is not sexually active
    b. 40-year-old with diabetes
    c. 38-year-old with breast cancer
    d. 48-year-old with emphysema

27. In which person should oral contraceptives be used with caution? (Select all that apply.)
    a. 32-year-old who smokes
    b. 45-year-old who does not exercise
    c. 38-year old with diabetes
    d. 28-year-old with epilepsy

28. What is the major risk associated with the use of leuprolide acetate for the treatment of endometriosis?
    a. depression
    b. decreased libido
    c. cardiac dysrhythmias
    d. potential loss of bone density

29. A client who has been taking Tri-Levlen for contraception reports a variety of side effects. Which clinical manifestations are due primarily to an excess of estrogen? (Select all that apply.)
    a. acne
    b. nausea
    c. fluid retention
    d. breast tenderness

30. A client who has been taking Tri-Levlen for contraception reports her current drug history. Which drugs will interact with her oral contraceptive? (Select all that apply.)
    a. phenytoin
    b. caffeine
    c. vitamins
    d. theophylline

31. Which laboratory value(s), if they changed in a client who has been taking Tri-Levlen for contraception, should be an area of concern?
    a. thyroid and liver function
    b. blood glucose
    c. triglycerides
    d. BUN

32. A client who has been taking Tri-Levlen for contraception calls and reports missing one pill. What is the nurse's best advice?
    a. "Skip this pill. Take the next pill at the normal time tomorrow."
    b. "Take the missed pill right away. Take tomorrow's pill at the usual time."
    c. "Discard the current pill pack and start a new package of pills."
    d. "Do a home pregnancy test and report the results."

33. The family planning nurse would be correct to tell a client to stop taking Tri-Levlen for contraception and notify her health care provider if she experiences which alteration?
    a. increased vaginal discharge
    b. severe headaches
    c. lighter/shorter periods
    d. menstrual cramping

34. Which alterations are known with danazol (Danocrine)? (Select all that apply.)
    a. It is a pituitary gonadotropin-inhibiting agent.
    b. Menses cease during therapy.
    c. Ovulation occurs during therapy.
    d. It has no estrogenic action.

35. What risk factor(s) decrease with the use of progestin in HRT?
    a. risk for endometrial hyperplasia
    b. risk of endometrial cancer
    c. risk of breast cancer
    d. risk of cervical cancer

36. What are the advantages of the Estraderm transdermal system? (Select all that apply.)
    a. less expensive than tablets
    b. applied 2 times per week for 3 weeks using rotation of sites
    c. drug absorbed directly into bloodstream
    d. results in less nausea and vomiting

37. Which statement(s) best describe(s) the combined birth control pills? (Select all that apply.)
    a. available in 24-day active pills
    b. available in 28-day active pills
    c. available as a chewable pill
    d. available without a prescription

38. Which medications are used to prevent and/or treat osteoporosis? (Select all that apply.)
    a. estrogen
    b. statins
    c. bisphosphonates
    d. SERMs

39. Which statement(s) best describe(s) HRT? (Select all that apply.)
    a. HRT may be used to prevent heart disease.
    b. HRT is indicated for the treatment of menopausal vasomotor symptoms.
    c. HRT should be used for the shortest period of time possible, at the lowest effective dose.
    d. Vaginal creams or rings may be used to treat urogenital atrophy.

Case Study

Select the best answer.

During her gynecology intake interview with the nursing case manager at her company's new health care clinic, C.W., age 55 years, states, "I seem to be having more discomfort when I have intercourse. I don't lubricate when I want and need to; if my husband hurries me, it is downright painful. This is probably my problem, but my husband thinks that after a 35-year marriage, I just don't really want to have sex any more."

The nurse compiles a few more facts about C.W. for review and consideration. In addition to her dyspareunia, C.W. has urinary frequency and urgency, leukorrhea, itching, thinning vaginal epithelium with a glazed-looking appearance, and minimal elasticity upon speculum examination.

C.W. is Caucasian, is very thin, and reports no periods for nearly 2 years. She has no history of vaginal infections, and her hygiene is excellent.

1. What is the most likely physiologic explanation for C.W.'s current experiences during intercourse?
    a. increased progesterone
    b. decreased progesterone
    c. increased estrogen
    d. decreased estrogen

2. Given the fact that C.W. has had no periods for more than a year, the nurse knows that menopause (has / has not) occurred. (Circle correct answer.) The nurse asks C.W. if she has considered exploring the use of HRT. C.W. responds that she has thought about it, listens to every news report that addresses the issue, but is afraid to take hormones unless she can perceive more benefits than potential liabilities for her personally. How might the nurse advise C.W.? (Select all that apply.)
    a. "The problems you're experiencing would be relieved or decreased by the use of HRT."
    b. "Your risks for the diseases associated with HRT increase with age anyway, so you might as well try it."
    c. "This is the only treatment currently available for the problems you're experiencing."
    d. "There is more than one method of delivery that will decrease the risks of using HRT."

3. While conducting an assessment of C.W. for other physical changes associated with menopause, what other physical characteristics might the nurse discuss with C.W.? (Select all that apply.)
    a. vascular changes
    b. experience of hot flashes
    c. enlargement of the breasts
    d. sleep disturbances
    e. changes in height

4. C.W.'s physical characteristics put her at particular risk for which alterations?
    a. spotting
    b. migraines
    c. fractures
    d. diabetes

5. Why is this risk an especially important consideration for C.W.?
    a. Bone mass loss occurs in the first 3-5 years postmenopause.
    b. Her decreased estrogen levels put her at risk for CAD.
    c. She is 55 years old.
    d. She does little to no physical exercise.

6. What priority benefits of HRT should the nurse discuss with C.W.? (Place in order of importance.)

   a. reduction in the incidence of coronary artery disease

   b. thicker vagina with increased moisture and lubrication with decreased discomfort

   c. decreased loss of bone density

   d. reduction of sleep deprivation and somatic discomforts

7. C.W. mentions, "If the estrogen is so beneficial, why does a person also have to take a medication with it that partially blocks these beneficial effects?" What is the best response?

   a. "The added medication minimizes the risk of endometrial hyperplasia, endometrial cancer, and breast cancer."

   b. "The added medication decreases the risk of osteoporosis."

   c. "The added medication minimizes the risk of CAD and breast cancer."

   d. "The added medication increases the level of vaginal moistness."

8. C.W. asks, "Do I need to swallow pills if I just want to get rid of these vaginal problems?" What is the nurse's best response?

   a. "You can use a local estrogen cream and it has the same effectiveness as the oral therapy."

   b. "The vaginal cream is only applied as needed, so it might be better for you."

   c. "The systemic approach is better to treat your vaginal problems and receive the cardiovascular and bone benefits."

   d. "The oral method of administration is easier to use than the vaginal cream."

9. The nurse reviews C.W.'s history for the presence of any factors that might contraindicate the use of estrogens. What factors should the nurse look for? (Select all that apply.)

   a. suspected or known breast cancer

   b. thrombophlebitis

   c. acute liver disease

   d. diabetes

10. C.W. elects to try HRT. Several months go by and the nurse receives a call from C.W. stating that she is having bleeding during the last week of her cycle that lasts a few days but does not quite resemble her former periods. She also says that she is having an occasional hot flash during this period and that she thought these would disappear with the therapy. What advice should the nurse provide? (Select all that apply.)

    a. "This is normal as you go through withdrawal bleeding."

    b. "If you experience headaches or visual changes, you should report them to your health care provider."

    c. "This is normal; we will just need to increase the amount of HRT you're currently taking."

    d. "You should increase your fluid intake to counter the loss of vascular fluid."

57 Drugs for Men's Health and Reproductive Disorders

Study Questions

Match the terms in Column I with the definitions in Column II.

Column I

___ 1. Anabolic steroids
___ 2. Androgens
___ 3. Hirsutism
___ 4. Spermatogenesis
___ 5. Virilization
___ 6. Antiantigens
___ 7. Cryptorchidism
___ 8. Gynecomastia
___ 9. Oligospermia
___ 10. Priapism

Column II

a. Low sperm count
b. Undescended testis
c. Breast swelling or soreness
d. Ongoing painful erection
e. Growth of facial hair, and vocal huskiness in women
f. Formation of spermatozoa
g. Steroid hormones related to the hormone testosterone
h. Testosterone
i. Blocks the synthesis or action of androgens
j. Increased hair growth

NCLEX Review Questions

Select the best response.

11. Which client should not receive sildenafil?
    a. 62-year-old with renal disease
    b. 68-year-old with cardiac disease
    c. 56-year-old with hepatic disease
    d. 58-year-old with CNS disorder

12. A 17-year-old male client receiving androgen therapy for hypogonadism asks the nurse what androgen therapy does. What is the nurse's best response?
    a. "It ensures the ability to respond sexually."
    b. "It ensures adequate sperm production."
    c. "It promotes larger stature through protein deposition."
    d. "It stimulates the development of secondary sex characteristics."

13. A 17-year-old male client receiving androgen therapy for hypogonadism observes that some of the football players at his school take hormones to help them bulk up. What is the nurse's best response?
    a. "This is safe as long as they use the proper dosage."
    b. "This can cause serious, often irreversible, health problems years later."
    c. "Most athletic organizations endorse this practice."
    d. "As long as they don't use other street drugs, this is probably safe."

14. A 17-year-old male client receiving androgen therapy for hypogonadism asks how often and for how long he must have his testosterone enanthate injection. How long should this client be on this therapy?
    a. daily for a month
    b. biweekly for 4 months
    c. biweekly for 4 years
    d. weekly for a year

15. In reviewing the current medications of a 17-year-old male client receiving androgen therapy for hypogonadism, what should the nurse be aware of?
    a. Androgens may decrease blood glucose levels in diabetics, so an insulin dose may need adjustment.
    b. Barbiturates potentiate androgens.
    c. There is no interaction with steroids.
    d. Androgens decrease the effect of anticoagulants.

16. During one of his clinic visits, a 17-year-old male client receiving androgen therapy for hypogonadism tells the nurse that his great-aunt said that she took male hormones. He asks you why they would be given to a woman. What is the nurse's best response?
    a. "Women are not treated with male hormones."
    b. "Women bodybuilders take androgens."
    c. "The doctor will explain this to you later."
    d. "Women with advanced breast cancer or severe menopausal symptoms may benefit from androgens."

17. Which clinical manifestations would indicate that a 17-year-old male client receiving androgen therapy for hypogonadism is receiving too much testosterone enanthate? (Select all that apply.)
    a. deepening of his voice
    b. continuous erection
    c. breast soreness
    d. urinary urgency

18. Before a 17-year-old male client can begin his androgen therapy regimen, which contraindications must be ruled out? (Select all that apply.)
    a. nephrosis
    b. hepatic insufficiency
    c. diabetes
    d. pituitary insufficiency

19. On one of his clinic visits, a 17-year-old male client receiving androgen therapy for hypogonadism tells you that his grandfather is taking antiandrogens. He asks you why these drugs are used. What are the indications for the use of antiandrogens? (Select all that apply.)
    a. cancer of the prostate
    b. male pattern baldness
    c. virilization syndrome in women
    d. precocious puberty in girls

Case Study

Select the best answer.

M.T., age 16 years, is the shortest boy in his class. His parents bring him to the endocrine clinic because of their concern.

1. Why would the treatment team explore family feelings before initiating treatment? (Select all that apply.)
    a. To determine if the treatment should be implemented
    b. To identify if the client is motivated to do the treatment
    c. To determine if the client has any contraindications
    d. To assess M.T.'s self-esteem

2.   What should the family be told about the effectiveness of androgen treatment for delayed growth?

   a.   It is very effective and will cause M.T.'s height to increase quickly.

   b.   There is much evidence that the treatment plays a role in promoting growth.

   c.   There is no evidence that this treatment is effective.

   d.   There is one drug that is effective in treating growth problems.

3.   How is an androgen selected for therapy?

   a.   It is based on the genetic makeup of the individual and family.

   b.   It is based on the amount of growth and sexual maturation desired.

   c.   It is based on the current height of the individual.

   d.   It is based on the time frame available until the epiphyseal plates close.

4.   Which body systems' functioning needs to be monitored during therapy?

   a.   gastrointestinal tract

   b.   endocrine, gastrointestinal, and renal systems

   c.   endocrine system only

   d.   central nervous system

5.   How long can this therapy be expected to last?

   a.   1 month

   b.   3-6 months

   c.   7-12 months

   d.   15 months

58 Drugs for Disorders in Women's Health, Infertility, and Sexually Transmitted Infections

Study Questions

Crossword puzzle: Use the definitions to determine the correct terms.

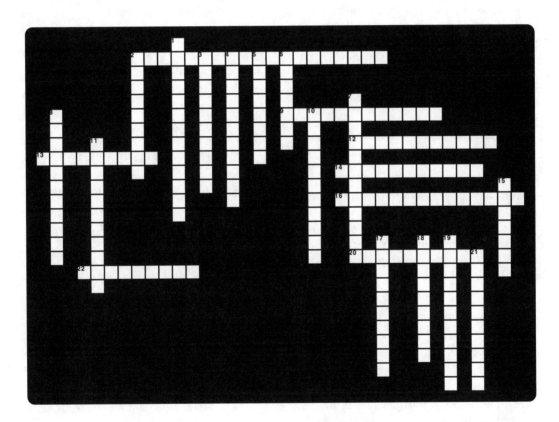

Across

2. Increased pigmentation and thickening of the skin (2 words)
9. Benign tumors in the uterus
12. Uterine bleeding greater than 80 mL or for more than 7 days occurring at regular intervals
13. What is in micronized progesterone that makes it contraindicated in some individuals (2 words)
14. Absence of ovulation
16. This type of drug suppresses ovulation and causes long-term endometrial atrophy
20. Absence of menses
22. Excessive hair growth

Down

1. Abnormal location of endometrial tissue outside the uterus
2. Drug used to treat a primary infection of genital herpes

3. An STI for which a vaccine exists (2 words)
4. Herb taken to relieve depression (3 words)
5. A disease that is transmitted transplacentally
6. Resistance to this hormone is a hallmark of polycystic ovary syndrome (PCOS)
7. Pelvic pain that is associated with the menstrual cycle
8. Type of underwear men should use to improve male fertility (2 words)
10. Inability to conceive a child after 12 months of unprotected sex
11. Cough medicine that can thin cervical mucus and can lead to conception
15. Treatment of endometriosis
17. Drug of choice for the treatment of syphilis
18. Herbal supplement that may help with some PMS symptoms as well as breast pain
19. Herb that prevents progesterone overproduction and inhibits prolactin release
21. Most effective risk-reducing behavior for avoidance of STIs

NCLEX Review Questions

Select the best response.

23. A 19-year-old client comes to the clinic complaining of dysuria and yellow-green discharge. Culture confirms *Neisseria gonorrhoeae*. Because the client has presented with a sexually transmitted infection, which test should the client be counseled to consider?
    a. fasting blood sugar
    b. liver function
    c. HIV test
    d. fertility workup

24. All recent sexual partners need to be informed of a client's gonorrhea, and until reculturing demonstrates cure, what should the client do to prevent further sexual disease transmission?
    a. Abstain or use condoms during sex.
    b. Ask partners to take antibiotics.
    c. Douche before intercourse.
    d. Only engage in anal intercourse.

25. A client has repeated gonorrhea and chlamydia infections as well as HPV and is being followed up at the infectious disease clinic. In teaching the client about the transmission of sexually transmitted infections, the nurse is aware that which sexual interaction can cause the most trauma?
    a. genital-genital
    b. genital-anal
    c. oral-genital
    d. mouth-to-mouth

26. A client with repeated gonorrhea and chlamydia infections as well as HPV asks how long she must abstain from sex. What is the nurse's best response?
    a. "Two months."
    b. "You may have sex using condoms."
    c. "Until the medication is finished."
    d. "Until your partner finishes his treatment."

27. A client asks if gonorrhea and syphilis are the same. What is the nurse's best response?
    a. "No, but if you have one, you should consider being tested for the other."
    b. "Yes, they are essentially the same."
    c. "No, syphilis cannot be cured."
    d. "No, gonorrhea has no serious effects."

28. A client with repeated gonorrhea and chlamydia infections as well as HPV says she might be pregnant. What is the risk to the fetus?
    a. If the client is treated now and avoids sexual risk, there is no risk to the fetus.
    b. The fetus will have an eye infection.
    c. The fetus will have a birth defect.
    d. The client will need a cesarean delivery.

29. A client wonders if her HPV will be cured. What is the best response by the nurse?
    a. "The lesion can be removed, but the HPV cannot be cured."
    b. "Cryotherapy will cure your HPV."
    c. "Medications can eliminate recurrences."
    d. "HPV cannot be cured, but it is not highly contagious."

30. A client would like to know how HIV is spread. What methods of transmission should be taught to the client? (Select all that apply.)

    a. contact with contaminated blood

    b. sexual contact

    c. urine

    d. breast milk

31. What reason is the most appropriate to justify the nurse asking a client with repeated gonorrhea and chlamydia infections as well as HPV if she would like to be tested for HIV? (Select all that apply.)

    a. STIs indicate possible risky behavior.

    b. Repeated infections suggest immune compromise.

    c. Early detection is the best hope for cure.

    d. Treatment will prevent her from passing it on.

32. A married couple has a fertility workup, and the wife has been prescribed clomiphene citrate. The nurse explains clomiphene citrate's action. How does the medication work to improve fertility?

    a. It stimulates ovulation.

    b. It replaces FSH.

    c. It stimulates LH.

    d. It normalizes prolactin levels.

33. A client asks about the side effects of clomiphene citrate. What is the nurse's best response?

    a. "It can cause decreased appetite."

    b. "Mild insomnia can occur while taking this drug."

    c. "You will experience breast discomfort."

    d. "You will need to drink more fluid as this drug will cause dehydration."

34. Which client(s) should not be placed on clomiphene citrate? (Select all that apply.)

    a. 33-year-old who is pregnant

    b. 26-year-old with fibroids

    c. 28-year-old with depression

    d. 35-year-old with diabetes mellitus

35. Which symptoms will hormone replacement therapy (HRT) for menopause address? (Select all that apply.)

    a. gastrointestinal disturbances

    b. vasomotor symptoms

    c. prevention of osteoporosis

    d. urogenital atrophy

36. Which is the correct method of administration of Lupron?

    a. Shake reconstituted product until clear; use 2-mL syringe.

    b. Reconstituted product is stable for 48 hours; use supplied syringe.

    c. Reconstituted solution is "milly;" use supplied syringe.

    d. Store product in refrigerator; use 2-mL syringe.

37. When teaching a client about the correct use of nafarelin acetate (Synarel nasal solution), which priority information should be provided? (Select all that apply.)

    a. Precise guidelines must be followed.

    b. Medication is expensive; need to plan for 6 months' expenses to avoid interruptions in therapy.

    c. Clear nasal passage and administer spray in one nostril only.

    d. Avoid use of nasal decongestant sprays.

38. Which change, if seen with Danocrine, is not related to the medication?

    a. weight gain

    b. rash

    c. decrease in breast size

    d. hot flashes

39. What are the chances of conception during a cycle while taking Danocrine?

    a. 4%

    b. 6%

    c. 8%

    d. 10%

Case Study

Select the best answer.

Tess and Tom, a married couple who are both 32 years old, are being evaluated for infertility.

1. Why is Tess's history of several episodes of gonorrhea while she was in college significant?
    a. The ovaries will decrease frequency of ovulation following repeated episodes of gonorrhea.
    b. Repeated antibiotics use decreases the thickness of the lining of the uterus so it is not able to support pregnancy.
    c. Repeated episodes of gonorrhea may have scarred the fallopian tubes.
    d. Gonorrhea will decrease the production of ova in the ovaries.

2. Because of her history, it is suggested that Tess consider HIV testing. How are HIV and gonorrhea interrelated? (Select all that apply.)
    a. HIV can more readily enter the cell through lesions caused by sexually transmitted infections.
    b. If a partner transferred the gonorrhea, he could have also transferred HIV.
    c. The gonorrhea virus is very similar to the HIV virus and it can mutate to HIV.
    d. Gonorrhea decreases the immune response and makes the client more susceptible to HIV.

3. It is determined that Tom's sperm count is within normal range, but Tess is not ovulating regularly. A course of clomiphene citrate is recommended. What side effects can Tess expect? (Select all that apply.)
    a. breast discomfort
    b. fatigue
    c. dizziness
    d. depression
    e. diarrhea

4. What adverse effects might require that the regimen be interrupted? (Select all that apply.)
    a. visual impairment
    b. ovarian hyperstimulation
    c. midcycle ovarian pain
    d. headaches
    e. cysts

5. How does a woman's basal temperature change throughout her ovulatory cycle?
    a. Ovulation is predicted by a 0.1° F drop in basal body temperature followed by a 1° F rise.
    b. Ovulation is predicted by a .5° F drop in basal body temperature followed by a 1° F rise.
    c. Ovulation is predicted by a 0.1° F increase in basal body temperatures followed by a 1° F decrease.
    d. Ovulation is predicted by a 0.5° F increase in basal body temperatures followed by a 1° F decrease.

6. When should a couple engage in coitus related to the time that the woman is ovulating?
    a. 4 days before ovulation to 3 days after
    b. 2 days before ovulation to 2 days after
    c. 5 days before ovulation to 1 day after
    d. 3 days before ovulation to 3 days after

7. What stresses might a couple experience during infertility therapy?
    a. Sex becomes a much larger part of their normal routine.
    b. Sex can become a chore and feel dehumanizing to one or both partners.
    c. Frequency of sex is decreased to only occur during ovulation.
    d. Sex can become uncomfortable related to its frequency.

8. What damage might be inflicted on the marriage if pregnancy is not achieved? (Select all that apply.)
    a. One or both partners may feel inadequate.
    b. One or both partners may have a decrease in self-esteem.
    c. One or both partners may become anorexic.
    d. One or both partners my begin blaming the other for failure to become pregnant.

59 Adult and Pediatric Emergency Drugs

Study Questions

Match the condition in Column I with the drug that treats it in Column II.

Column I

_____ 1. Anaphylactic shock
_____ 2. Angina pectoris
_____ 3. Asystole
_____ 4. Extravasation
_____ 5. Hypoxemia
_____ 6. Torsades de pointes
_____ 7. PVCs
_____ 8. Atrial fibrillation
_____ 9. Increased intracranial pressure
_____ 10. Profound bradycardia with hypotension
_____ 11. PSVT

Column II

a. Magnesium sulfate
b. Diltiazem
c. Atropine sulfate
d. Mannitol
e. Phentolamine
f. Lidocaine
g. Nitroglycerin
h. Epinephrine
i. Oxygen
j. Adenosine

Match the drug in Column I with its classification in Column II.

Column I

_____ 12. Isoproterenol
_____ 13. Epinephrine
_____ 14. Lidocaine
_____ 15. Norepinephrine
_____ 16. Verapamil
_____ 17. Mannitol
_____ 18. Diltiazem
_____ 19. Albuterol
_____ 20. Furosemide

Column II

a. Antidysrhythmic, class IB
b. Diuretic
c. Calcium channel blocker
d. Catecholamine
e. Beta-adrenergic agonist

NCLEX Review Questions

Select the best response.

21. Sublingual nitroglycerin may be prescribed for chest pain. What is the most important vital sign to assess before giving this drug?
    a. temperature
    b. blood pressure
    c. heart rate
    d. respiratory rate

22. Following administration of IV morphine to treat chest pain associated with acute myocardial infarction, what is the most important aspect of client monitoring?
    a. measurement of central venous pressure
    b. measurement and strict recording of intake and output
    c. assessment of respiratory status
    d. documentation of neurologic function

23. Which is an emergency drug indicated for the treatment of symptomatic bradycardia?
    a. lidocaine
    b. atropine
    c. naloxone
    d. epinephrine

24. When monitoring a client with an isoproterenol (Isuprel) infusion, the nurse must be alert to the development of dangerous adverse effects. Which ones may require slowing or discontinuing drug administration?
    a. tachycardia and cardiac ectopy (PVCs and ventricular tachycardia)
    b. bradycardia and hypotension
    c. bradycardia and hypertension
    d. respiratory depression and cardiac ectopy

25. In which category is the drug verapamil?
    a. calcium channel blocker
    b. beta blocker
    c. cardiac glycoside
    d. nitrate

26. Which is a dangerous adverse effect of IV procainamide administration?
    a. respiratory depression
    b. hypertension
    c. hypotension
    d. urinary retention

27. What is amiodarone IV used to treat?
    a. atrial dysrhythmias
    b. ventricular dysrhythmias
    c. a and b
    d. none of the above

28. What is the best indication for sodium bicarbonate?
    a. metabolic alkalosis
    b. metabolic acidosis
    c. respiratory alkalosis
    d. respiratory acidosis

29. The client is admitted to the neurosurgical floor with a closed head injury. Mannitol is ordered to decrease intracranial pressure. Through which mechanism does mannitol exert its pharmacologic effects?
    a. cerebral vasoconstriction
    b. peripheral vasodilation
    c. loop diuresis
    d. osmotic diuresis

30. Methylprednisolone (Solu-Medrol) is a controversial adjunctive therapy in the treatment of acute spinal cord injury. The nurse must be aware that the loading dose of this drug must be given within how many hours of the injury?
    a. 2
    b. 4
    c. 6
    d. 8

31. The client is receiving labetolol IV, a drug typically prescribed to treat which alteration?
    a. severe anxiety
    b. hypotension
    c. severe hypertension
    d. cardiac arrest

32. For which type of shock should dopamine be administered when a client experiences hypotension? (Select all that apply.)

    a.   neurogenic shock

    b.   hypovolemic shock

    c.   septic shock

    d.   cardiogenic shock

33. Through which mechanism does dobutamine elevate blood pressure?

    a.   vasoconstriction

    b.   vasodilation

    c.   increasing cardiac output

    d.   positive alpha effects

34. The client has a diagnosis of septic shock. A norepinephrine drip is infusing through a central IV line. The bag of norepinephrine is almost empty. For which reason should the nurse make it a priority to prepare a new bag?

    a.   Hypertensive crisis can result if the infusion is interrupted.

    b.   Profound hypotension can occur if the infusion is abruptly discontinued.

    c.   The client is at high risk for bradycardia and heart block.

    d.   The organisms responsible for septic shock will proliferate.

35. For which reason is dextrose 50% most commonly prescribed?

    a.   as a maintenance infusion to keep a vein open

    b.   to increase urine output

    c.   to treat hyperglycemia

    d.   to treat insulin shock

36. What is the proper method of administering adenosine?

    a.   slow IV push

    b.   diluted in 50 mL of normal saline and infused via an electronic pump over 30 minutes

    c.   rapid IV push as a bolus

    d.   via a nebulizer

37. What is a priority nursing action after administration of a total IV lidocaine dose of 3 mg/kg to an adult?

    a.   A continuous infusion of lidocaine must be initiated to maintain a therapeutic serum level.

    b.   A therapeutic serum level will be achieved and maintained.

    c.   It is recognized that a lidocaine overdose has occurred.

    d.   Additional bolus doses must be administered to achieve a therapeutic serum level.

38. To administer epinephrine 0.3 mg for IM injection, which solution should the nurse select?

    a.   1:10,000 solution of epinephrine

    b.   1:100 solution of epinephrine

    c.   1:1000 solution of epinephrine

    d.   1:1 solution of epinephrine

39. To administer epinephrine 1 mg for IV injection, which solution should the nurse select?

    a.   1:10,000 solution of epinephrine

    b.   1:100 solution of epinephrine

    c.   1:1000 solution of epinephrine

    d.   1:1 solution of epinephrine

40. The lowest adult dose of atropine for heart block or symptomatic bradycardia is 0.5 mg IV. What happens at lower dosages?

    a.   Vagal activity is completely blocked.

    b.   Paradoxical bradycardia can occur.

    c.   Miosis occurs.

    d.   The client is at high risk for tachycardia.

41. Flumazenil is used to reverse the effects of which drug?

    a.   narcotics

    b.   antipsychotics

    c.   benzodiazepines

    d.   paralytic agents

42. Magnesium sulfate is indicated for treatment of which alteration? (Select all that apply.)

    a. torsades de pointes

    b. hypomagnesemia

    c. hypermagnesemia

    d. ventricular tachycardia

43. Furosemide exerts its effects on pulmonary edema through which mechanisms?

    a. venodilation and diuresis

    b. bronchodilation and antiinflammatory actions

    c. vasoconstriction and diuresis

    d. bronchodilation and diuresis

44. Which of the following statements best describe(s) epinephrine? (Select all that apply.)

    a. Epinephrine is a catecholamine.

    b. Indications for epinephrine include asystole and ventricular fibrillation.

    c. The action of epinephrine is enhanced if it is infused through alkaline solutions such as sodium bicarbonate.

    d. Metabolic acidosis decreases the effectiveness of epinephrine.

45. Which priority nursing intervention(s) should be implemented when caring for a client with a nitroprusside infusion? (Select all that apply.)

    a. The solution must be protected from light.

    b. Thiocyanate levels should be monitored.

    c. A blue or brown color to the solution is typical.

    d. Continuous blood pressure measurement is required.

46. Which clinical manifestation(s) is/are commonly associated with atropine administration? (Select all that apply.)

    a. dry mouth

    b. urinary retention

    c. mydriasis

    d. miosis

Case Studies

Select the best answer.

Case Study 1

T.M., an acutely ill 64-year-old man, is brought to the emergency department by his family to be treated for "the flu." His initial vital signs are as follows: BP 70/40 mm Hg, heart rate 140 beats/min, respiratory rate 32 breaths/min, and temperature 40.2 °C PO. After examination and diagnostic studies, T.M. is diagnosed with pneumonia and septic shock.

A triple-lumen subclavian line is inserted for administration of fluids and IV medications and for measurement of central venous pressure (CVP). His initial CVP reading is 3 cm of H_2O. A 2000 mL normal saline fluid bolus is infused rapidly, which elevates his CVP to 9 cm of H_2O. His BP increases to 86/60 mm Hg, and his heart rate decreases to 110 beats/min. A dopamine infusion is initiated at 5 mcg/kg/min and titrated to 8 mcg/kg/min to achieve a systolic BP of >100 mm Hg. He is medicated with acetaminophen for fever. T.M. will be admitted to the ICU for placement of a pulmonary artery catheter and further aggressive management.

1. Why were IV fluids given to raise blood pressure before initiating dopamine? (Select all that apply.)

    a. The client's hypovolemia should be treated before starting the dopamine infusion.

    b. The IV will help increase the urine output from the client.

    c. Starting dopamine after fluid intake is better to prevent more fluid loss through urine output.

    d. Hypovolemia must be improved before starting dopamine as this will increase the level of vasoconstriction.

2. What are the beneficial pharmacologic effects of dopamine at the dose range in the case study? (Select all that apply.)

    a. increased blood pressure

    b. increased heart rate

    c. increased cardiac output

    d. decreased blood glucose levels

3. How should dopamine be administered for precise dosing?
   a. through titrating the dosage frequently
   b. using a flowmeter
   c. using an electronic infusion pump
   d. using a buretrol

4. What are priority nursing assessments and interventions when monitoring a client receiving a dopamine infusion? (Select all that apply.)
   a. continuous monitoring of heart rate and blood pressure
   b. monitoring intake and output
   c. monitoring for tachycardia, dysrhythmias, myocardial ischemia, and nausea and vomiting
   d. monitoring blood glucose levels
   e. not discontinuing the infusion abruptly

5. What actions should be taken if a dopamine infusion should infiltrate and produce tissue extravasation? (Select all that apply.)
   a. Discontinue the IV and restart the infusion at another site.
   b. Irrigate the infusion and then continue the medication.
   c. Request a central line be inserted.
   d. Use phentolamine at the site to reduce tissue damage.

6. T.M. had a heart rate of 140 beats/min on arrival. Are either verapamil or adenosine indicated in this case to treat the client's tachycardia?
   a. Yes, these medications will decrease the high heart rate.
   b. Yes, these medications will increase blood pressure, which will decrease heart rate.
   c. No, these medications will actually increase the client's heart rate.
   d. No, these medications will not be needed when the hypovolemia and fever have resolved.

Case Study 2

C.S., a 56-year-old man, is admitted to coronary care step-down after a 3-day critical care unit stay for an inferior wall myocardial infarction. After dinner, C.S. summons nursing assistance for complaints of severe substernal chest pain with radiation into his left arm. He has an IV of D_5W infusing at KVO. He is receiving O_2 at 4 L by nasal cannula. C.S. has a PRN order for nitroglycerin (NTG) 0.4 mg SL for chest pain.

1. Should the NTG 0.4 mg SL be administered in this case?
   a. No, the client should receive morphine.
   b. No, the client should have his O_2 increased.
   c. Yes, as this drug will increase vessel dilation.
   d. Yes, this drug will increase urine output, which will decrease fluid volume.

2. What data should the nurse collect before administering the NTG? (Select all that apply.)
   a. heart rate and blood pressure
   b. a fuller description of the chest pain
   c. evaluation of the client's troponin levels
   d. blood glucose levels

C.S. continues to complain of severe chest pain after three NTG tablets, 5 minutes apart. The health care provider is notified. Morphine sulfate, 2 mg IV push, is ordered, which may be repeated at 5-minute intervals until chest pain is relieved or until 10 mg has been administered.

3. If respiratory depression occurs as a result of the morphine, what drug should be available to reverse the effects?
   a. atropine sulfate
   b. romazicon
   c. naloxone
   d. oxygen

C.S. is transferred back to the critical care unit. IV NTG is ordered to be started at 10 mcg/kg/min and titrated to relieve chest pain while keeping systolic BP >100 mm Hg.

4.   What are pertinent nursing considerations when administering IV nitroglycerin? (Select all that apply.)

   a.   Continuously monitor heart rate and blood pressure.

   b.   Be sure to titrate the dosage on an electronic infusion pump.

   c.   Monitor intake and output.

   d.   Monitor client for ECG changes.

5.   What actions should the nurse take if systolic BP falls to 96 mm Hg? (Select all that apply.)

   a.   Decrease the amount of morphine sulfate given for chest pain.

   b.   Decrease the rate of infusion of the NTG.

   c.   Increase the rate of infusion of the NTG.

   d.   Increase the rate of fluid volume infused.

6.   What should be done if the client's blood pressure drops precipitously to 75 mm Hg? (Select all that apply.)

   a.   Call the physician.

   b.   Discontinue the NTG.

   c.   Elevate the head of the bed to a high-Fowler's position.

   d.   Place the client's head down and elevate his legs.

C.S.'s chest pain is relieved with the NTG infusion. He remains comfortable over the next 3 hours until his cardiac monitor alarms for a low heart rate of 38 beats/min. C.S. is found to be diaphoretic with a blood pressure of 60 mm Hg by palpation. The nurse turns off the NTG infusion.

7.   What is the drug of choice for symptomatic bradycardia?

   a.   morphine sulfate 5 mg

   b.   atropine sulfate

   c.   dopamine

   d.   epinephrine

8.   By which action does this drug exert its effects?

   a.   increasing the heart rate by stimulating the vagus nerve to fire

   b.   increasing the heart rate by blocking the effects of the vagus nerve

   c.   decreasing the blood pressure by blocking the baroreceptors

   d.   decreasing the blood pressure by stimulating the baroreceptors

Answer Key

CHAPTER 1— Drug Action: Pharmaceutic, Pharmacokinetic, and Pharmacodynamic Phases

Crossword Puzzle

Across
1. pharmaceutic
5. pharmacogenetic
6. pharmacokinetic
7. tachyphylaxis
10. half life
11. protein binding

19.

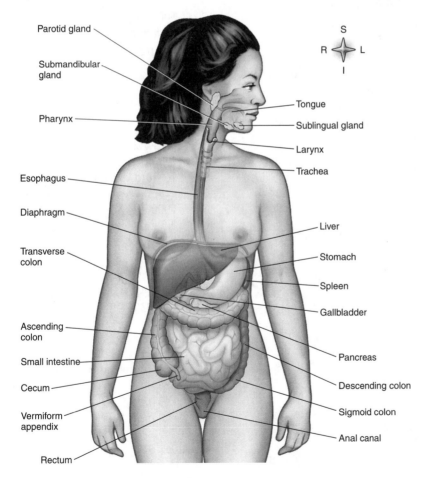

Parotid gland

Submandibular gland

Pharynx

Esophagus

Diaphragm

Transverse colon

Ascending colon

Small intestine

Cecum

Vermiform appendix

Rectum

S
R —|— L
I

Tongue

Sublingual gland

Larynx

Trachea

Liver

Stomach

Spleen

Gallbladder

Pancreas

Descending colon

Sigmoid colon

Anal canal

Down
1. pharmacodynamic
2. antagonist
3. toxicity
4. receptor
8. agonist
9. placebo

12. e
13. d
14. b
15. a
16. f
17. c
18. c

20. b
21. d
22. b
23. a
24. c
25. b
26. d
27. b
28. c
29. b
30. b
31. a
32. a
33. d
34. b
35. c
36. a
37. a, b, c
38. b
39. c
40. b, c, d
41. a, b, d
42. deltoid muscle
43. protein-binding percentage
44. hepatic metabolism; bile; feces; lungs; saliva; sweat; and breast milk
45. (1) stimulation or depression, (2) replacement, (3) inhibition or killing of organisms, and (4) irritation
46. d
47. c
48. a
49. b

Case Study
1. b
2. a, b, c
3. d
4. b

CHAPTER 2—
Nursing Process and
Client Teaching

1. a
2. a
3. b
4. a
5. c
6. a
7. d
8. c
9. c
10. a
11. d
12. b
13. a
14. b
15. a
16. b
17. a
18. a
19. b
20. a
21. c
22. c
23. c
24. d
25. b
26. d
27. a
28. d
29. a, b, c, e
30. b, c, d
31. a, c, d
32. d
33. a, b, c, d
34. a, b, d, e

CHAPTER 3—
Medication Safety

1. c
2. f
3. j
4. g
5. a
6. h
7. b
8. d
9. e
10. i
11. d

12. f
13. e
14. b
15. a
16. c
17. a
18. a
19. b
20. a
21. b
22. a
23. c
24. d
25. a
26. e
27. b
28. b
29. c
30. b
31. a
32. b
33. b, c, d, e
34. a, b, c

CHAPTER 4—
Medication
Administration

1. enteric-coated; timed-release
2. fine-sized particle
3. semi- or high Fowler's
4. 50
5. 20
6. c
7. a
8. b
9. ventrogluteal
10. vastus lateralis
11. deltoid
12. gluteal
13. dorsogluteal
14. c
15. b
16. a
17. a
18. d
19. a
20. a
21. a, b, c, d
22. c
23. a, b

CHAPTER 5—
Medications and
Calculations

Section 5A
1. b
2. f
3. g
4. c
5. k
6. l
7. m
8. r
9. d
10. e
11. h
12. q
13. p
14. i
15. o
16. a
17. n
18. j
19. a, 1000 mg; b, 1000 mL; c, 1000 mcg
20. 3000 mg
21. 1500 mL
22. 100 mg
23. 2.5 L
24. 0.25 L
25. 0.5 g
26. 4 pints
27. 32 fl. oz
28. 48 fl. oz
29. 2 pints
30. 16 fluid drams
31. grams to milligrams
32. 1000 mg; 15 gr
33. 0.5 g; 7 ½ gr
34. 100 mg; 1 ½ gr
35. 60 or 64 mg
36. $\frac{1}{150}$ gr
37. 1 L; 1 qt
38. 8 fl. oz; 1 medium-sized glass
39. 1 oz; 2 T; 6 t
40. 1 t
41. 15 (16) minim; 15 (16) drops
42. 1 ½ oz; 9 t
43. 150 mL; 10 T

Section 5B
1. d

2. b
3. a
4. 250 mg per 5 mL
5. d
6. d; b
7. a; b
8. d; b
9. d
10. b
11. b; a
12. b

Section 5C

1. c
2. b; c
3. a; b
4. a
5. c
6. a; a
7. a; d
8. c; c
9. c; c
10. d
11. b; c
12. a; a
13. a
14. b
15. c
16. c
17. b
18. b
19. b
20. e
21. b
22. a

Section 5D

1. b, c, d, e
2. c, d
3. self-sealing rubber tops; reusable if properly stored
4. b, c
5. is not
6. units
7. a
8. c
9. b
10. b
11. c
12. d
13. b; c
14. a
15. c

16. Withdraw 36 units of Humulin L insulin.

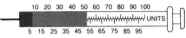

17. First withdraw 8 units of Humulin R (regular) insulin and then 44 units of Humulin N (NPH) insulin. Total: 52 units of insulin.

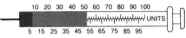

The regular insulin (Option C) should be drawn up first.

18. b
19. a; a
20. b
21. c; c
22. b
23. c
24. b
25. 2.7, 3; c
26. 1.8, 2; a
27. d
28. c
29. 2, 2.6; b
30. c; d; b
31. b
32. c

Section 5E

1. a, b, c
2. c
3. 10-20 gtt/mL; 60 gtt/mL
4. microdrip set
5. keep vein open; 250-mL IV bag
6. $D_5\%W$
7. NSS or 0.9% NaCl
8. $D_5\frac{1}{2}$NSS or 5%/0.45% NaCl
9. D_5LR or 5%D/LR
10. small; short
11. calibrated cylinder with tubing; intermittent IV drug administration
12. volumetric
13. uniform concentration of the drug
14. 27-28 gtt/min
15. c; 31-32 gtt/min
16. a; 83 gtt/min

17. 1000 mL; 2500 mL; 100 mL/hr; macrodrip set; 16-17 gtt/min
18. e; 27-28 gtt/min
19. c; c
20. 10 mL of sterile water; 1 g = 10 mL; b
21. 6.6 mL; 2 g = 8 mL; b
22. c; b
23. 4 mL of sterile water; 1 g = 4 mL; c; c
24. a; c
25. 7.5 mL; c
26. 1.6 mL; b
27. c; c
28. a
29. b; b
30. b; b

Section 5F

1. b, c
2. b; d
3. a; b
4. c
5. a; b
6. b
7. b
8. b; a; e
9. 0.87; c
10. a; a
11. b; a
12. a; b
13. a; b
14. 2 mL, 2 mL; a; b
15. a; b

CHAPTER 6— The Drug Approval Process

Crossword Puzzle

Across
3. digitalis
6. misfeasance
8. nonfeasance
10. codeine
11. brand

Down
1. VIPPS
2. malfeasance
4. iron
5. heroin
7. generic

9. amphetamines
12. b
13. d
14. c
15. a
16. d
17. b
18. c
19. a
20. d
21. d
22. a
23. b
24. c
25. c
26. a
27. d
28. b
29. b
30. b
31. a
32. a
33. c
34. a, b
35. a, c
36. a, b, c
37. a, b, d
38. a
39. b

CHAPTER 7—
Cultural and
Pharmacogenetic
Considerations

1. e
2. f
3. b
4. a
5. d
6. c
7. a
8. d
9. a
10. b
11. d
12. a, b, c
13. b, c, d

Case Study
1. c
2. c
3. b
4. a, b, d

5. c
6. c

CHAPTER 8—
Drug Interactions
and Over-the-Counter
Drugs

Crossword Puzzle

Across
3. amphetamines
6. absorption
8. distribution
9. excretion

Down
1. FDA
2. biotransform
4. two
5. synergistic
7. OTC

10. c
11. d
12. a
13. b
14. e
15. a
16. b
17. a, d
18. f
19. f
20. a, d
21. b
22. b
23. b
24. c
25. c
26. a
27. b
28. d
29. c
30. a
31. b
32. b
33. b
34. a, c, d
35. a, b, c, d
36. a, d, e
37. a, b, c, d

CHAPTER 9—
Drugs of Abuse

Crossword Puzzle

Across
2. drug addiction
6. relapse
7. cocaine
9. nicotine
11. cue-induced cravings

Down
1. drug misuse
2. drug abuse
3. detoxification
4. intoxication
5. tolerance
8. abstinence
10. bupropion

12. b
13. a
14. d
15. c
16. b
17. d
18. d
19. a
20. a
21. c
22. a
23. a, b, e
24. a, b, c

CHAPTER 10—
Herbal Therapy with
Nursing Implications

1. d
2. a
3. e
4. b
5. c
6. g
7. f

```
P U R Y S T P J B W Q S A
I E H R Z X A J M I Y B N
T I N C T U R E Z P I I X
D A T W E X T R A C T S U
L D U E R E A O I L B X W
W V F D A O M T Y R N O L
N H R S Q U N U E Q P P I
W K L M P Z A H A R C U R
```

8. syrup
9. tea
10. tincture
11. extracts
12. oil
13. herbs
14. d
15. g
16. h
17. j
18. a
19. f
20. b
21. c
22. e
23. i

Crossword Puzzle

Across
2. sage
7. saw palmetto
9. evening primrose
10. cranberry
11. garlic
12. milk thistle

Down
1. dong quai
3. valerian
4. ginger
5. bilberry
6. feverfew
8. peppermint

24. c
25. a
26. b
27. d
28. b
29. b
30. b, c, d
31. b, d
32. a, b, e
33. a, b, c
34. a, b, c

Case Study
1. a, c, d
2. a, b
3. b
4. c

CHAPTER 11—
Pediatric Pharmacology

1. fewer; lower
2. age; health status; route of administration
3. 1; 3
4. body fluid composition; tissue composition; protein-binding capability
5. 2 years; higher
6. e
7. d
8. a
9. b
10. c
11. b
12. a
13. c
14. a
15. a, b, d, e
16. b, c, d
17. a, b, c

Case Study
1. b
2. b, d
3. a, b, c

Chapter 12—
Geriatric Pharmacology

Crossword Puzzle

Across
2. absorption
4. distribution
6. diuretics
8. polypharmacy
10. nonadherence

Down
1. digoxin

3. biotransformation
5. kidneys
7. laxatives
9. adherence

11. a
12. a
13. d
14. b
15. c
16. b
17. b
18. d
19. c
20. b
21. a
22. b
23. a, c, e
24. a, b, d
25. a, b, d
26. a, b, c

Case Study
1. a
2. b, c, d
3. a
4. a, d

CHAPTER 13—
Medication Administration in Community Settings

1. professional; legal; regulatory
2. avoid
3. general; diet; self-administration; side effects; cultural considerations
4. safety
5. original labeled; child-safe
6. personal beliefs
7. traditional; folk

8. d
9. a
10. a, c
11. a
12. b
13. c
14. a, b, c, d, e, f, g, h
15. a, b, c
16. a, c, d

Case Study
1. a, b, c
2. a, b, c
3. a, b, c

CHAPTER 14—
The Role of the Nurse in Drug Research

1. d
2. a
3. g
4. b
5. c
6. f
7. e
8. i
9. j
10. h
11. k
12. e
13. a
14. g
15. f
16. d
17. c
18. b
19. c
20. b
21. d
22. c
23. b
24. b
25. d
26. c
27. a, c, d
28. b, c, d, e, f

Case Study
1. a
2. c, d

CHAPTER 15—
Vitamin and Mineral Replacement

1. a
2. b
3. b
4. a
5. a
6. a
7. a
8. a
9. b
10. b
11. a
12. d
13. c
14. e
15. a
16. b
17. d
18. c
19. d
20. b
21. a
22. c
23. d
24. a
25. c
26. a
27. b
28. a, b, d
29. b
30. a, b, c
31. d
32. d
33. a
34. c
35. b, c
36. a, b, c
37. a, c, d

CHAPTER 16—
Fluid and Electrolyte Replacement

1. d
2. f
3. b
4. e
5. a
6. c
7. c

8. a
9. d
10. e
11. b
12. a
13. d
14. d
15. c
16. a
17. a
18. d
19. d
20. c
21. d
22. a, b, d
23. b
24. a
25. b
26. c
27. b
28. b
29. a
30. c
31. b
32. b
33. c
34. a
35. c
36. a
37. b
38. d
39. c
40. d
41. a, b, d
42. a
43. a, b, c, d
44. b, c, d
45. a, b, c
46. d
47. b
48. a, b, c

Case Study
1. c
2. a
3. a, b
4. a, b
5. a
6. c
7. c
8. c
9. a, b, d

CHAPTER 17—
Nutritional Support

Crossword Puzzle

Across
3. hypoglycemia
4. elemental
5. air embolism
6. infection
7. pneumothorax
9. polymeric

Down
1. hyperglycemia
2. hyperalimentation
3. hypervolemia
8. hydrothorax

10.

11. d
12. a
13. b
14. c
15. a
16. b
17. d
18. b
19. b
20. c
21. c
22. b
23. d
24. c
25. a, b, c
26. a, c, d
27. d, b, e, c, a
28. a, b, c
29. b, c, d

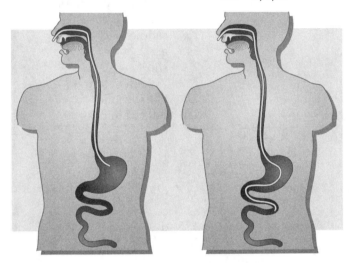

Nasogastric   Nasoduodenal/nasojejunal

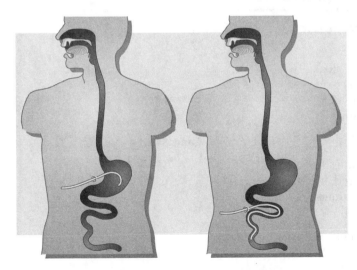

Gastrostomy   Jejunostomy

CHAPTER 18—
Adrenergic Agonists and Adrenergic Blockers

1. c
2. d
3. b
4. e
5. a
6. smooth
7. adrenergic
8. sitting up
9. do
10. sympatholytics
11. Regitine
12. Minipress
13. beta blocker
14. hypertension
15. asthma; hypotension
16. antagonists (The two drugs could counteract each other—as *antagonists*—thus negating a therapeutic action.)
17. d
18. c, a
19. a
20. a
21. b
22. d
23. c
24. d
25. b
26. b
27. a
28. a
29. b
30. d
31. d
32. c
33. c
34. b
35. b, d
36. d
37. a, b, e

Case Study
1. b
2. a, c
3. b
4. a, b, c
5. b, c, d
6. a, b, c

CHAPTER 19—
Cholinergic Agonists and Anticholinergics

1. c
2. e
3. d
4. h
5. a
6. b
7. f
8. g
9. b
10. a
11. b
12. c
13. a
14. b
15. a
16. a, d
17. c
18. a
19. c
20. a, b, c
21. c
22. a
23. a, b, d
24. d
25. b
26. c
27. b
28. b, c, e, f
29. b, c, d, e

Case Study
1. a, d
2. c
3. a, b, c
4. a
5. b
6. a, b, c

CHAPTER 20—
Central Nervous System Stimulants

Crossword Puzzle

Across
4. dependence
6. ADHD
9. anorexiants
10. analeptics

Down
1. amphetamines
2. phenylpropanolamines
3. methylphenidate
5. narcolepsy
7. hyperkinesis
8. armodafinil

11. a, b, c
12. a, b, c
13. a, b, d, e
14. b
15. d
16. a, b, c
17. b
18. a
19. d
20. b
21. a
22. c
23. a, b, c
24. b
25. d
26. a, c
27. a, e

Case Study
1. b
2. a, c, d
3. a, b, d
4. a, b, c
5. a, b, c
6. a, b, c

CHAPTER 21—
Central Nervous System Depressants

Crossword Puzzle

Across
1. saddle block
2. nitrous oxide
3. hangover
5. insomnia
6. kava kava
7. benzodiazepines
8. local anesthetic
12. balanced anesthesia
13. barbiturates

Down
1. spinal block
4. epidural block
9. sedation

10. caudal block
11. flurazepam
14. sedative-hypnotics; general and local anesthetics; analgesics; narcotic analgesics; anticonvulsants; antipsychotics; antidepressants
15. rapid eye movement; non-rapid eye movement
16. sedation
17. may
18. ultra-short
19. central nervous; pain; consciousness
20. surgical; analgesia; excitement or delirium; medullary paralysis
21. spinal
22. respiratory distress or failure
23. saddle block
24. are
25. short
26. Zolpidem tartrate
27. Flumazenil
28. esters; amides
29. d
30. f
31. e
32. a
33. b
34. c
35. d
36. d
37. d
38. a
39. a
40. a, b
41. d
42. d
43. b
44. a, b, c
45. a, b, d, e
46. a, c

Case Study
1. a, b, c, d, e
2. c
3. c
4. a, b, c

CHAPTER 22—
Anticonvulsants

Crossword Puzzle

Across

2. atonic
3. petit mal
4. myoclonic
7. convulsions
9. partial
11. teratogenic

Down

1. grand mal
2. anticonvulsants
5. clonic
6. anoxia
8. seizure
10. EEG

12. 1%
13. EEG
14. idiopathic
15. generalized; partial
16. preventing; do not
17. are not
18. phenytoin
19. over-the-counter
20. intramuscular
21. d
22. a
23. b
24. c
25. c
26. d
27. a
28. a
29. b
30. a, b, c
31. a, b, d
32. c
33. a
34. d
35. a
36. a, b, c
37. a, b, d
38. b, c, d, e

Case Study

1. b
2. b
3. c
4. c

CHAPTER 23—
Drugs for Neurologic Disorders: Parkinsonism and Alzheimer's Disease

1. c
2. a
3. d
4. e
5. b
6. dopamine; acetylcholine
7. dopamine
8. levodopa
9. carbidopa
10. Aricept (donepezil)
11. enhance
12. selegiline
13. liver
14. ethopropazine; orphenadrine
15. b
16. d
17. b, c
18. b
19. a
20. c
21. a, b, c
22. a, b, c
23. b, c, e
24. a
25. d

Case Study

1. a, b, c
2. b, c
3. c
4. c
5. a, b, d

CHAPTER 24—
Drugs for Neuromuscular Disorders: Myasthenia Gravis, Multiple Sclerosis, and Muscle Spasms

Crossword Puzzle

Across

1. acetylcholine
4. myasthenic crisis

5. edrophonium
8. hemiplegia
9. ptosis
10. fasciculations

Down

2. neostigmine
3. cholinergic crisis
4. miosis
6. myelin sheath
7. dantrium

11. d
12. a
13. b
14. a
15. d
16. a
17. a
18. b, c, d
19. b
20. a, b, c
21. d

Case Study

1. c
2. d
3. a
4. a
5. a, b, c

CHAPTER 25—
Antiinflammatory Drugs

1. e
2. d
3. f
4. i
5. c
6. b
7. a
8. g
9. h
10. injury; infection
11. redness; heat; swelling; pain; loss of function
12. delayed
13. does
14. higher (or increased)
15. 24
16. b
17. a
18. b
19. a, b, d

20.	d
21.	c
22.	a
23.	b
24.	c
25.	a, c, d
26.	a, b, c
27.	c
28.	a
29.	b
30.	a
31.	a, c
32.	c
33.	a, c, d, e
34.	a, b, c, e
35.	b, c, d, e

Case Study

1. c
2. d
3. c
4. a
5. a, b, c, d
6. a, b, c

CHAPTER 26—
Nonopioid and Opioid Analgesics

Crossword Puzzle

Across
3. nociceptors
6. opioid
7. MAOI
8. NSAIDs
9. analgesics
10 nonopioid

Down
1. prostaglandins
2. fenoprofen
4. hepatonecrosis
5. viral
11. CNS; peripheral nervous system
12. respirations; coughing
13. antitussive; antidiarrheal
14. head injury; respiratory depression
15. side effect; health care provider
16. IV
17. d

18.	d
19.	a
20.	a, b, c
21.	d
22.	c
23.	c
24.	b
25.	b
26.	d
27.	a, b, c
28.	b
29.	a, b, c
30.	a
31.	a, b, e, f
32.	a
33.	d
34.	c
35.	b
36.	c

Case Study

1. a, d
2. b
3. a, c, d
4. b
5. b
6. b
7. a, b, d
8. a
9. b, d

CHAPTER 27—
Antipsychotics and Anxiolytics

1. e
2. d
3. f
4. g
5. a
6. h
7. b
8. c
9. thought processes; behaviors; dopamine
10. dihydroindolones; thioxanthenes; butyrophenones; dibenzoxapines
11. drowsiness
12. pruritus; photosensitivity
13. decrease
14. are not
15. tolerance
16. sedative-hypnotics

17.	c
18.	a
19.	a
20.	b
21.	b
22.	c
23.	b
24.	d
25.	b
26.	b
27.	b
28.	c
29.	a
30.	b
31.	b
32.	c
33.	a
34.	a
35.	c
36.	b
37.	b
38.	d
39.	c
40.	c
41.	d
42.	b
43.	b
44.	c
45.	a, b
46.	a, b, c

Case Study

1. b
2. c
3. d
4. a

CHAPTER 28—
Antidepressants and Mood Stabilizers

```
T C S R V R N M J R D M J A H J H
R I Y Y V X R S A N O D J J Y E B
A N O D U O I A N N O Y N J Y V O
P I M J L R W L D I K Q P B I I
L K F X S J G Q M O H C T W V T F
N M D S K W V O B N P I L W O C B
M A G W I G D V D L Q T X K A U
J O T R I C Y C L I C S B U J E K
Y I Z Y M P F R F J A K P H C R V
Q S Q M U H G O U I D O F U C C X
L S T N A S S E R P E D I T N A Q
```

1. bipolar
2. SSRIs
3. MAOIs

4. manic
5. antidepressants
6. reactive
7. tricyclics
8. a
9. a
10. b
11. d
12. c
13. b

Crossword Puzzle

Across
4. St. John's wort
6. major
8. reactive
10. bipolar
11. bedtime
12. tyramine

Down
1. imipramine
2. lithium
3. ginseng
4. St. John's wort
5. imipramine
7. feverfew
9. two to four

14. d
15. b
16. c
17. a
18. a, b, c
19. c
20. a
21. b
22. c
23. a
24. a, c, d
25. a, b, d
26. b
27. c
28. a
29. a, c, e
30. a, b, c, d

Case Study
1. d
2. a, b, c, d
3. c
4. a, b, d
5. a, b, c, d

CHAPTER 29— Penicillins and Cephalosporins

Crossword Puzzle

Across
3. cross-resistance
6. bacteriostatic
7. methicillin
10. acquired resistance
11. immunoglobulins
12. natural resistance

Down
1. nosocomial infections
2. nephrotoxicity
3. culture and sensitivity
4. superinfection
5. antibacterial
8. penicillin
9. bactericidal

13. e
14. g
15. f
16. h
17. a
18. b
19. c
20. d
21. a
22. b
23. a, b, c
24. b
25. a
26. d
27. d
28. c
29. a
30. a
31. d
32. a, b, d
33. a
34. b
35. a
36. a, b, d, e
37. a, c, d
38. c
39. b
40. c
41. a

Case Study
1. c
2. b

3. a, b
4. c
5. a, b, c

CHAPTER 30— Macrolides, Tetracyclines, Aminoglycosides, and Fluoroquinolones

1. g
2. b
3. f
4. a
5. c
6. f
7. a
8. e
9. h
10. g
11. e
12. d

Crossword Puzzle

Across
3. tetracycline
4. erythromycin
5. vancomycin
7. azithromycin
8. spectinomycin
9. protein synthesis
10. glycylcyclines

Down
1. nephrotoxicity, ototoxicity
2. ketolides
6. bactericidal

13. b
14. a
15. a
16. c
17. a, b, c
18. a, b, d, e
19. a, b, c, d
20. b, c, d, e
21. b
22. b
23. c
24. b
25. c
26. a, b, c, d

Case Study
1. a
2. a, b, c
3. b
4. a
5. a, b, c, d

CHAPTER 31—
Sulfonamides

```
W J Q I O K D N F A B U L H N R Q
W D P E N I C I L L I N O K R H K
B L R Y E D R M C P S D D O V P A
L K C O V N V E E A U L G Y Q N M
M C R C C E R M V F C L J M E C T
P A A N Y Y I U A I F I U S Q X Y
V X B J D S S C D C D F L S K K E
E Q A R G I N C R E A S E O N W S
B Q A R E N O T L Q V U Z D B D L
Y N C I T A T S O I R E T C A B E
R T R I M E T H O P R I M C J C F
```

1. folic acid
2. penicillin
3. trimethoprim
4. are not
5. is not
6. liver; kidneys
7. bacteriostatic
8. increases
9. a
10. b
11. b
12. a
13. a
14. d
15. a
16. b
17. b
18. a, b, c
19. a
20. a, c, d, e
21. b, c, e

Case Study
1. a, b, c, d
2. c
3. a, b, c

CHAPTER 32—
Antituberculars, Antifungals, Peptides, and Metronidazole

Crossword Puzzle

Across
2. gram-positive
3. first-line drugs
4. vagina
8. lungs
9. hepatotoxicity
10. IV
11. bactericidal

Down
1. rifabutin
5. amphotericin B
6. streptomycin
7. fluconazole

12. a
13. a
14. b
15. a
16. a
17. b
18. b
19. b
20. a
21. d
22. a
23. a
24. b
25. c
26. a, b, c
27. b
28. a
29. c
30. a, b
31. c
32. d
33. a
34. b
35. a, b, c
36. c
37. a
38. c, d
39. b
40. a, b, c
41. a, c, d, e
42. a, b, d, e

Case Study
1. a, b, c, d

2. b
3. c
4. a, c
5. a, c

CHAPTER 33—
Antivirals, Antimalarials, and Anthelmintics

```
E D I R O L H C O R D Y R U V O J
C Y T O M E G A L O V I R U S Z W
R T M C H E N I D A T N A M I R R
V A R I C E L L A F R E L K N C M
I G O X E L P M I S S E P R E H S
S K L S O H D A G C A X N X G U D
Z O G R N R X D T V R E T A G G D
U J R E W O L S A I S R P Q D D T
T B H R U X T O X I C I T Y R A R
X R E P L I C A T I O N T D M O
B W H E R P E S Z O S T E R M O F
```

1. replication
2. is not
3. slower; toxicity
4. rimantadine hydrochloride; renal; hepatic
5. herpes simplex type I; herpes zoster; varicella (zoster); cytomegalovirus
6. type A
7. c
8. e
9. a
10. b
11. d
12. c
13. c
14. a
15. b
16. c
17. a, b, c
18. a, c, d
19. d
20. a
21. a, b, d
22. a, c, d
23. a
24. d
25. a, b, c
26. b, c
27. d
28. a, b, c
29. a, c, e
30. a, c, e
31. a, b, c, d

Case Study
1. c
2. a, b, c
3. a, b
4. a, b, c
5. b

CHAPTER 34—
Drugs for Urinary Tract Disorders

Crossword Puzzle

Across
1. acute pyelonephritis
4. urinary stimulants
7. bacteriostatic
8. acute cystitis

Down
2. cranberry
3. *Pseudomonas aeruginosa*
5. nitrofurantoin
6. bactericidal

9. b
10. a, b, d
11. b
12. b, c, d
13. a, c, d
14. b
15. b
16. a, b, c
17. a
18. a, b, c
19. c
20. a
21. a, c, d, e
22. a, b, d
23. a, c, d, e

Case Study
1. c
2. a, b
3. a, c, d
4. a, b, c

CHAPTER 35—
HIV- and AIDS-Related Drugs

Crossword Puzzle

Across
3. cell-mediated

6. nucleoside analogues
7. efavirenz
8. non-nucleoside analogues
10. innate
11. viral load

Down
1. reverse transcription
2. tenofovir
4. acquired
5. budding
9. adherence

12. c
13. a
14. c
15. c
16. b
17. a, b, d
18. a, b, c
19. a
20. d
21. a
22. a
23. b
24. a
25. a, b, c
26. a, b, d
27. b
28. d
29. c
30. a, b, d
31. a, b, c
32. c
33. b
34. b
35. a, b, c, d
36. a, b, c, d
37. c
38. d
39. a
40. a, c, d
41. a, b, c

Case Study
1. c
2. b
3. a, b, c, d
4. a, b, c, d

CHAPTER 36—
Vaccines

Crossword Puzzle

Across
3. seroconversion
5. anaphylaxis
7. passive
8. pathogen

Down
1. attenuated viruses
2. recombinant
4. vaccine
6. antibodies

9. a
10. a, b, d
11. d
12. d
13. a
14. c
15. c
16. b
17. a
18. b
19. d
20. a
21. c
22. d
23. c
24. d
25. c
26. a
27. c
28. d
29. b
30. a
31. c
32. a, c, d

Case Study
1. c
2. a, b, c
3. a
4. c
5. a

CHAPTER 37—
Anticancer Drugs

Crossword Puzzle

Across
3. cytoprotectant

5. nonspecific
7. dose dense
8. specific
10. adjuvant therapy
11. combination
12. growth fraction

Down
1. palliative
2. multidrug resistance
4. antineoplastic
6. vesicant
9. apoptosis

13. h
14. j
15. a
16. d
17. i
18. c
19. g
20. b
21. f
22. e
23. a
24. d
25. c
26. c
27. a
28. d
29. d
30. a
31. d
32. a
33. a
34. c
35. c
36. d
37. a
38. d
39. c
40. c
41. d
42. c
43. a
44. b
45. d
46. b
47. a
48. c
49. a
50. d
51. c
52. c
53. c

Case Study
1. c
2. a
3. c
4. b
5. a, b, c, d, e

CHAPTER 38—
Targeted Therapies to Treat Cancer

1. growth factor
2. signal transduction
3. phosphorylation
4. transcription factors
5. cyclins
6. proteasome; degradation
7. targeted; cellular receptors; enzymes; pathways
8. d
9. b
10. d
11. a
12. a
13. d
14. c
15. c
16. a, b, c, d
17. a, c, d

Case Study
1. d
2. a, b, d
3. c
4. b
5. a, b, c, d

CHAPTER 39—
Biologic Response Modifiers

Crossword Puzzle

Across
2. oprelvekin

4. nadir
5. absolute neutrophil count
6. interleukin
8. pegylation
9. interferon
10. tumoricidal
11. sargramostim
12. myelosuppression
13. hybridoma technology

Down
1. colony stimulating
3. erythropoietin
7. thrombocytopenia

14. b
15. c
16. a
17. d
18. e
19. a, b, d
20. a
21. b
22. a, b, c
23. d
24. b
25. b
26. a
27. a, b, c
28. a, b, c
29. a, b, d
30. a, b, d

Case Study
1. b
2. b
3. b

CHAPTER 40—
Drugs for Upper Respiratory Disorders

1. c
2. a
3. d
4. b

5. common cold; acute rhinitis; sinusitis; acute tonsillitis; laryngitis
6. common cold
7. two to four
8. constricted
9. sedation
10. urinary
11. rebound
12. six
13. antitussives
14. water or fluids
15. are not
16. minimal
17. b
18. c
19. d
20. a
21. c
22. a
23. c
24. a, c, d
25. b
26. a
27. a, b, c, d
28. a, b, c, e
29. a, b, d, e
30. b, d

Case Study
1. b
2. a
3. a
4. a, b, c
5. d
6. a, b, c

CHAPTER 41— Drugs for Lower Respiratory Disorders

1. d
2. f
3. b
4. c
5. a, b
6. b
7. b
8. cyclic adenosine monophosphate (cAMP)
9. epinephrine
10. beta$_2$-adrenergic agonists
11. nonselective
12. cAMP

13. increases
14. synergistic
15. shorter
16. methylxanthine/xanthine; asthma
17. glucocorticoids
18. prophylactic; histamine
19. rebound bronchospasm
20. beta$_2$
21. montelukast (Singulair)
22. evening
23. 10 mg adult; 5 mg child without food
24. mucolytic
25. antibiotic
26. b
27. a, c, d
28. c
29. c
30. b
31. d
32. a, b, c
33. a, b, d
34. b, c, d
35. a, b, c
36. a, c, d
37. b, c, d
38. c
39. d
40. b
41. a, b, d, e
42. b, c, d, e
43. a, b, d, e

Case Study
1. d
2. c
3. a, b, c, d
4. a, c
5. a, b, d, e

CHAPTER 42— Cardiac Glycosides, Antianginals, and Antidysrhythmics

Crossword Puzzle

Across
1. hypercapnia
2. preload
3. antianginal
6. repolarization
8. depolarization

10. hypokalemia
11. afterload
12. bradycardia
13. antidysrhythmics

Down
1. hypoxia
4. nitrates
5. ischemia
7. glycoside
9. tachycardia

14. weakens; enlarges
15. increase
16. pump
17. digitalis glycosides
18. increase; decrease
19. positive inotropic action (increases heart contraction); negative chronotropic action (decreases heart rate); negative dromotropic action (decreases conduction of the heart cells); and increased stroke volume
20. decrease
21. it undergoes first-pass metabolism by the liver
22. 2-5 minutes; repeated every 5 minutes three times
23. headache
24. beta blockers
25. verapamil (Calan)
26. reflex tachycardia; pain
27. stressed (or exerted)
28. at frequent times daily with increasing severity
29. is at rest
30. spasm
31. reduction of venous tone or coronary vasodilator
32. hypoxia; hypercapnia
33. fast sodium channel blockers; beta blockers; calcium channel blockers; also drugs that prolong repolarization
34. alcohol; cigarettes
35. b
36. a
37. b
38. a
39. c
40. d
41. b
42. a

43. d
44. b
45. d
46. b
47. a
48. d
49. a, c, d
50. b
51. b
52. d
53. c
54. d
55. c
56. d
57. a
58. b
59. a, b, c, d
60. c
61. a, b, d
62. d
63. a, b, c, d
64. a, b, d
65. a, b, c, d
66. a, c
67. c
68. a, b, c
69. c
70. b
71. a
72. b
73. b
74. c
75. a, b, c
76. a, b, c
77. a, d, e
78. b, c, e
79. a, c, d

Case Study
1. a, b, c
2. a, b
3. a, c, d
4. a, b, c, d

CHAPTER 43—
Diuretics

Crossword Puzzle

Across
3. natriuresis
6. osmolality
7. mannitol
8. hyperkalemia

9. diuresis
10. hypertension
11. hyperkalemia
12. oliguria

Down
1. carbonic anhydrase inhibitor
2. furosemide
4. aldosterone
5. hyperglycemia

13. hypokalemia
14. hypomagnesemia
15. hypercalcemia
16. hypochloremia
17. minimal loss
18. hyperuricemia
19. hyperglycemia
20. cholesterol, LDL, and triglycerides are elevated
21. b, c, d
22. b
23. c
24. b
25. b
26. c
27. a, c, d
28. a
29. a
30. a
31. d
32. b
33. d
34. a
35. d
36. a, b, c, e
37. a, b, c
38. a, c, d
39. a, b, d
40. a, b, d
41. c
42. a, c, d
43. a, b, c, e

Case Study
1. b
2. a
3. b
4. c
5. a, b, d, e
6. b
7. c

CHAPTER 44—
Antihypertensives

Crossword Puzzle

Across
1. atrium
2. diuretics
8. salt restriction
9. coughing

Down
1. angiotensin II blockers
3. African Americans
4. prazosin
5. calcium blockers
6. nitroprusside
7. blood pressure

10. sympatholytics: centrally acting; peripherally acting; alpha₁ blocker; alpha-beta blocker
11. beta blockers; calcium blockers; ACE inhibitors; also diuretics
12. prehypertension; stage I; stage II
13. beta blockers; ACE inhibitors; also A-II blockers
14. diuretics
15. stage II
16. diminished; lowered
17. cardioselective
18. decrease very-low-density lipoprotein (VLDL) and LDL; increase HDL
19. c
20. d
21. b
22. e
23. f
24. g
25. b
26. b
27. b
28. a
29. d
30. a, c, d
31. c
32. a
33. d
34. d
35. b
36. d
37. b

38. d
39. a
40. b
41. d
42. b
43. c
44. b
45. a
46. a, b, c
47. d
48. b
49. a
50. c
51. b
52. c
53. b
54. b, c
55. a, b, c
56. b, d

Case Study

1. b
2. c
3. a
4. d
5. a, b, c, d
6. c
7. a, c, d, e
8. a, b, c
9. b, c, d
10. a, b, d

CHAPTER 45—
Anticoagulants, Antiplatelets, and Thrombolytics

```
J B S J A G G R E G A T I O N U O
V M L K I N W P O F L W Y W W I L
A S S Y L O N R B I F Q H E D
D V T N G M X L U S P C G X Z T U
Q F S R B W A R L K C Q U U H S S
B T L K O H B P V D G H Z I H I E
Q S R A P K V W D Q C G F S Q A
W T P N Q F E J W G L V D M I O U
T A N T I C O A G U L A N T D U
Q F Y X K C K P Y M K H H H B A W
J F U C I T Y L O B M O R H T G Y
```

a. aggregation
b. anticoagulant
c. fibrinolysis
d. ischemia
e. thrombolytic
f. stroke
g. INR

h. LMWH
i. DVT
j. PT

1. artery; vein
2. clot formation
3. do not have
4. venous thrombus that may lead to pulmonary embolism
5. subcutaneously; intravenously
6. standard heparin; lower the risk of bleeding
7. warfarin
8. decrease
9. 4 to 6
10. plasminogen; plasmin
11. hemorrhage
12. fondaparinux (Arixtra)
13. c
14. d
15. a
16. a
17. e
18. d
19. f
20. b
21. f
22. c
23. d
24. c
25. d
26. a
27. d
28. b
29. b
30. d
31. a
32. c
33. b
34. a, b, c
35. a, b, d
36. b, c, d
37. a
38. a, b, d
39. a, c, d
40. b, d, e, f
41. a, b, c, d, e

Case Study

1. c
2. a
3. a
4. d

5. a, b, c, d, e
6. a, b, c, d

CHAPTER 46—
Antihyperlipidemics and Peripheral Vasodilators

Crossword Puzzle

Across
3. weeks
5. chylomicrons
8. nicotinic acid
10. gastrointestinal

Down
1. ginkgo biloba
2. exercise
4. homocysteine
6. HDL
7. clofibrate
9. fat

11. b
12. c
13. a
14. a
15. b
16. d
17. c
18. a
19. a
20. b
21. c
22. c
23. c
24. b
25. c
26. b
27. a
28. a, b, c, d
29. a, d, f
30. a, c
31. a

Case Study

1. c
2. b
3. c
4. a
5. c
6. d
7. a, d
8. b, c, d, e

CHAPTER 47—
Drugs for Gastrointestinal Tract Disorders

1. f
2. d
3. e
4. b
5. g
6. c
7. a
8. a, b
9. a, b, d, e
10. c
11. d
12. a, b, c
13. b
14. b, d
15. b
16. c
17. c
18. a
19. c
20. a, c, d
21. c
22. a, b, c
23. c
24. a, b, c, d
25. c
26. d
27. b
28. b
29. a
30. a, b, c, d
31. b
32. d
33. c, d
34. a, c, d
35. a, b, d
36. a, c, d
37. a
38. c
39. d
40. a, b, c
41. b
42. b
43. a, b, c
44. a, d, e
45. b, c, d, e

Case Study
1. a, b, c, d, f
2. a

3. d
4. a
5. a, b
6. a, b
7. a, b, d

CHAPTER 48—
Antiulcer Drugs

1. h
2. i
3. f
4. c
5. g
6. d
7. j
8. b
9. a
10. e
11. c
12. c
13. a
14. d
15. c
16. e
17. b

CHAPTER 49—
Drugs for Eye and Ear Disorders

18. d
19. c
20. a
21. a
22. a, b, d
23. b
24. b
25. c
26. b
27. a
28. d
29. a
30. a, b, c
31. b, c, d
32. a, d, e
33. b, c, d

Case Study
1. a
2. c
3. c
4. a
5. a, b, c, e
6. c
7. c
8. a, c
9. a, b, c

```
C X C P I A I R U N A L K L W G Z C G M G P A A U N D Z Q Z F R
L N F E A I S X L A G O G D K K Y X P K V N P V S O P R Z D R I
S R O T I B I H N I E S A R D Y H N A C I N O B R A C L T E M Z
U E A S M S T V R P Z P D S D E U E I X X W A N E T L Q Q H L W
A Y D L F O I J C W D U S Z V H B Z T D N Y E M M J V L B Y N Y
K R E N M X N T E A R S B Q U P T E P C P R T G L G O L K D S P
L R S I E C T C I N C R E A S E T O B Z D V P B T O Q K D R N O
T S F L S I R M S V A M O C U A L G X L E T C J S U I J G A Q M
S B K U A I A J H C I Y Q B B L J Z I J O Z H M I L W F X T Y T
N T J W E J O T W Z I T D Y K T M H F D O O O C C V Y P C I H K
I U X A R Z C I T R D T C O B H C F D S S T D V Z W H Y U O S U
Q W V A C C U T O I S V E N B B U N C E I S E S T C X A M N B H
N J Z V N Z L M I N B C V R U N N R S C C J B J U C L E P C P P
R D V Y I D A M A S W W E W U J G W S H C R H M K G C N F F Y I
L N P O E P R Y V B V N C A R I N I I B U N E L A Y A S Y R V Y
X L T Q S S B R R J A Q P I P K D O E I F O H A P X K R I D R O
E E B T E M F X G K L S E V S Y W E C R E Y W U S X Z T G Y D Q
Z C L R T W I P Z Q E A Y J X P D R J R O W F B I E R S P J O S
O B U L Q L B Z V N B D T U Y X D A Q Z Y F V X P L W G I Y V W
L Q X E W H C E A C Y C L O P L E G I C S K T O N U W I X W T F
```

1. foreign body
2. tears
3. intraocular
4. diuretics; (open-angle) glaucoma
5. decrease
6. anuria; dehydration
7. blood sugar
8. cycloplegics
9. children
10. increase
11. conjunctivitis
12. carbonic anhydrase inhibitors
13. increase
14. carbonic anhydrase inhibitors
15. osmotics
16. e
17. d
18. f
19. a
20. b
21. c
22. a
23. c
24. c
25. b
26. b
27. d
28. a, c, d
29. a, b, d
30. a, b, d
31. a, b, d
32. a, b, d
33. a, c, d

Case Study
1. b
2. c
3. b
4. a
5. a, b
6. a, b, c, d
7. a, b, c

CHAPTER 50—
Drugs for Dermatologic Disorders

1. c
2. d
3. b
4. a

5. epidermis
6. dermis
7. subcutaneous tissue
8. sebaceous gland
9. hair shaft
10. blood vessel
11. sweat gland
12. fatty tissue
13. e
14. f
15. a, b, c
16. a
17. a
18. c
19. b
20. c
21. a
22. a
23. a
24. b
25. a, b, d
26. a, b, d
27. d
28. d
29. a, b, d
30. c, d
31. a, b, c

Case Study
1. b
2. a
3. b
4. d
5. a, b, c, d
6. a, b, c, d
7. a, b, c
8. a, b, c

CHAPTER 51—
Endocrine Drugs: Pituitary, Thyroid, Parathyroid, and Adrenal Disorders

1. f
2. i
3. j
4. a
5. n
6. h
7. b
8. m
9. o

10. c
11. g
12. d
13. k
14. l
15. e
16. b
17. b
18. a
19. b
20. a
21. b
22. b
23. a
24. b
25. b
26. a
27. d
28. e
29. h
30. c
31. b
32. f
33. g
34. a
35. c
36. a, c, d
37. a, b, c
38. a
39. a, b, d
40. b
41. b
42. b
43. a, b, d
44. a, b, c
45. c
46. c
47. b
48. a
49. a, b, c, d
50. a, c, e
51. a, c, d, e

Case Study
1. a
2. b
3. b, c
4. a
5. b
6. a, b, c, d

CHAPTER 52—
Antidiabetics

1. f
2. h
3. k
4. j
5. b
6. e
7. i
8. g
9. a
10. c
11. d
12. a, b, d
13. a, b, d
14. d
15. d
16. a, b, c, d, e
17. a, b, d, e, f
18. are not
19. a, b, c, d, e, f
20. a, b, c, d, e
21. c
22. e
23. a
24. b
25. f
26. g
27. d
28. b
29. a
30. c
31. e
32. f
33. b
34. a
35. b
36. c
37. b
38. d
39. a, c, d
40. b
41. c
42. a, b, d
43. a, b, d
44. c
45. b
46. a
47. d
48. b
49. d
50. b, c, d
51. d
52. b
53. c
54. b
55. d
56. b
57. b, c, d
58. a, c, d, e
59. a, b, c, e

Case Study
1. a, b
2. a
3. d
4. a, b, c, d, e
5. a, b, c, d
6. a, b, c

CHAPTER 53—
Female Reproductive Cycle I: Pregnancy and Preterm Labor Drugs

1. g
2. f
3. j
4. i
5. a
6. b
7. d
8. e
9. h
10. c
11. are not
12. a, b
13. do not
14. does
15. slower
16. b
17. a, b, c
18. b, c
19. c
20. b
21. a, b, c
22. a, b, d
23. c
24. will not
25. b
26. a, b, d, e
27. a, b, d
28. b, c
29. a
30. d, e
31. c
32. c
33. g
34. b
35. d
36. h
37. f
38. d
39. a, b, c
40. b, c, d
41. b
42. b
43. b
44. a
45. a, b, d
46. b, c, d
47. a, b, c
48. a, c, d
49. a
50. c
51. a, c, d
52. c
53. a, c, d

Case Study
1. a, c, d, e
2. a
3. a
4. a, b, c, d
5. a, b, c, d
6. decrease
7. a, b
8. b
9. c
10. b

CHAPTER 54—
Female Reproductive Cycle II: Labor, Delivery, and Preterm Neonatal Drugs

Crossword Puzzle

Across
1. somatic
4. regional
5. kappa
7. ripening
8. Bishop score
9. meperidine
10. contraction
11. visceral

Down
1. surfactant
2. intrathecally
3. Pitocin
6. uterine inertia

12. c
13. a
14. c
15. a, b, d
16. a
17. c
18. d
19. b
20. a
21. d
22. c
23. c
24. d
25. d
26. b
27. d
28. c
29. a, b, d
30. c
31. c
32. c
33. a, c, d
34. a, c, d
35. a
36. d
37. a, b, c
38. b, c, d
39. a, b, d, e
40. d, e
41. a, c, e

Case Study
1. a
2. a, b, c
3. a, b, c, d
4. c
5. a
6. a
7. c
8. a
9. c
10. b

CHAPTER 55— Postpartum and Newborn Drugs

Crossword Puzzle

Across
1. puerperium
2. erythromycin
4. congenital rubella
6. urticaria
7. folliculitis
8. episiotomy

Down
1. phytonadione
3. benzocaine
5. lactation

9. a, b, c
10. b
11. d
12. b, c
13. a, b
14. c
15. b
16. a, b, c
17. a, c, d
18. a
19. a

Case Study
1. b, c, d, e
2. antibodies; antigen; antibody; nonsensitized; prevent; sensitized; antibody; antigen
3. positive; antibodies; antigen; negative; negative; 72
4. a
5. d
6. a, b, c

CHAPTER 56— Drugs for Women's Reproductive Health and Menopause

Crossword Puzzle

Across
5. venous thromboembolism
10. progestin
13. menorrhagia
15. dysmenorrhea
17. osteoporosis
18. oophorectomy
19. methotrexate
20. mittelschmerz

Down
1. oligomenorrhea
2. dyspareunia
3. morning after
4. chloasma
6. ethinylestradiol
7. menopause
8. mifepristone
9. menarche
11. the minipill
12. candida
14. amenorrhea
16. misoprostol

21. b, d, e
22. a, c
23. a, b, c, d
24. a, b, d
25. a, b, d
26. c
27. a, c, d
28. d
29. b, c, d
30. a, b, d
31. d
32. b
33. b
34. a, b, d
35. d
36. b, c, d
37. a, b, c
38. a, c, d
39. b, c, d

Case Study
1. d
2. has not; a, d
3. a, b, d, e
4. c
5. a
6. a, c, d, b
7. a
8. c
9. a, b, c
10. a, b

CHAPTER 57— Drugs for Men's Health and Reproductive Disorders

1. g
2. h
3. j
4. f
5. e
6. i
7. b
8. c
9. a
10. d
11. b
12. d
13. b
14. b
15. a
16. d
17. b, c, d
18. a, b, d
19. a, b, c

Case Study

1. a, b, c, d
2. d
3. b
4. b
5. b

CHAPTER 58— Drugs for Disorders in Women's Health, Infertility, and Sexually Transmitted Infections

Crossword Puzzle

Across

2. acanthosis nigricans
9. leiomyomatas
12. menorrhagia
13. peanut oil
14. anovulatory
16. progestational
20. amenorrhea
22. hirsutism

Down

1. endometriosis
2. acyclovir
3. hepatitis B

4. St. John's wort
5. syphilis
6. insulin
7. dysmenorrhea
8. boxer shorts
10. infertility
11. guaifenesin
15. danazol
17. penicillin
18. cranberry
19. chasteberry
21. abstinence

23. c
24. a
25. b
26. b
27. a
28. a
29. a
30. a, b, d
31. a, b, d
32. a
33. c
34. a, b, d
35. b, c, d
36. c
37. a, b, c
38. b
39. a

Case Study

1. c
2. a, b
3. a, b, c, d
4. a, b, c, e
5. b
6. a
7. b
8. a, b, d

CHAPTER 59— Adult and Pediatric Emergency Drugs

1. h
2. g
3. c, h
4. e
5. i
6. a
7. f
8. b
9. d

10. c
11. j
12. e
13. d
14. a
15. d
16. c
17. b
18. c
19. e
20. b
21. b
22. c
23. b
24. a
25. a
26. c
27. c
28. b
29. d
30. d
31. c
32. a, c, d
33. c
34. b
35. d
36. c
37. a
38. c
39. a
40. b
41. c
42. a, b
43. a
44. a, b, d
45. a, b, d
46. a, b, c

Case Study 1

1. a, d
2. a, c
3. c
4. a, b, c, e
5. a, c, d
6. d

Case Study 2

1. c
2. a, b
3. c
4. a, b, d
5. a, b
6. a, b, d
7. b
8. b

Appendix A
Basic Math Review

Objectives

- Convert Roman numerals to Arabic numbers
- Convert Arabic numbers to Roman numerals
- Solve problems with fractions
- Solve ratio and proportion problems
- Convert percentages to decimals, fractions, and ratios and proportions
- Complete the math review test with a grade of 80% or higher

Key Terms

Arabic numbers	proportion
dividend	ratio
divisor	Roman numerals
least common denominator	

Introduction

Principles of basic mathematics surround us each day; they are part of life. Knowledge of arithmetic and how to do basic mathematical calculations is needed in everyday living and throughout one's nursing career.

Keep in mind that your goal is to prepare and administer medications in a safe and correct manner. The following recommendations are offered:

- **Think.** Focus on each step of the problem. This applies to simple as well as difficult problems.
- **Read accurately.** Pay particular attention to the location of the decimal point and the operation to be done (i.e., addition, subtraction, multiplication, division).
- **Picture the problem.**
- **Identify an expected range for the answer.**
- **Seek to understand the problem**, not merely the mechanics of how to do it.

The basic math review describes arithmetical operations that form the foundation that nurses use to calculate ordered dosages of medications. Specific information includes converting Roman and Arabic numerals; addition, subtraction, multiplication, and division of fractions and decimals; and solving percentage and ratio and proportion problems.

Number Systems

Arabic and Roman are the two systems of numbers associated with drug administration.

The *Arabic System* is expressed in numbers 0, 1, 2, 3, 4, 5, 6, 7, 8, and 9. Each has a place value reading from right to left. For example, the number 123 has 3 in the one's place, 2 in the ten's place, and 1 in the hundred's place. Each successive numeral indicates a value ten times more than the preceding one.

The *Roman System* is expressed by selected capital or lowercase letters (e. g., I, V, X, i, v, x). The Roman letters may be changed to equivalent Arabic numbers:

The equivalents are:

Roman Numerals		Arabic Number
I	i	1
V	v	5
X	x	10
L	l	50
C	c	100
D	d	500
M	m	1000

Roman numerals are commonly used when writing drug dosages in the Apothecary System. The Roman numerals are written in lowercase letters (e.g., i, v, ix). The lowercase letters may be written with a line above the letters (e.g., $\bar{\text{i}}$, $\bar{\text{v}}$, $\bar{\text{ix}}$) and a dot above each (e.g., i, ii, iii).

Roman numerals may appear in combination, such as xi and ix. Addition and subtraction are used to read multiple Roman numerals.

Expressing Roman numerals:

#1. When the first Roman numeral is greater than (>) the following numeral(s), then ADD them together.

  Examples: xiii = 10 + 3 = 13
       vi = 5 + 1 = 6

#2. When the first Roman numeral is less than (<) the following numeral(s), then SUBTRACT the first number from the second.

  Examples: ix = 10 − 1 = 9
       XL = 50 − 10 = 40

#3. Numerals are never repeated more than three times in a sequence.

  Examples: iii = 3
       xxx = 30

#4. When a smaller numeral is between two numerals of greater value, the smaller numeral is subtracted from the numeral following it.

> *Examples:* xix = 10 + (10 − 1) = 19
>
> mcmxci = 1000 + (1000 − 100) + (100 − 10) + 1 = 1000 + (900) + (90) + 1 = 1991

Practice Problems I

Express the following as Arabic numbers:

1.	XVI	_____		4.	XXII	_____
2.	XC	_____		5.	L	_____
3.	XIV	_____		6.	MXL	_____

Express the following as Roman numerals:

7.	100	_____		10.	259	_____
8.	36	_____		11.	85	_____
9.	30	_____		12.	60	_____

Fractions

A fraction is one or more of the equal parts of a unit. In the fraction ½, the 2 is the denominator and indicates into how many parts the whole is divided. The 1 is the numerator and indicates how many of the equal parts are taken.

The value of a fraction depends mainly on the denominator, and when it increases, the value of the fraction decreases because it takes more parts to make a whole. For example: with the fractions ⅓ and 1/12, the larger value is ⅓ because three parts make the whole, whereas for 1/12 it takes 12 parts to make a whole.

Proper, Improper, and Mixed Fractions

A **proper faction** has a numerator less than the denominator.

> *Examples:* ¾, ⅞, ½

An **improper fraction** has a numerator equal to or greater than the denominator.

> *Examples:* 8/6, 11/11, 6/3

An improper fraction may be changed to a whole or mixed number by dividing the numerator by the denominator.

> *Examples:* 8/6 = 1 2/6 or 1⅓
>
> 11/11 = 1
>
> 6/3 = 2

A **mixed number** is a whole number and a fraction (e.g., 2⅛, 3⅓, 6½). Mixed numbers can be changed to improper fractions by multiplying the denominator by the whole number, then adding the numerator.

> *Examples:* 2½ = 1 17/8; 3⅓ = 10/3; 6½ = 13/2.

Addition and Subtraction of Fractions

To ADD fractions with the same denominator, add the numerators, keep the same denominator, and reduce to lowest terms.

Examples: $\frac{1}{2} + \frac{1}{2} = \frac{2}{2} = 1$

$\frac{3}{8} + \frac{7}{8} = \frac{10}{8} = 1\frac{2}{8} = 1\frac{1}{4}$

$\frac{5}{6} + \frac{4}{6} = \frac{9}{6} = 1\frac{3}{6} = 1\frac{1}{2}$

To ADD fractions with different denominators, change to fractions having the least common denominator (LCD), which is the smallest whole number that contains the denominator of each of the fractions. Divide the LCD by the denominator of each fraction and multiply both terms of the fraction by the quotient.

Example: $\frac{1}{6} + \frac{3}{8} + \frac{3}{4} + \frac{5}{12}$

Twenty-four is the smallest number that yields a whole number when divided by denominators in the example: 6, 8, 4, and 12. Then multiply both numerator and denominator by the same number. Then add as you would with fractions of the same denominator and reduce to lowest terms.

$\frac{1}{6} = \frac{4}{24}$

$\frac{3}{8} = \frac{9}{24}$

$\frac{3}{4} = \frac{18}{24}$

$\frac{1}{2} = \frac{10}{24}$

$\frac{44}{24} = 1\frac{17}{24}$

To SUBTRACT fractions with the same denominator, subtract the smaller numerator from the larger, keep the denominator, and reduce to lowest terms.

Example: $\frac{9}{10} - \frac{1}{10} = \frac{8}{10} = \frac{4}{5}$

To SUBTRACT fractions with different denominators, change fractions to LCD, subtract the numerator, and keep the denominator.

Examples: $\frac{5}{6} - \frac{1}{3} = \frac{5}{6} - \frac{2}{6} = \frac{3}{6} = \frac{1}{2}$ (LCD = 6)

$\frac{5}{8} - \frac{1}{4} = \frac{5}{8} - \frac{2}{8} = \frac{3}{8}$ (LCD = 8)

Multiplying Fractions

To MULTIPLY fractions:

a)   multiply the numerator

b)   multiply the denominator

c)   reduce fraction to lowest terms

Example 1: $\frac{1}{3} \times \frac{3}{8} = \frac{3}{24} = \frac{1}{8}$

Answer is $\frac{3}{24}$, which is reduced to $\frac{1}{8}$. To reduce to lowest terms, 3 goes into both numbers evenly (i.e., $3 \div 3 = 1$ and $24 \div 3 = 8$).

Example 2: $\frac{1}{8} \times 4 = \frac{1}{8} \times \frac{4}{1} = \frac{4}{8} = \frac{1}{2}$

A whole number is considered the numerator over one ($\frac{4}{1}$). Four divided by eight ($4 \div 8$) = ½. ($0.5 = \frac{5}{10} = \frac{1}{2}$).

Dividing Fractions

To DIVIDE fractions, invert the second fraction (or divisor) and then multiply.

Example 1: $\frac{1}{2} \div \frac{1}{4} = \frac{1}{2} \times \frac{4}{1} = \frac{4}{2} = 2$

Example 2: $\frac{9}{10} \div \frac{1}{3} = \frac{9}{10} \times \frac{3}{1} = \frac{27}{10} = 2\frac{7}{10}$

Decimal fractions: To change fractions to decimals, divide the numerator by the denominator (e.g., $\frac{1}{2} = 1:2 = 0.5$; $\frac{1}{8} = 0.125$).

Practice Problems II

1. Which has the greatest value, $\frac{1}{6}$ or $\frac{1}{8}$?

2. Reduce improper fractions to whole or mixed numbers:

    a. $\frac{16}{4} =$ c. $\frac{7}{3} =$

    b. $\frac{36}{6} =$ d. $\frac{21}{8} =$

3. Add fractions:

    a. $\frac{1}{10} + \frac{3}{10} =$ c. $\frac{1}{16} + \frac{5}{8} =$

    b. $\frac{1}{8} + \frac{3}{24} =$

4. Subtract fractions:

    a. $\frac{7}{9} - \frac{1}{9} =$ c. $2\frac{1}{4} - 1\frac{3}{8} =$

    b. $\frac{3}{8} - \frac{1}{16} =$

5. Multiply fractions:

    a. $\frac{3}{8} \times \frac{1}{6} =$

    b. $6\frac{1}{4} \times 2\frac{1}{3} =$

6. Divide fractions:

    a. $\frac{1}{3} \div 2 =$ c. $4\frac{1}{2} \div 4 =$

    b. $\frac{7}{8} \div \frac{1}{3} =$ d. $6\frac{3}{5} \div 3 =$

7. Change each fraction to a decimal:

    a. $\frac{1}{3} =$ c. $\frac{3}{10} =$

    b. $\frac{3}{5} =$

Decimals

Decimals are referred to as (1) whole numbers and (2) decimal fractions. The following number, 1234.8765, is an example of the division of units for a whole number with a decimal fraction.

Decimal fractions are written in tenths, hundredths, thousandths, and ten thousandths. Decimal fractions are rounded off to tenths after solving problems using decimals. To round off in tenths, when the hundredth column is five or greater, the number in the tenth column is increased by one (e.g., 0.47 = 0.5, 0.12 = 0.1).

Decimal fractions are an integral part of the metric system. Tenths refers to the first decimal place 0.1 or $\frac{1}{10}$; hundredths, the second decimal place 0.01 or $\frac{1}{100}$; and thousandths, the third decimal place 0.001 or $\frac{1}{1000}$; When a decimal fraction is changed to a fraction, the denominator is based on the number of digits to the right of the decimal point (first = 10; second = 100; third = 1000).

Examples:
1.   0.9 = $\frac{9}{10}$ or 9 tenths
2.   0.33 = $\frac{33}{100}$ or 33 hundredths
3.   0.444 = $\frac{444}{1000}$ or 444 thousandths

Multiplying Decimals

To multiply decimal numbers, multiply the multiplicand by the multiplier as you would two numbers. Identify how many numerals are to the right of the decimals in both numbers. Counting from right to left, mark off the same number of spaces in the answer. Round off to tenths.

Example: 1.65   multiplicand
                <u>4.4</u>   multiplier
                660
                <u>660</u>
                7.260

Answer: 7.3. Since 6 is greater than 5, the "tenth" number is increased by 1.

Dividing Decimals

The decimal point in the divisor is moved to the right to make a whole number. The decimal point in the dividend is then moved to the right an equal number of decimal spaces. Carry number to two places beyond the decimal point.

Example: 3.69 ÷ 1.2   or $\frac{3.69}{1.2}$ dividend
                                              divisor

$$
\begin{array}{r}
3.075 \\
1.2\overline{)3.6900}
\end{array} = 3.1 \quad \text{dividend}
$$

divisor

$$
\begin{array}{r}
36 \\ \hline
90 \\
84 \\ \hline
60
\end{array}
$$

Practice Problems III

1.   Multiply   a.   4.7 × 0.284

                      b.   6.1 × 1.052

2.   Divide   a.   74 ÷ 3.6

                      b.   18.7 ÷ 0.41

3. Change the decimals to fractions:
    a.   0.21 =
    b.   0.02 =
    c.   0.068 =

Ratio and Proportion

A **ratio** is the relationship between two numbers and is expressed with a colon separating the numbers (e.g., 3 : 4 [3 is to 4]). A ratio is another way of expressing a fraction (e.g., 3 : 4 = 3/4). Proportion is the relationship between two ratios and is expressed with a double colon or equal sign separating the ratios (e.g., 3 : 4 [:: or =] 6 : 8). The middle numbers of the proportion example are called *means* and the end numbers are called *extremes*. The product of the means equals the product of the extremes.

Example 1:

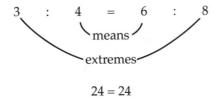

$$24 = 24$$

When the value of one number of the proportion is not known, it is represented by an "X". To solve for "X", the means are multiplied and the extremes are multiplied. The number with the X is always the divisor. Check: substitute the answer for "X"

Examples:

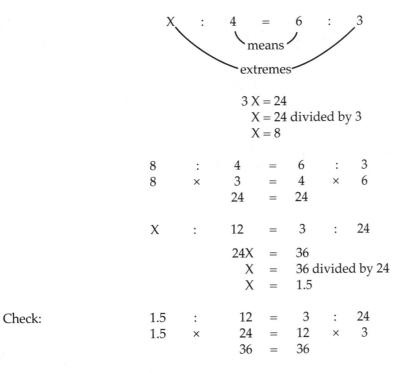

$$3 X = 24$$
$$X = 24 \text{ divided by } 3$$
$$X = 8$$

8	:	4	=	6	:	3
8	×	3	=	4	×	6
		24	=	24		

X	:	12	=	3	:	24

$$24X = 36$$
$$X = 36 \text{ divided by } 24$$
$$X = 1.5$$

Check:

1.5	:	12	=	3	:	24
1.5	×	24	=	12	×	3
		36	=	36		

The ratio and proportion problem may be set up as a fraction. Cross multiply to solve for X or to prove the computation.

	Example:	Ratio and proportion	X	:	4	=	3	:	1
					X	=	12		

	Fraction		$X/4$	=	$3/1$	
			X	=	12	

	Check:		$12/4$	=	$3/1$	
			12	=	12	

Practice Problems IV

Solve for "X":

1.   2   :   20   ::   5   :   X

2.   0.8   :   100   ::   X   :   1000

3.   Change the ratio and proportion to a fraction:

                    1   :   3   ::   X   :   18

4.   It is 1500 miles from New York City to Miami, Florida. Your car uses one gallon of gasoline per 32 miles on average. How many gallons of gasoline are required for the trip?

Percentage

Percent means parts of 100; thus 4% means four parts of 100 and 0.4% means 0.4 parts (less than 1) of 100. A percent may be expressed as a fraction, a decimal, or a ratio.

Example:

Percent	Fraction	Decimal	Ratio
20	$20/100$	0.20	20 : 100
0.5	$0.5/100$	0.005	0.5 : 100

To change percent to decimal, move the decimal point two places to the LEFT. Unless noted otherwise, the decimal point is assumed to be after the number (e.g., 20% = 20.%).

Practice Problems V

Change each percent to a fraction, a decimal, and a ratio

Percent	Fraction	Decimal	Ratio
1			
$3/4$			
300			

Answers

Practice Problems I

1. $10 + 5 + 1 = 16$

2. $100 - 10 = 90$

3. $10 + 4 = 14$

4. $10 + 10 + 2 = 22$

5. 50

6. $1000 + (50 - 10) = 1040$

7. C

8. XXXVI

9. XXX

10. CCLIX

11. LXXXV

12. LX

Practice Problems II

1. $\frac{1}{6}$ has the greater value; there are six parts in a whole and not eight.

2. a. 4   b. 6   c. $2\frac{1}{3}$ d. $2\frac{5}{8}$

3. a. $\frac{1}{10} + \frac{3}{10} = \frac{4}{10} = \frac{2}{5}$

   b. $\frac{1}{8} + \frac{3}{24} = \frac{3}{24} + \frac{3}{24} = \frac{6}{24} = \frac{1}{4}$

   c. $\frac{1}{16} + \frac{5}{8} = \frac{1}{16} + \frac{10}{16} = \frac{11}{16}$

4. a. $\frac{7}{9} - \frac{1}{9} = \frac{6}{9} = \frac{2}{3}$

   b. $\frac{3}{8} - \frac{1}{16} = \frac{6}{16} - \frac{1}{16} = \frac{5}{16}$

   c. $2\frac{1}{4} - 1\frac{3}{8} = \frac{9}{4} - \frac{11}{8} = \frac{18}{8} - \frac{11}{8} = \frac{7}{8}$

5. a. $\frac{3}{48} = \frac{1}{16}$

   b. $\frac{25}{4} \times \frac{7}{3} = \frac{175}{12} = 14\frac{7}{12}$

6. a. $\frac{1}{3} \times \frac{1}{2} = \frac{1}{6}$

   b. $\frac{7}{8} \times \frac{3}{1} = \frac{21}{8} = 2\frac{5}{8}$

   c. $\frac{9}{2} \times \frac{1}{4} = \frac{9}{8} = 1\frac{1}{8}$

   d. $\frac{33}{5} \times \frac{1}{3} = \frac{33}{15} = 2\frac{3}{15} = 2\frac{1}{5}$

7. a. 0.33   b. 0.60   c. 0.30

Practice Problems III

1. a. $1.3348 = 1.33$

   b. $6.4172 = 6.42$

2. a. 20.5

   b. 45.6

3. a. $\frac{21}{100}$

   b. $\frac{2}{100}$

   c. $\frac{68}{1000}$

Practice Problems IV

1. $2X = 100$
   $X = 50$

2. $100\,X = 800$
   $X = 8$

3. $\frac{1}{3} = \frac{X}{18}$
   $3X = 18$
   $X = 6$

4. 1 gal : 32 mi :: X gal : 1500 mi
   $32\,X = 1500$
   $X = 46.875$ gal
   $X = 47$ gallons

Practice Problems V

	Percent	Fraction	Decimal	Ratio
1.	1	$\frac{1}{100}$	0.01	1 : 100
2.	$\frac{3}{4}$	$\frac{0.75}{100}$	0.0075	0.75 : 100
3.	300	$\frac{300}{100}$	3.00	300 : 100

Appendix B
Prototype Drug Chart

Prototype Drug Chart   **Generic Name:**_____

Drug Class: **Dosage:**

Trade Name:

Pregnancy Category:

Contraindications: **Drug-Lab-Food Interactions:**

Caution:

Pharmacokinetics: **Pharmacodynamics:**

Absorption: *Onset:*

Distribution: *Peak:*

Metabolism: *Duration:*

Excretion:

Therapeutic Effects/Uses:

Mode of Action:

Side Effects: **Adverse Reactions:**

                                             Life-Threatening Reactions: